The Sleeper Agent

The Rise of Lyme Disease, Chronic Illness and the Great Imitator Antigens of Biological Warfare

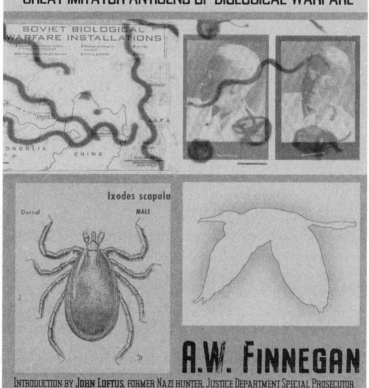

A.W. Finnegan

Introduction by John Loftus, former Nazi hunter, Justice Department Special Prosecutor

Published by:
Trine Day LLC
PO Box 577
Walterville, OR 97489
1-800-556-2012
www.TrineDay.com
TrineDay@icloud.com

Library of Congress Control Number: 2023943059

Finnegan, A.W.
—1st ed.
p. cm.

Epub (ISBN-13) 978-1-63424-382-7
Trade Paperback (ISBN-13) 978-1-63424-381-0
1. Biological warfare. 2. Biological Warfare history. 3. Biological weapons. 4.. Biological weapons Soviet Union History. 5. Lyme Disease history. 6. Tick-Borne Diseases history. 7. Erich Traub (1906-1958). I. Finnegan, A.W.. II. Title

FIRST EDITION
10 9 8 7 6 5 4 3 2 1

Printed in the USA
Distribution to the Trade by:
Independent Publishers Group (IPG)
814 North Franklin Street
Chicago, Illinois 60610
312.337.0747
www.ipgbook.com

A little neglect may breed mischief...
for want of a nail, the shoe was lost;
for want of a shoe the horse was lost;
and for want of a horse the rider was lost.
                    – Benjamin Franklin, *Poor Richard's Almanack*

"*The power of biological weapons is ten times more than the nuclear power. Unless we act fast with an open mind, any one of them can extinct the human race.*"
                    – Amit Ray, *Nuclear Weapons Free World - Peace on the Earth*

In the field of biological weapons, there is almost no prospect of detecting a pathogen until it has been used in an attack.
                    – *Barton Gellman*

DEDICATION

I want to dedicate this book to all the injured and sick people in the world, afflicted and affected by these horrific diseases, who struggle to cope and know the 'why' behind their suffering. Why they are brushed aside and neglected by physicians and the medical establishment? Why they suffer and what is the cause of it? Why they can't seem to recover no matter what they do? Why they have no answers and no official recognition of their suffering and most of all, a very real disease.

I dedicate this book to all Lyme and chronic disease activists who genuinely sought and fought for change in the hopes of dealing with this terrible nine-headed hydra of immune tolerance and all of its classic manifestations and co-infecting agents. I thank the girls who worked in TruthCures and those who began to shine light on immune tolerance. A very special **thank you to Jena Blair and Laura Hovind** for teaching me the basics of immune tolerance when I was coming to the realization of what my disease was, and through this were the keys that opened so many other doors critical to the rest of the story.

I want to dedicate this book to John Loftus, for having the compassion to reveal these dark secrets festering underneath Western civilization with many victims, unwarned and unprepared for the steady rise and proliferation of mystery diseases, chronic diseases that evade a diagnosis or admission of illness. This was a courageous and honorable deed that allowed for this entire book to be written. Without John Loftus, none of the keys that unlock so many other doors in the history of biological warfare and bioterrorism, would have been opened. We thank you for your courage, care, and compassion to do what is right at considerable risk, but nonetheless heroic.

Finally, I dedicate this book to Anne and Dan Benjamin, for their work and intelligence on Dr. Traub, with their desire to have this case on war criminals in Paperclip to be 're-opened.' A line of life work I never would have predicted myself to have taken on, the arduous, meticulous work of pasting together the history of some truly sinister intentions they initially took on and discovered. Though I never met them, this book carried on the torch of Light they shined in dark places with their brilliance to achieve and uncover some of the unspeakable evils that lurk in this world.

CONTENTS

FOREWORD

I am honored that Adam Finnegan asked me to write an introduction to his brilliantly researched history of the "stealth weapons" of biological warfare, and their relationship to Lyme disease. All the credit for this goes to Adam Finnegan. He has collected hundreds if not thousands of scientific publications and retrieved formerly classified documents from archives around the world. His meticulously documented footnotes will be a valuable guide to researchers for many years to come.

Stealthy bioweapons are those that do not cause mass fatalities but slowly weaken our immune systems until we collapse from the slow emergence of dormant diseases. There are many such illnesses that slumber inside each of us. Some, like herpes simplex, are thought to be relatively benign. But others, like Guillain Barre, are potentially serious diseases that have been suppressed by our immune systems over the generations but are now emerging in record numbers.

Some diseases like cancer, have always been with us but have previously affected only a small percentage of our population. In the last few decades, something has caused cancer to afflict Americans in unprecedented numbers. America is one of the wealthiest nations on Earth, but it also has the highest rates of cancer in the world. The latter fact has baffled the biological sciences.

It is Adam's hypothesis that the massive rise in cancer are the by-product of man-made, biological weapons that stealthily attack our immune systems in a manner that is not easily detectable. These stealthy bioweapons cause a rapid elimination of antibodies, so our doctors cannot rely on standard lab tests to detect ongoing infections. In some cases, such as Lyme disease, the antibodies vanish within weeks. In other cases, such as Rabbit Fever, a bacterial infection transmitted by ticks, the underlying bioweapon can be engineered to disappear within two hours.

The absence of antibody detection deprives the medical community of the ability to diagnose these stealth epidemics. Diagnosis is further hindered by the fact that stealth bioweapons can manifest themselves in the form of dozens of different diseases. By attacking our immune systems, stealthy bioweapons compromise our immune systems and slowly awaken the diseases that are latent within each of us.

Biowarfare scientists understand that our own natural defenses can become the most powerful weapon to destroy us. In some cases – like the October 1918 "second wave" mutation of the "Spanish flu" influenza – young, healthy soldiers infected with the new influenza variant had strong immune systems that released such a "cytokine storm" of anti-pneumonia fluids into their lungs that they turned blue and literally drowned in their own bodies. It was a shockingly deadly pandemic, killing between 50 and 100 million worldwide.

But the greatest percentage of Spanish flu victims were found among the enemy armies of Germany and Bolshevik Russia. They sincerely but erroneously believed that their millions of casualties must be the result of a biological weapon. Upon that one mistake, a century of secret biological warfare research commenced.

Defecting Soviet, and then Russian scientists, have told that inconvenient truth to the CIA and MI6 for decades. Tragically, their warnings were ignored because Adam's collection of formerly classified documents has demonstrated that the Russians have been consistently testing their stealth bioweapons on the American people for the last fifty years.

At first glance, a layman might be horrified to think that even if 10 percent of what Adam has discovered is true, it will stand conventional virology on its head. It is indeed shocking, but I believe his evidence stands for itself. I have personally verified more than 70% of what Adam has written from my own access to classified archives and my discussions with biological warfare experts.

According to Ken Alibek, the former head of the Russian biowarfare program, who defected to the United States, there was a clandestine "Tripartite Agreement" among Russia, Britain, and the US not to expose each other's bioweapons violations because of their international ban. According to my own sources in the NATO intelligence community, this impunity from exposure emboldened the Russians to continue their secret biological experiments in ways that may result in continuing damage to American public health for generations to come.

Unlike nuclear weapons, stealthy biological weapons of mass destruction have been used again and again, not just in America but around the world. I've read about the deployment of banned bioweapons in the Top-Secret files of the NATO intelligence agencies.

The great tragedy is that much of this information could have been revealed when I was called as an expert witness before the

House Judiciary Committee in 1985. But under extreme pressure from the Reagan administration, Senator Barry Goldwater, and other Republican politicians with ties to the House and Senate intelligence committees, Roman Mazzoli, the Democratic Sub-Committee Chairman of the House Judiciary Committee, blocked my testimony about bioweapons being unleashed on the US.

The point man for the pressure was a former Justice Department Acting Assistant Attorney General named Mitch McConnell who threatened Mazzoli's Congressional seat if he didn't block my testimony. Mazzoli ultimately agreed to betray his party and the nation, and he even refused to hold executive sessions where I could've testified.[A]

This meant that I could not discuss any classified information during my public testimony before Congress. President Ronald Reagan's Deputy Assistant Attorney General, Richard Keegan, directly threatened that if I disclosed any classified information in public, I would lose my law license and be banished to prison.

My expert sources in biowarfare had warned me that bioweapons had been unleashed on Americans, but none of them would testify before Congress after they witnessed the reprisals I had endured in the 1980s after I exposed Nazi war criminals working for the US Government.

But American law places a thirty-year expiration date on classified files. In 2017, 32 years after I testified to Congress. I asked Adam Finnegan (himself a victim of Lyme disease – like me) if he would volunteer to see whether or not any of the aforementioned intelligence material was accessible to the public. The Freedom of Information Act had been an utter waste of time with regards to this intelligence information I sought, but Adam absolutely astonished me by obtaining obscure scientific papers from Russian, German, British and American archives.

The documents uncovered by Adam will come as a bit of a shock to the CIA and the western medical establishment: The Russians have been genetically modifying the DNA of viruses and bacteria for almost a century.

The Russians, and for that matter the Nazis, bypassed the intricate study of mapping DNA genomes by using "serial passages" to create untraceable genetic mutations in hundreds of laboratory animals, which were usually mice. Serial passages are conducted by in-

---

A   Mazzoli's own Congressional staff informed me. They told me that he had been threatened with defeat unless he restricted my testimony about Nazis in America. The staff said there were "a lot of Germans and Ukrainians in his congressional district but very few Jews."

fecting animals with a virus or bacteria and passing the infected animals through a series of alternating the biological agents in animal blood and egg fluids and further adapting it to additional animals. After dozens of such serial passages the end product is a new hybrid.

Serial passages can produce attenuated or weakened vaccine strains capable of eliciting immune responses without virulence or, conversely, producing much greater virulence than the original virus or bacteria. The process of serial passages can also produce a virus or bacteria that is capable of infecting other species of animals or even humans, whereas the original virus didn't have that capability.

Serial passages can achieve laboratory viral and bacterial mutations in a few weeks that would take decades to develop in nature. Unlike the modern western process of genetic splicing of RNA and DNA, serial passages are invisible even under an electron microscope and look exactly like natural evolution.

It is as if the Russians had developed advanced moon rockets in the 1930s and then successfully covered it up for almost a century. The evidence of this Russian technique for the creation of genetically altered stealth diseases has been sitting unread in our classified archives all along. Read the documents Adam discovered and judge for yourself.

Before you put his book down, let me explain how I came to learn independently that most of what Adam has written is all too true.

In the 1980s, my primary focus was on Nazi war criminals in America – not Russian stealth weapons. My first book, *The Belarus Secret*, recently republished by TrineDay as *America's Nazi Secret*, discuses classified files concerning Nazi war criminals who were hidden in America by British intelligence agents and were secretly working for the Soviets.[B]

My manuscript was subject to a protracted CIA review in the early 1980s, but it was eventually cleared for publication by government censors. Before my book ever came out, and before the government censors could change their minds, I exposed the secret Nazi connection on a rare double segment of *60 Minutes* that won the 1982 Emmy Award for outstanding investigative journalism.

For a brief time, I was a very minor celebrity. The publicity attracted the attention of like-minded people in the intelligence community

---

B   *The Belarus Secret* was the Alfred Knopf Nominee for the Pulitzer Prize in history (now republished by Trine Day as *America's Nazi Secret*). My manuscript was written in 1981 and declassified in 1982. My beloved friend and co-author of two later books is Mark Aarons of Sydney Australia who forayed behind the Iron Curtain where my security clearances forbade me from setting foot. I do not think I could possibly have carried on for so long or achieved so much without his advice and support.

who admired my integrity in exposing classified corruption through lawful means. At the time, I had a Q clearance from the Department of Energy that allowed for access to data on nuclear weapons design, manufacture, or usage.

Since I was the only lawyer that many intelligence personnel knew with a Q clearance and other ultra-level security clearances, they descended on me to tell me about other intelligence scandals to see if I could have them declassified as well through the CIA's Pre-Publication Review Committee. For the last several decades, I have been a pro bono attorney serving professional intelligence officers from the Western secret services. I protect their identities under the attorney-client privilege of confidentiality as I attempt to make their stories lawfully declassified.

In the early 1980's, I was approached by someone quite senior in the intelligence community who was privy of my Q-level security clearance because he also had a Q clearance. He told me intricate details about several near disasters that only someone with a Q clearance for nuclear weapons would know. I recall him describing an incident where the US Air Force accidentally dropped an atom bomb on North Carolina, and almost all of the Permissive Action Link (PALs), a series of security devices for nuclear weapons, had failed. Luckily, the final PALS activated to stop the nuclear detonation. But the detonation was a much closer call than the media realized.

My new Q source then began to tell me about similar scandals involving biological weapons. He told me of an experiment where light bulbs full of "harmless" germs were released inside the New York subway system. It was thought to be a test of harmless "simulants" to determine how far a real biological weapon could be spread by passing subway cars. For obvious reasons, the public was shielded from this information.

My new Q source then edified me about a real nightmare. After World War II, German scientists had been brought to the US by a high-ranking British intelligence agent, who had been the British liaison to US for nuclear secrets, which meant he had TOP SECRET clearances. However, American codebreakers began to focus on political activities of the high-ranking, British intelligence agent, eliciting suspicions that he might be working for Soviet intelligence. Their suspicions were confirmed in 1951 when the British agent defected to Moscow. He had been part of a cell that penetrated the MI6, the British version of the CIA. Three of the cell members worked in the British Embassy in Washington DC after 1949. All three later defected to Russia and acknowledged they had been spying for the Russians throughout WWII and afterwards.

After I received permission from the CIA to publish a brief addition to my book about Lyme disease, I became overwhelmed with additional sources from the intelligence community. The handful of horror stories turned into a torrent of disclosures about Russian biological warfare. The intelligence community had a much wider view of history than the public, because so much of our modern history has been classified.

In order to win the battles for declassification, I was required to prove that at least some mention of a topic had appeared somewhere in the public domain. Several volunteers tried to assist me in finding open-source documents about the British spy cell and the Nazi/Soviet scientists the spy cell recruited, but in the 1980's our requests under the Freedom of Information Act were almost always declined for reasons of "national security." I wondered what possible national security interest would be left for America to protect the British spies?

As I augured into that quandary, I discovered the unvarnished truth about the Freedom of Information Act bulwark we encountered. During the Korean War, the British and the Canadians convinced the CIA to collude with them in a series of clandestine biological attacks on North Korea and on Chinese cities across the Yalu River.[C] The North Koreans complained to the United Nations that they were being hit by "feather bombs" that gently delivered infected insects on top of the snow. The US denied everything in the UN, but the denials were problematic, because captured American pilots had confessed to dropping the illegal biological bombs.

President Dwight Eisenhower's Secretary of State John Foster Dulles and CIA Director Allen Dulles claimed it was a Chinese propaganda ploy. But decades later, a pair of Canadian scholars blew the whistle on the Eisenhower administration by exposing their country's role in the American, British and Canadian biowarfare in North Korea. The scholars meant well, but their limited exposé, based on declassified records, only scratched the surface, because it did not mention the Soviets, the world's most perfidious patron of illegal biological weapons.

Author Linda Hunt has unparalleled expertise on biowarfare, and she's the giant upon whose shoulders all future biowarfare researchers have stood. She was first to warn the world about the dangers posed by Operation Paperclip scientists. Operation Paperclip recruited top

C   The Office of Policy Coordination, led by Alan Dulles and Frank Wisner, ran the bug bomb program under the cover of the propaganda section PP of OPC inside the State Department. After Eisenhower's election, both the PP propaganda section and the PM paramilitary section of OPC were merged with the clandestine services division of the CIA, then called the Directorate of Plans, later the Directorate of Operations.

Nazi scientists and brought them to the US, even though many of the scientists were Nazi war criminals, and among the scientists was an evil genius who's responsible for Lyme disease.

When I initially contracted Lyme disease, I thought my discomfort was due to an old army parachute accident: I didn't have a clue that a new and unidentified illness was slowly attacking my immune system. I came down with everything from full blown colon cancer to a bewildering array of bacterial and fungal infections that the Veterans Administration misdiagnosed as a terminal illness, and then wrote off my condition as a "fever of unknown origin."

Adam Finnegan has performed a great and brave service writing this book and elucidating the nefarious origins of Lyme disease. Moreover, his assembly of documents on the history of stealth bioweapons is unparalleled. Without his collection of documents, the stories that my clients told me over the last half of the century could have been lost to history.

It is, indeed, terrifying to embrace Adam's conclusions, but we must deal with our fears by recognizing the facts. Adam's conclusions follow a pattern of Russian scientific research in stealthy biowarfare experiments.

America owes Adam a debt of great gratitude for forcing us to ask ourselves fact-based questions about what is responsible for the decline of Americans' health when compared to other modern countries He has devoted years of his life without renumeration in the hope of helping others. I hope that he receives some type of grant or funding to continue his remarkable research. Years from now, I would not be surprised if he is the first non-physician to be nominated for the Nobel Prize in medicine.

– John Loftus, 2023

PREFACE

From the moment I pulled that black-legged tick from my lower back and caught a simultaneous inner ear/respiratory infection in 2016, this book was set in motion. Of course, I didn't know it yet. I had no plans to initiate an extensive study in the science and immunology of the complex state of *immune tolerance*, which is the basis of chronic disease. I had no interest to spend endless days, sometimes 18 hours a day, on sites like PubMed, Archive, WorldCat, and library archives of almost every government agency relevant to the topic.

However, even before this, there was a process that had to unfold, and had I not met certain individuals with key pieces and answers to the overall puzzle, that process could have never been initiated. It was several weeks after that tick bite, and what seemed like a simultaneous viral infection that was going around, which me and several friends also caught, that I began to get strange symptoms I had never experienced and were unlike any symptom of any illness I have ever experienced in my life. Strange headaches and migrating pains of all kinds have permanently remained, filling my head and sinus area with the most intense pressure. I started seeking medical attention, thinking that whatever it was, must have had some easily explainable, curable answer. This assumption would prove to be seriously mistaken.

What started as a diagnosis of viral labyrinthitis which I was told would subside in several weeks, turned into a chronic, systemic disease that has thoroughly hexed me ever since. I sought medical attention from a variety of other specialists, all of whom had no answers, no help to offer, and no concern for my suffering, that, in their mind, was non-existent. The medical system I had relied on for so long had completely failed me, and this would remain so indefinitely, because the myriad of health problems at play in the state of chronic disease, are generally not picked up by any of the conventional approaches, diagnostics, and medical technologies used by regular health care providers.

It would seem unlikely to the uninitiated, not familiar with the science of immune tolerance and the work of Dr. Erich Traub, that such a debilitating disease could possibly exist that produces no abnormal blood work, little to no outward signs of disease, and negative results for many of the diseases that could be implicated, and thus, cases like mine, just one of millions with the same story, are cast into medical exile, left to fend for themselves.

I began to study, learn, and amass extensive research over many years to find the cause of my disease, I obtained copies of the infectious disease testing of tick-borne diseases, and later tests by the alternative IgX that goes by the pre-Dearborn standard, as the 1994 Dearborn standard excludes the large majority who get the immunosuppressive form of the disease. The IgX came back with positive reactivity for Lyme disease (*Borrelia burgdorferi*), *Mycoplasma pneumoniae*, reactivated Epstein-Barr Virus (EBV), and reactivated human herpesvirus 6 (HHV-6), an encephalitis virus that many people have in latent form, much like herpes-simplex virus and EBV, but there are additional tick-borne co-infections that produce little to no antibodies and thus, no positive result.

Unlike the disinterested healthcare physicians, I initially sought, I had a vested interest in my physical health, something the public health agencies had no consideration for. The unfortunate majority with conditions like mine don't fit into their box of definitions for reportable diseases since they standardized tests that bury those cases.

I have the researchers and activists at TruthCures.org to thank for my introductory and preliminary understanding of immune tolerance, and the mechanisms at play in chronic disease. Had these exceptional women not worked tirelessly to get this information out to people, I may have never been able to open all the other doors in the story with a scientific context. This would have never allowed me to understand the context of Dr. Traub's work on immune tolerance and slow-virus infections, particularly the mechanics of reactivated Epstein-Barr Virus, which Lymphocytic choriomeningitis (LCM virus) became a model of. Yet, that was only half of the equation in uncovering the story as it is laid out in the following pages.

I was given one additional key that unlocked many additional doors from a historical context, by a good friend and true American hero, former Justice Department federal prosecutor and retired Nazi hunter, John J. Loftus. It was his clues that led me to the Russian connections, which at first, challenged my worldview, thinking there was no way they could have been able to pull off the amount of progress and full-spectrum dominance in this perpetual war with biological weaponry, now in motion for over a century. But I gave these leads a chance, and they have not stopped producing new leads ever since.

I was already familiar with Michael C. Carroll's work, *Lab 257: The Disturbing Story of the Government's Secret Plum Island Germ Laboratory,* a major inspiration of which I would later revisit, and a book that my source had also been one of the primary sources for, John Loftus had been the first to reveal the connection between Lyme Disease and biological warfare in his early book *The Belarus Secret,* and Erich Traub was already a point of interest from before I had many of the additional pieces of the puzzle.

The game of biological warfare is a very esoteric war since no country wants to look like Germany did after the first world war with the use of chemical and biological weapons against their enemies. Not to worry though, as it is my hope that you, the reader, will read this work and begin your initiation into the understanding of stealth biological warfare, the strategic weapons that tire, exhaust, and overwhelm their targets, so slowly that the country barely understands what hit them, until it's too late…

Preliminary Discussion:

THE ART OF GERM WEAPONS

THE FIVE ANGLES OF BIOLOGICAL WARFARE

*If you want to understand Biological Warfare you must figuratively
stand on your head. Biological Warfare is an upside-down science, an
inversion of nature.*

– Theodore Rosebury [1]

1. *There are two classes of biological weapons, those that act-quickly and
typically kill (tactical bioweapons), and those that act slowly to disable,
tire and exhaust (strategic bioweapons). Strategic bioweapons are stealthy
and hard to track, diagnose, and treat. Although not typically fatal, they
are far more successful than tactical bioweapons in the long-term, used
strategically and on larger nations or groups of people.*

Many have made the argument that a biological warfare agent that
can remain inapparent or have long incubation periods would not make
much sense.[2] However, this idea can and will be deconstructed and
shown to be wrong. In order to understand the purpose of a bioweapon that slowly incubates and does not kill but slowly wears down the
enemy, we must explain the classification of the two kinds of biological
weapons. This will allow one to realize the deeper context and value of
strategic weapons as a class of stealth disablers. These agents and the
antigen associated with them are the central focus of this book.

Attacks with slow-acting strategic bioweapons are carried out
against civilians rather than armies of the target nation. Strategic attacks involve attacking the population of a nation itself. Strategic biological weapons were brought up in testimony by General Douglas
MacArthur to congress on June 09, 1969, listing the term incapacitating antipersonnel agents:

Incapacitating Antipersonnel Agents

A number of diseases cause virtually no mortality, and the agents of these diseases are generally termed incapacitating. Some mortality might be caused in individuals with preexisting illness or those suffering from malnutrition or radiation sickness. Q Fever, Chikungunya virus, and Venezuelan Equine Encephalitis are examples.[3]

Furthermore, the desire for synthesizing new agents that do not naturally exist and act as strategic bioweapons targeting the immune system were brought up in the same congressional hearing, noting:

Within the next 5 to 10 years, it would probably be possible to make a new infective microorganism which could differ in certain important aspects from any known disease-causing organisms. Most important of these is that it might be refractory to the immunological and therapeutic processes upon which we depend to maintain our relative freedom from infectious disease.[4]

On the one hand, there are bioweapons that cause fast-acting, maximum damage on the target in a short amount of time. These are tactical bioweapons and are the common example of what most people think of as a biological warfare agent. Where these agents are used, the damage is apparent, the afflicted are easy to spot, diagnose, track, and the disease outbreak can be contained very quickly for this reason.

In opposition to these tactical bioweapons are the slow-acting, stealth bioweapons, used for a long-term strategy of *tire and exhaust*. In this case, the target will develop chronic, debilitating mystery diseases that disable the immune system and plague the individuals affected.[5] These can in many ways be thought of as economic weapons that affect the ability to work and puts extreme strain on the healthcare systems to the point of being completely overwhelmed. The burden can vary but oftentimes it will be considerable and those affected will become debilitated, and this adds significant burden to both the economy and the public health system.[6] Other aspects of these weapons are their ability to cause mental illnesses and this burden can put an immense strain on the population of a target nation. This is because the agent is oftentimes what is termed *neurotropic*.

You will hear this term *neurotropic* throughout the book. This term can be defined as the quality of an agent to colonize and deteriorate the brain and central nervous system. You may also hear of other *tropisms*, implying a destructive effect, such as to the heart and cardiovascular system, in which case, *cardiotropic* would be the term describing the quality of that agent.

The suffix *-trope* and its adjective form *-tropic* are defined etymologically as *"that which turns," from Greek tropos "a turn, direction, course, way,"* and I often think of this quality synonymously with *Atropos*, one of the 3 Greek Fates who cuts the cord of life at death, thus turning one away from life, implying a destructive effect.

When millions of people are infected and sick with complicated diseases that debilitate and cause mental illnesses, someone has to take care of them, or at the very least, their ability to contribute to society is greatly diminished or even harmful to it. This causes a serious strain on the economy and public health system, overwhelmed by the burden of an enemy they cannot easily define or see.[7]

The work of the German virologist and bioweaponeer, Dr. Erich Traub, is central to this story. He is the doorway to understanding strategic bioweapons. His studies of Lymphocytic Choriomeningitis Virus (LCM) and what is termed *immune tolerance,* are at the center of this book.

You will hear the term *immune tolerance* throughout this book. It is central to the theme of stealth disablers and the life work of Erich Traub. We can define immune tolerance as follows:

> A state of unresponsiveness to a specific antigen or group of antigens to which a person is normally responsive. Immune tolerance is achieved under conditions that suppress the immune reaction and is not just the absence of an immune response.[A]

In the simplest of terms, the term *"immune tolerance"* can be thought of as chronic immunosuppression, an impaired immune system that leaves the individual sick and worn out. The early studies of immune tolerance and LCM virus by Erich Traub taught us that a devious infection can be present, actively causing a chronic, slow disease while appearing healthy with no abnormal bloodwork, little to no antibodies or inflammation, but left the victim feeling horrible and incapacitated, and this is where the dynamic began to turn in favor of stealth disablers that destroy the immune system as effective weapons in a long-term strategy.[8] It was a disease marked by slow, chronic health problems and invasion of the central nervous system. One can think of the way inflammation causes swelling, as the immune system

---

A   Definition from MedicineNet.com author: Medical Author: William C. Shiel Jr., MD, FACP, FACR)

is doing all it can to keep these toxic pathogens out of the brain, organs, and cardiovascular system.

When the immune system is suppressed and forced into tolerating these pathogens, it cannot keep the pathogens out of the brain and central nervous system, and this has a terrible effect on the overall health and mental well-being of the individual.[9] They are plagued by slow, chronic neurodegenerative diseases and mental health problems in the same manner as Traub's LCM virus.

Moreover, Traub found that the LCM virus maintains itself from one generation to the next, passing down through generations, causing cancer to skyrocket in the subsequent generations.[10] LCM virus mimics other latent viruses humans commonly have within them, like Epstein-Barr Virus (EBV).[11] These latent viruses are reactivated by different forms of physical stress and immune deficiencies, which you will see later in this book with Traub's LCM Virus. Many of these viruses are carcinogenic and *neurotropic* when reactivated into an active infection.[12]

Another central theme of this book is that latent germs and viruses can be reactivated into more destructive forms and actually cause new outbreaks of disease, and this will be explained when we reach the chapters about Erich Traub. In the present book, you will be taught the esoteric science of *immune tolerance* and its contribution to chronic disease, mental illness, and cancer. Now let us proceed to the next angle in the art of germ weapons.

2. Biological warfare is a dirty business, and always needs the "cover" of benign, well-meaning research to hide its more nefarious activities. A spade is never called a spade, a weapon is never called a weapon.[13]

The second inner teaching of biological warfare tells us that biological warfare, like chemical warfare, is a dirty game. It is looked at in the same disdain that accompanies drug trafficking and human experimentation. It is an unacceptable practice in the global community.[14] It is extremely undesirable for a nation to be caught in a public political scandal over the use of unconventional chemical or biological weapons like Germany had during the First World War after using chemical and germ warfare.[15]

Germany used chemical weapons on their opponents during World War I, as well as biological weapons in the years leading up to the war and well into it, infecting military cavalry and medical horses with glanders and anthrax,[16] and these horses would be used not only as cavalry horses, but also to produce serum and vaccines,[17] an act intended for humans indirectly. This allowed the Spanish Flu virus to mutate to a far more dangerous virus in subsequent waves.

As a result of using unconventional weapons in WWI, Germany was sanctioned and ordered to pay reparations that were economically crippling, taking them 92 years to pay off their debt for those deeds,[18] and paved the way for the rise of the Third Reich to form and bring about the Second World War.

This aspect becomes one of several major reasons why it is done in such a secretive, concealed manner, always hiding weapons work under the "cover" of something with a more nonthreatening, benign purpose like medical prophylactics, vaccines, biotherapeutics, agricultural research and veterinary problems.[19]

They will not call a weapon a weapon on paper or in discussion, they simply do not make this mistake. The failure to understand this invariably results in a dead-end street for researchers trying to paste together the history of the biological weapons game. This is a pre-requisite concept if one is to understand the contents of this book.

The work is often conducted through scientific research in the academic and corporate sector, and by everyday scientists and most of the work is published in scientific journals. Dr. George Merck presented this concept in written testimony to congress in 1946 with the following:

> While the military developments cannot be disclosed in the interest of national security, the research contributed significant knowledge to what was already known concerning the control of diseases affecting humans, animals, and plants. Arrangements have been made whereby this information of value to humanity as a whole will be made available to the public from those sources responsible for the work. This will be accomplished through reports before scientific bodies, publication in scientific journals and other means by which advances in science and medicine are disseminated in peacetime.[20]

3. There is essentially no difference between offensive and defensive research other than the true intentions of those who conduct it.

The third teaching of biological warfare tells us that there is essentially no difference in offensive or defensive research other than the intention of those utilizing it. That is to say, the kind of research utilized in weaponizing pathogens is often similar to those claiming to use the same research to defend against it. In modern times, *gain-*

of-function research became a more well-known term for raising the virulence of various pathogens claiming it was for the purpose of research to defend against it.

In 1972, a new treaty was proposed called the Biological and Toxin Weapons Convention (BTWC) to update the 1925 Geneva Protocol that banned the use and stockpiling of biological weapons. In the new treaty, it allowed defensive research and as a result, many offensive biological weapons programs actually expanded because they could claim it was for defensive purposes and it would lawfully be covered under that treaty. As Soviet bioweaponeer Igor V. Domaradskij said in his memoir *Biowarrior: Inside the Soviet/Russian Biological War Machine*:

> With the signing of the BTWC, biological defense was no longer a priority; under cover of the treaty, and unknown to the rest of the signatories, a greatly expanded and ambitious bioweapons program would rapidly take root in the USSR. [21]

4. Biological warfare is a clandestine warfare, waged through secret acts of sabotage that can be written off as a natural outbreak, since no country wants to get caught using a weapon banned by international treaties, but every country wants to reap the rewards of using them without getting caught.

The fourth inner teaching of biological weapons tells us that biological warfare is a clandestine form of warfare that is mostly fought through intelligence channels, espionage, sabotage, covert acts of bioterrorism, and the like. It would rely on operatives or assets that work in areas that cross many domains, such as the scientific and academic communities, the public health system, the corporate sector, and so on.[22]

Bioterrorism is usually carried out in ways that can be claimed a natural outbreak and the target will have a hard time proving it an act of bioterrorism. The reason is this: if the intended damage can be inflicted on the target without any suspicion or knowledge of intentional acts of bioterrorism, the attack can be met without the fear of repercussions or military response. Every country wants to sow the perceived advantages of using such unconventional weapons, but no country wants to get caught using them and end up like Germany after the First World War.

5. The animal kingdom and animal disease are a vast reservoir of new human pathogens in endless varieties and before the advent of modern genetic engineering, genetic engineering was done through the use of animal passages to bring about desired mutations.

What the reader should also know before we embark on this journey through the secret history of biological weapons, is that before the advent of modern genetic engineering technologies to modify biological agents, selective animals were used in what is called *serial passages* using certain animals or combinations of animals. This involves running the agent through an animal and allowing the disease to unfold, and then re-isolating the agent and running it through another animal, in repeated sequence until it mutated to a desired outcome. This allowed for distinct and desired mutations, which became a fine art for Erich Traub.

Directed in this way, it brought desired mutations and characteristics with varying *tropisms*, for example, mouse passages were used to impart neurotropic qualities in humans. Birds and egg passages were often used to adapt agents to humans due to the similarity between the human and avian immune system.[23,24]

Many of the animal diseases can be modified to infect humans, and the factors that make this necessary are fusion proteins and *Mycoplasma*, components that suppress the host defenses and provide opportunities for pathogens to mutate and adapt themselves to new hosts.[25] Animal disease also gave an advantage to create new agents pathogenic to man that had never been seen in humans before and would confuse diagnosis.[26]

One desirable characteristic of using animal passages even after the advent of genetic engineering technology became available was that animal passages would be untraceable and left no fingerprints of tampering with genetic engineering technology. It would mean that the agents created could always be written off as some form of mutation that occurred as a natural event from wild animals.

The idea that most of the animal diseases affecting animals are limited to animals and not a threat to humans is liable to change at any time.[27] While it is acknowledged that some disease agents infect both animals and humans, such as brucellosis, anthrax, avian influenza, among others, many diseases considered solely animal diseases can and do change to infect humans and other hosts it otherwise did not, and it is for this reason that many disease agents considered not a danger to humans could actually play more prominent roles in the spread of disease in the United States and abroad.[28]

For instance, Foot-and-Mouth Disease Virus (FMD), Vesicular Stomatitis Virus (VSV), and Newcastle Disease Virus (NDV), are considered animal diseases, and not generally applied in human pathology. However, animal disease served not only as a good cover, but

19

a reservoir of disease to draw from and adapt to humans to become dangerous human pathogens.[29]

Vesicular Stomatitis Virus, for example, generally a virus causing disease in cattle and swine, infected a lab worker at Plum Island in the mid-1950s, with additional exposures at the Beltsville Experiment Station and the University of Wisconsin.[30]

Foot-and-Mouth Disease, a virus closely related to poliovirus that causes blistering around the hoofs and mouth of an animal, is generally considered a disease of cattle and ruminants only, but has also infected humans in the past, even if rare, but due to their ability to mutate rapidly, FMD had potential to be weaponized to take to human hosts and become a human pathogen.

Albert Demnitz, the director of the German IG Farben subsidiary, Behringwerke AG, published a paper on the question of FMD's ability to infect human hosts.[31] Furthermore, much of Erich Traub's career as a bioweaponeer centered around turning animal diseases to human pathogens.[32] During World War II at the Insel Riems facility in Germany, Traub's colleague, Heinz Röhrer, adapted FMD to mice, causing it to mutate and take on *neurotropic* properties more closely resembling polio, and it was termed "*mouse polio.*"[33]

Following the war, Traub further adapted this *neurotropic* FMD to chickens, first on Insel Riems under Russian captivity, as well as during his time in the United States and Colombia.[34] Adapting these agents to chickens appears to be the point where it adapts itself more easily to human hosts, and as we previously mentioned, there is a close relationship between the immune system of the bird and the human.[35, 36]

DECODING THE ART OF PLAGUE AND PESTILENCE

With the five angles of biological warfare and the art of germ weapons having now been imparted to the reader, the deeper elements and context of this war can now be understood in a more realistic sense as hostile acts of intelligence and elements of war.

Finally, as controversial an idea as this is, vaccines have always been and will continue to be a target for directed acts of bioterrorism.[37] Sabotage and the problematic nature of the vaccines themselves make it an excellent channel for attack. It targets the source materials, production, and distribution of vaccines which can be manipulated for purposes of sabotage. This will be explained by the former KGB agent turned defector Alexander Kouzminov in later chapters.

Even as far back as the Civil War, the Confederates accused the North of deliberately infecting soldiers with vaccino-syphilis from contaminated smallpox vaccines,[38] and in the years preceding the First World War, horses became a target for infecting with bacterial germs, knowing that horses would be used to produce serums and vaccines for humans.[39] This may have likely been some of the unseen elements that contributed to the spread and mutation of the Spanish Influenza of 1918,[40] a situation that became the model to emulate for future activities in biological weapons and their use.[41]

To further complicate this picture, vaccines meant to protect can also impart permanent, long-term health effects that fall in the category of *immune tolerance* and chronic disease, along with the psychiatric and neurological outcomes that present as mental illness.[42] I understand that this topic has become controversial and politicized, but it cannot be avoided in this book because it is intricately interwoven into the story and the science of *immune tolerance* and chronic immunosuppression. We only have one immune system and it is not indestructible or built to handle the stress of endless inoculations of every kind, as antigen/spike protein is very toxic and serves as the weapon itself in the strategic class of bioweapons.

Many of us have a false understanding of immunology and infectious disease because of the public health system and biodefense being dishonest about many of the factors surrounding these agents and the diseases they cause. This book will challenge the paradigms of immunology and infectious disease for most of those reading this book, but these concepts have been discussed in the scientific literature since the days of Erich Traub, though most of them have been ignored when it comes to the public health system providing healthcare. His work demonstrated how one can be quite sick even though they appear healthy with no abnormal bloodwork.

I ask the reader to forgive me if at times it is hard to understand, but I have taken a highly complex science and history and explained it in as simple terms as I possibly could. To leave many of these aspects out to make it easier for the reader to understand would mean leaving out extremely crucial evidence of the case I am trying to make, and I only have one chance to make my case.

Endnotes

1   Rosebury, Theodore. *Peace of Pestilence: Biological Warfare and How to Avoid it.* Whittley House, McGraw-Hill Book Co., New York, Toronto, London. (1949)

2   Zimmerman, B. E., & Zimmerman, D. J. (2003). Killer germs: microbes and diseases that threaten humanity. Contemporary Books., pp. 202, *"And why, pray tell, would any government purposely design a biological warfare germ that had an asymptomatic incubation period averaging nine years?"*

3   U.S. Congress. Committee on Appropriations. Department of Defense Appropriations for Fiscal Year 1970: Hearings before the Subcommittee of the Committee on Appropriations, United States Senate, Ninety-first Congress, First Session, on H.R. 15090, an Act Making Appropriations for the Department of Defense for the Fiscal Year Ending June 30, 1970, and for Other Purposes. 91st Cong., 1st sess. Cong. (OCoLC) 624466202. Washington: U.S. G.P.O., 1969. See Pt. 1, pp. 891.

4   U.S. Congress. Committee on Appropriations. Department of Defense Appropriations for Fiscal Year 1970: Hearings before the Subcommittee of the Committee on Appropriations, United States Senate, Ninety-first Congress, First Session, on H.R. 15090, an Act Making Appropriations for the Department of Defense for the Fiscal Year Ending June 30, 1970, and for Other Purposes. 91st Cong., 1st sess. Cong. (OCoLC) 624466202. Washington: U.S. G.P.O., 1969. Part 5, Research, Development, Test, and Evaluation. pp. 129

5   Martin, W J. "Severe stealth virus encephalopathy following chronic-fatigue-syndrome-like illness: clinical and histopathological features." *Pathobiology : Journal of Immunopathology, Molecular and Cellular Biology* vol. 64,1 (1996): 1-8. doi:10.1159/000163999

6   Consider: Johnson, H. (2006). *Osler's web: inside the labyrinth of the chronic fatigue syndrome epidemic.* iUniverse.

7   Another good example: Murray, P. (1996). *The widening circle: one mother's story of battling Lyme Disease and becoming a medical pioneer.* St. Martin's Press.

8   Traub, E. Observations on immunological tolerance and "Immunity" in mice infected congenitally with the virus of lymphocytic choriomeningitis (LCM). Archiv Fur Die Gesamte Virusforschung, 10(3), 303-314. doi:10.1007/bf01250677. (1960).

9   Kahan, Shannon M, and Allan J Zajac. "Immune Exhaustion: Past Lessons and New Insights from Lymphocytic Choriomeningitis Virus." *Viruses* vol. 11,2 156. 13 Feb. 2019, doi:10.3390/v11020156

10   Traub, E. Can LCM virus cause lymphomatosis in mice? Archiv Fur Die Gesamte Virusforschung, 11(5), 667-682. doi:10.1007/bf01243307. (1962).

11   Kimura, Hiroshi, and Jeffrey I Cohen. "Chronic Active Epstein-Barr Virus Disease." Fr*ontiers in Immunology* vol. 8 1867. 22 Dec. 2017, doi:10.3389/fimmu.2017.01867

12   Sausen, Daniel G et al. "Stress-Induced Epstein-Barr Virus Reactivation." *Biomolecules* vol. 11,9 1380. 18 Sep. 2021, doi:10.3390/biom11091380

13   Domaradskij Igor Valerianovich., and Wendy Orent. *Biowarrior: Inside the Soviet/Russian Biological War Machine.* Prometheus, 2003, pp. 111-112

14   Thus, the Geneva Convention of 1925, and the later Biological Weapons and Toxin Convention (BWTC), with worldwide participation.

15   History.com Editors. (2010, February 9). Germans introduce poison gas. History.com. https://www.history.com/this-day-in-history/germans-introduce-poison-gas

16   Landau, Henry. *The Enemy Within: The Inside Story of German Sabotage in America.* Putnam, 1937

17   *Popular Science.* "Exhibition - Living Factories, 'How New York City's Health Department Makes Serums and Vaccines for the U.S. Army.'" U.S. National Library of Medicine. Nation-

al Institutes of Health, December 21, 2016. https://www.nlm.nih.gov/exhibition/fromdnato-beer/exhibition-living-factories.html

18   Blakemore, Erin. "Germany's World War I Debt Was So Crushing It Took 92 Years to Pay Off." History.com. A&E Television Networks, June 27, 2019. https://www.history.com/news/germany-world-war-i-debt-treaty-versailles

19   Domaradskij Igor Valerianovich., and Wendy Orent. *Biowarrior: Inside the Soviet/Russian Biological War Machine*. Prometheus, 2003, pp. 111-112

20   War Bureau of Consultants Committee, and George W. Merck. 1945. Report to the Secretary of War by Mr. George W. Merck, Special Consultant for Biological Warfare. Report to the Secretary of War by Mr. George W. Merck, Special Consultant for Biological Warfare. National Acadamy of Science (NAS) Online Collections. Retrieved from: http://www.nasonline.org/about-nas/history/archives/collections/organized-collections/1945merckreport.pdf

21   Domaradskiï Igor Valerianovich., and Wendy Orent. *Biowarrior: Inside the Soviet/Russian Biological War Machine*. Prometheus, 2003, pp. 111-112

22   Kouzminov, Alexander. *Biological Espionage: Special Operations of the Soviet and Russian Foreign Intelligence Services in the West*. Manas Publications, 2006.

23   Weill, Jean-Claude et al. "A bird's eye view on human B cells." *Seminars in Immunology* vol. 16,4 (2004): 277-81. doi:10.1016/j.smim.2004.08.007

24   Kohonen, P., et al. Avian Model for B-Cell Immunology ? New Genomes and Phylotranscriptomics. Scandinavian *Journal of Immunology*, 66(2-3), 113–121 (2007). doi:10.1111/j.1365-3083.2007.01973.x

25   See: Traub, E. & K. Beller. Stand und Aussichten der Erforschung des ansteckenden Katarrhs der Luftwege beim Pferd. [The Position and Outlook in Research on Infectious Respiratory Catarrh of the Horse]. Z. Veterinark, 53: 88-97. (1941). [Translated to English by A. Finnegan, 2019], see: Aho, K, and R Pyhälä. 1974. "Agglutinins against Human Erythrocytes Modified by Newcastle Disease Virus in Mycoplasma Pneumoniae Infections." *Clinical and Experimental Immunology*. U.S. National Library of Medicine. August 1974. https://www.ncbi.nlm.nih.gov/pmc/articles/PMC1554100/, see: Clark, Jason. "Mycoplasmas - Identifying Hosts for a Stealth Pathogen." *Veterinary Journal* (London, England : 1997), U.S. National Library of Medicine, Nov. 2005, https://www.ncbi.nlm.nih.gov/pubmed/16266841, see: Naot, Yehudith. "Mycoplasmas as Immunomodulators." Rapid Diagnosis of Mycoplasmas, 1993, pp. 57–67., doi:10.1007/978-1-4615-2478-6_6.

26   Patterson, W.C., Mott L.O., Jenney E.W. A study of vesicular stomatitis in man. *J Am Vet Med Assoc*. 1958 Jul 1;133(1):57-62. PMID: 13549332.

27   Meyer, K F. "The animal kingdom, a reservoir of human disease." *Annals of Internal Medicine* vol. 29,2 (1948): 326-46. doi:10.7326/0003-4819-29-2-326

28   Meyer, K. F. "The Zoonoses in Their Relation to Rural Health by K.F. Meyer, George Williams Hooper Foundation, University of California, San Francisco." World Health Organization, World Health Organization, 1 Jan. 1970, https://apps.who.int/iris/handle/10665/103756

29   Rahman, Md Tanvir et al. "Zoonotic Diseases: Etiology, Impact, and Control." *Microorganisms* vol. 8,9 1405. 12 Sep. 2020, doi:10.3390/microorganisms8091405

30   Callis, J. J., et al. "Isolation of Vesicular Stomatitis Virus from an Infected Laboratory Worker." *Am J Vet Res.* , vol. 16, no. 1, Oct. 1955, pp. 623–626.

31   Demnitz, Albert. "„Kann Der Erreger Der Maul-und Klauenseuche Auch Beim Menschen Das Bild Der Maul-und Klauenseuche Hervorrufen?'" *Nachrichten Der Giessener Hochschulgesellschaft*, 1952, 21-29. Accessed July 26, 2019. http://geb.uni-giessen.de/geb/volltexte/2014/10598/pdf/NaGiHo_Bd_21_1952_21_29.pdf

32   Traub, E., Schneider, B., Zuchtung des Virus der Maul- und Klauenseuche im bebruteten Huhnerei. [Breeding of the Virus of Foot-and-Mouth Disease Virus in Chicken Embryos].

Z Naturforsch B. May-Jun; 3 (5-6):178-87. (1948)

33   Eberle, Henrik. "Ein Wertvolles Instrument": Die Universität Greifswald Im National-sozialismus. Bohlau Verlag, 2015, pp. 542

34   Traub, E., Schneider, B., Zuchtung des Virus der Maul- und Klauenseuche im bebru-teten Huhnerei. [Breeding of the Virus of Foot-and-Mouth Disease Virus in Chicken Embryos]. Z Naturforsch B. May-Jun; 3 (5-6):178-87. (1948) [Translated to English by A. Finnegan (2019)] also: Traub, E., & Capps, W. I. Experiments with chick embryo-adapted foot-and-mouth disease virus and a method for the rapid adaptation. National Naval Medical Center. Bethesda, MD. (1953) U.S. NAVY Project NM. NMRI Memorandum Report. Project NM 000 018.07

35   Weill, Jean-Claude et al. "A bird's eye view on human B cells." *Seminars in Immunology* vol. 16,4 (2004): 277-81. doi:10.1016/j.smim.2004.08.007

36   Kohonen, P., et al. Avian Model for B-Cell Immunology ? New Genomes and Phy-lotranscriptomics. *Scandinavian Journal of Immunology*, 66(2-3), 113–121 (2007). doi:10.1111/j.1365-3083.2007.01973.x

37   Kouzminov, Alexander. Biological Espionage: *Special Operations of the Soviet and Russian Foreign Intelligence Services in the West.* Manas Publications, 2006.

38   Carus, "The History of Biological Warfare"; Paul E. Steiner, *Disease in the Civil War: Natural Biological Warfare in 1861–1865* (Springfield, IL: C.C. Thomas, 1968); William B. Davis, "Report on Vaccination," in *Transactions of the Twenty-Fifth Annual Meeting of the Ohio Medical Society* (Columbus, OH: Nevins and Myers, 1870), 131–166

39   *Popular Science.* "Exhibition - Living Factories, 'How New York City's Health Department Makes Serums and Vaccines for the U.S. Army.'" U.S. National Library of Medicine. National Institutes of Health, December 21, 2016. https://www.nlm.nih.gov/exhibition/fromdnato-beer/exhibition-living-factories.html

40   Gates, F. L. "A Report On Antimeningitis Vaccination And Observations On Agglu-tinins In The Blood Of Chronic Meningococcus Carriers." *Journal of Experimental Medicine*, vol. 28, no. 4, 1918, pp. 449–474., doi:10.1084/jem.28.4.449

41   Traub, E. & K. Beller. Stand und Aussichten der Erforschung des ansteckenden Katarrhs der Luftwege beim Pferd. [The Position and Outlook in Research on Infectious Respiratory Catarrh of the Horse]. Z. Veterinark, 53: 88-97. (1941). [Translated to English by A. Finnegan, 2019]

42   Croft, P B. "Para-infectious and post-vaccinal encephalomyelitis." *Postgraduate Medical Journal* vol. 45,524 (1969): 392-400. doi:10.1136/pgmj.45.524.392

24

Chapter One

A Pretext for Biological War

The Early History of Biological Warfare & the Importance of Animal Disease

My father taught me many things here – he taught me in this room. He taught me – 'keep your friends close but your enemies closer.'
– Michael Corleone, The Godfather Part II

T o understand the climate of biological warfare, one needs only to look back at the chain of events that sparked it all - a continuous escalation of international tensions that led to deployment of biological weapons in times of war. The biological war is never apparent on its face. It is more esoteric, hidden in layers of plausible deniability, provocation, and what looks like natural outbreaks of disease.

Infectious diseases are not like conventional weapons of artillery. It must be remembered that we are not dealing with innate substances like a chemical or poison. These are living organisms. Organisms that survive in the face of incredible adversity, adapt, reorganize, reproduce, infect and spread. It does not discriminate between the intended target and the side who unleashes it. The organism will invade anything it can grab a hold of. It does not care about the politics of war.

The Pretext for Biological War (1700-1925)

B iological warfare, like chemical warfare,[1] is not new. In its more primitive forms, it had varying degrees of employment and success, and occurred for as long as man has been in existence. For example, a decomposing corpse could be thrown into a village's drinking well, contaminating their water source with deadly or crippling microbes.[2] Cattle hides infected with an unknown disease could be shipped over to an enemy nation to infect the merchants and customers.[3]

The United States had established itself in times of great struggle, war, and bloodshed.[4] What is not generally known is that biological warfare, albeit primitive, had a significant role in the early ages of the United States, and Britain had likely used similar tactics with other rivals.

The extent of this is highly obscure, but there are early reports suggesting Britain had been employing biological warfare on the American continent very early on, from at least the late 18th Century, in 1763, when America was establishing itself as the United States.

This happened at Fort Pitt during Pontiac's Rebellion, when the Delaware tribe launched attacks on the settlements and forts along the western frontier of the northern tier of British colonies. The British used smallpox as a weapon. A letter from William Trent, partner in the Indian trading company Levy, Trent & Company, describes the intent to deliberately spread smallpox to the attacking tribesmen.[5] The infected blankets were recorded by a Captain Ecuyer's June 1763 ledgers, billed by Levy, Trent & Company to the British Crown.[6]

The charge was also made in the early days of Australian colonization, in a research paper by biodefense advisor Seth Carus, detailing the British once again intentionally spreading smallpox to the aborigines to protect their colonies from native hostilities or attacks, much like that described on the North American continent.[7]

Most noteworthy attempts by the British to infect the American Continental Army were noted during the Revolutionary war, described by author Elizabeth Fenn, *Biological Warfare in Eighteenth Century North America: Beyond Jeffrey Amherst*, in which smallpox was yet again employed by the British to infect the Continental Army, by the words of first American President George Washington, one of the first to be quoted on the deliberate use of biological weapons against America:

> "The small pox rages all over the Town," wrote George Washington from his headquarters in nearby Cambridge on December 14. "Such of the [British] Military as had it not before, are now under inoculation—this I apprehend is a weapon of Defence, they Are useing against us."
>
> In fact, Washington already suspected that the British, in an effort to infect the vulnerable Continental Army, had inoculated some of the refugees leaving the city. On December 3, 1775, four deserters had arrived at the American headquarters "giving an account that several persons are to be sent out of Boston, this evening or to-morrow, that have been lately inoculated with the small-pox, with design, probably, to spread the infection, in order to distress us as much as possible." It was,

according to Washington's aide-de-camp, an "unheard-of and diabolical scheme." Washington at first regarded the report with disbelief. "There is one part of the information that I Can hardly give Credit to," he wrote. "A Sailor Says that a number of these Comeing out have been inoculated, with design of Spreading the Smallpox through this Country & Camp."[8]

In later years, halfway into the 19th Century, or the 1850's, Britain may have equally employed primitive biological warfare against Ireland, by spreading the potato blight that decimated potato yields during the Irish Famine, a staple in food source for many of the Irish natives. Potato blight (*Phytophthora infestans*), is a fungus that infects the nightshade family of plants, which encompasses tomatoes, potatoes, eggplants, tobacco, among many more.

Britain had been in deep conflict with the Irish just prior to the famine, and an attack that cannot be linked with absolute certainty to the attacking nation, makes an extremely effective tool for an overall attack strategy. What is telling, however, is the fact that Britain sent minimal aid or assistance to Ireland, despite being in a position to do so, while expecting them to be subservient to British rule. Later activity by British planes in the Second World War dropping insects to spread the potato blight in Germany would reinforce this idea.[9]

As if the suspicious activities surrounding the spread of smallpox and potato blight were not enough, there is evidence to suggest Britain was also carrying out additional attacks on the American and Australian livestock with contagious bovine pleuropneumonia (*Mycoplasma mycoides*), a devastating disease on livestock, which occurred simultaneously in each country after cattle from Britain had been sent into each respective country.

The similarity of circumstances suggests that deliberate sabotage may have been instigated by the British, economically motivated by the fear of Her contemporaries reaching prosperity and abundance without Britain's inclusion. Both countries were, at the time, in the middle of a gold rush.

The American incident was discussed 100 years later in an American USDA conference, "Report of the Meetings on Foreign Animal Diseases Attended by State and Federal Regulatory Officials During February and March 1955," ironically, on a ship named the *SS George Washington*:

> About 100 years ago, a British vessel with the name of George Washington docked in the Port of New York, almost opposite

the window of our office at Broadway. On this ship were some cattle which had been brought along to furnish milk and food for the crew members and passengers. The particular cow that furnished the milk had gone dry so that the master of the vessel proceeded to take the cow off the ship to a rural district then known as The Bowery where he traded this cow for a fresh cow. This transaction being done he returned to the ship and sailed away. The cow he traded, however, was infected with contagious pleuropneumonia which spread rapidly over the United States, particularly the eastern seaboard and as west as Ohio, and for a number of years this particular disease was the scourge of the infant livestock industry in the United States.[10]

Interestingly, Australia experienced outbreaks with contagious bovine pleuropneumonia from infected cattle imported from Britain under similar circumstances, at approximately the same time. An article published by the Commonwealth Scientific and Industrial Research Organization (CSIRO) of Australia, "Contagious Bovine Pleuropneumonia Eradication," described the introduction of the disease in close parallel to that in America.[11] This reflects precisely the same approach used with smallpox on the same two countries at strategic times.

SPREADING THE DISEASE

The antagonism between Germany and the United States before the years of the First World War may have been strengthened by antagonism in which Foot-and-Mouth Disease Virus (FMD) and the glanders bacteria played a considerable part. My source John Loftus laid out a memo for this writing, based on testimony from his sources, to describe the war from the perspective of one who has held the highest clearance and has seen many files unbeknownst to those without the proper clearance, that British Intelligence had infected horses and livestock with disease, destined for Germany from the United States. The result caused Germans to think the strike was an attack by the Americans:

> Before America's entry into WWI, the British secret service used hoof and mouth disease [and other diseases] to infect American [cattle and] horses that were going to be shipped to Germany. The use of draft animals to pull artillery and supply carts was still in widespread use in WWI. When America

[sided with Britain against Germany before the War], German agents retaliated by spreading glanders throughout many herds of American horses. Captured German agents later confessed these attacks to US intelligence, but the matter was classified.[12]

Early reports listed in articles of *The New York Times* suggest England was sending the United States diseased cattle while openly blaming the United States for trading infected livestock. In *The New York Times* article from August 3, 1883, "No Trace of Foot and Mouth Disease in this Country. Report of the Treasury Cattle Commission – the Only Cases of the Disease Known Imported from England." In this article, Britain accused the United States of shipping cattle from their ports infected with FMD.[13]

Another hint came the following year in the article, "Cattle Importations from England," where cattle from Britain are found to be the only source of FMD in American livestock, and the suspension of importation of cattle from Britain was put into effect.[14]

In 1895, an article discusses American and English horses being imported into Germany for racing and horse-breeding.[15] However, in 1898, Germany began to notice horses they purchased from the Americans were diseased, and it is at this point that discussion of whether or not to stop importing horses from the United States reached an open discussion, evident in *The New York Times* article dated February 11, 1898, "American Horses in Germany. No Quarantine to be Imposed Yet."[16]

Two years later, reports begin to surface that suggest the horses being shipped to Germany were infected and potentially the source of serious epidemics in Germany at the time. In an article dated March 15, 1900, *The New York Times* published, "Germans Object to American Horses," voicing defiance of the importation of American horses.[17]

Meanwhile, agents operating in New Orleans were infecting horses that were being sent to South Africa during the Boer wars, in a strange article dated April 25, 1901, titled "Boers Inoculating Horses? Agents, Disguised as Cattleman, Said to Have Caused Diseases in Animals Shipped from New Orleans," in a way much similar to the manner my source John Loftus suggested the British had done to horses and cattle destined for Germany.[18]

Furthermore, two additional articles report further details behind the supposed Boer Agents' infecting the animals with glanders, in an article from April 28, 1901, "Doubts that Boers Inoculated Horses," and the Department of Agriculture officials thought it was actually done by someone aboard the ship. It even reveals that the British agents did not press for a further inquiry saying, "[t]*here has been no examination of the horse shipments by the department's representatives, as the British agents never have requested such inspection.*"[19]

The second article floats the idea once more on June 21, "Diseased British Mules. Pro-Boer Sympathizers Said to Have Inoculated Animals Shipped from New Orleans," circulating the story despite the earlier statement that the British agents failed to request further inquiry. The British were claiming that this activity was being "*constantly committed,*" with the British responding by refusing American cattle from Louisiana.[20]

Interestingly enough, barely two weeks prior, Britain halted their importation of meat-supplies contracted with American companies, "American Beef Barred from British Army. All but Home-Bred Product Excluded from Contracts. Chicago Packers Fear Step Will Seriously Cripple Business – Ask Washington for Help," which suspiciously takes place just as the supposed Boer agents started infecting animals in the United States.[21]

This Boer incident being referred to reflected a suit brought in New Orleans court by representatives from the Boer army appealing to the United States to stop shipments of horses and mules to British armies in South Africa.[22] Just several months later, horses in the same state began dying off in large numbers from anthrax, sometimes called charbon disease, in *The New York Times* article from July 5, "Horses Dying in Mississippi. Charbon Has Carried off Practically All the Animals in Some Localities," in a highly fatal form.[23]

A month later, American horses sold to the Mexican Army are also found to be sick with a "peculiar disease," noted in an article, "American Horses Sick- Those Purchased for Mexican Army Develop a Peculiar Disease," from August 4, in Mexico City, describing a fatal disease killing many of them.[24]

Horses were big business at the time, as Britain was purchasing large stocks of horses and mules for the Boer War in South Africa. It was noted that British Agents had a large operation in America with the transport of horses, noted in a December article, "Animals for British Army" from 1901.[25]

It was likely at this point, horses going to Germany were deliberately infected and blamed on the United States. Interestingly, several British agents were charged with fraud at this time from the purchase of bad animals, noted in the article, "British Army Officers Charged with Fraud. Said to Have Bought Broken-Down Animals and Divided Profits. £15,779,000 for Transport. House of Commons Votes That Amount After Bitter Debate — Report on War Office Reorganization." [26]

By June of 1901, a major viral epidemic was spreading in the Northeastern states, "Horses have the grip. It Is Estimated that 10,000 Are Suffering from the Disease. In Several Hospitals 75 Per Cent. of the Horses Have It -- Work Animals the Principal Sufferers." [27] This factor will become relevant in the next chapter describing events of the First World War.

Just several years prior to all of this activity, Britain had isolated the virus of influenza, noted in *The British Medical Journal* of March 1898 in publication, "Isolation in Influenza," [28] where the isolation of the specific components of diseases with infectious cargo much smaller than bacteria, were starting to become known and isolated.

As far back as 1890, British scientific advances were already starting to note the correlation between influenza and bacterial pneumonia, as a viral and bacterial synergy. *The British Medical Journal* from the February 1890 issue published "Influenza and Pneumonia," [29] detailing the link between the two. Eight years after influenza was isolated, surface the first records describing what later became known as Newcastle Disease Virus, a virulent form of avian influenza, surfaces in Scotland, in a Gaelic poem, "Call nan Cearc," or "The Loss of the Hens," by John Campbell, describing its clinical picture of outward symptoms, discussed in published article, "Some Observations on the Epizootiology Of Newcastle Disease." [30]

Like smallpox, FMD was likewise an early tool of the British. Outbreaks of FMD hit New England in 1902, which caused the Department of Agriculture officials to put forward the idea of stopping imports due to the outbreaks. They eventually imposed a federal quarantine and prohibition on the export of New England cattle to other countries and states, initiating the setup of the USDA's Bureau of Animal Industry (BAI) to lead an eradication program and serve as the experimental arm of the USDA to stomp out the cattle plagues of FMD in the country. This was reported in "Annual Report of the Bureau of Animal Industry for the Year 1902: Volume 19, Foot-and-Mouth Disease," by D. E. Salmon, D. V. M. [31]

Britain was already publicly denouncing American cattle as tainted or infected with FMD and pleuropneumonia, the very agents they have been implicated using. This blatant antagonism surfaces in an article, on July 4, 1903, "Distrust American Cattle: Foreign Nations Afraid That Oriental Diseases Will Be Brought in from Philippines." [32]

Indeed, records would corroborate the claim that someone was infecting the animals onboard these ships as they were setting out to sea, and the British agents would have had the means and motive to do so. It is also interesting to note the concern described in the newspaper article, about exotic diseases the Americans might have imported from the Philippines, since British occupation in these regions brought with it the sudden appearance of highly virulent and pathogenic avian virus diseases like Newcastle Disease Virus (ND-V),[33] and a more destructive form of glanders known as melioidosis.[34]

By 1903, the United States was taking significant measures to reassure Germany of the safety of their meat imports from America, shown in article, "Safeguarding Meat Supply. Prompt Work of Government Experts in Stamping Out Epidemic Among Cattle," on October 20, 1903, indicating that events took place which American importations had arrived infected with disease.[35]

In the years prior, Germany's Friedrich Loeffler and Dr. Robert Frosch took up a heavily-funded research project to identify the pathogen causing Foot-and-Mouth Disease. The disease was decimating Germany's livestock in the years prior. My source John Loftus already revealed the British using FMD to infect American cattle heading to Germany, while Germany thought it was an attack by the Americans, whom they were doing business with. Germany had been pushed for the first time to respond. FMD originally occurred in Britain, along with contagious bovine pleuropneumonia. Both of these appear to have been used as attacks against the Americans under nefarious British activities.

My source John Loftus cites the claim by his sources that a coronavirus was isolated by the British program as early as 1904, as a classified matter, though it wouldn't be publicly identified and named coronavirus until 1968, and this is not to be confused with the recent SARS-CoV-2.[36] Back then it would have been known under a more basic name, such as infectious coryza, croup, grippe, or catarrhal fever, and years later it was known as avian infectious bronchitis and avian infectious laryngotracheitis.[37] Considering that other respiratory viruses like influenza were at the time being isolated, it would corroborate the claim.

If Britain had been isolating infectious pleuropneumonia-like organisms (PPLOs) like *Mycoplasma mycoides* and respiratory viruses from the start of the 20th century like influenza, Newcastle Disease Virus (NDV), and coronavirus, it would certainly corroborate the story, since the disease emerged in Australia and the United States right after the official emergence of Newcastle Disease in the Dutch East Indies in the Javanese islands.[38] Older descriptions of Newcastle Disease Virus (NDV), show up in Scotland in 1898, landing just several years before the revelation of the isolation of a coronavirus in 1904.[39]

The viral and bacterial synergy of combined infections would also come into play in the early development of germ weapons. British research at the time indicates they were aiming for an influenza and pneumonia-like synergy. After the initial viral infection, bacterial agents deal the fatal blow to finish them off.

In 1908, British researcher William Hunting published an extensive work on the disease of glanders, called *Glanders: A Clinical Treatise*, describing infections with both chronic and acute forms of the disease. In it, he notes that the disease commonly develops following viral influenza if the person suffers from a latent form of glanders.[40]

Glanders also becomes quite relevant in the British activities leading up to the First World War and beyond. Most notable is the fact that British research at the time demonstrates considerable foreknowledge of combined infections. Later in the same treatise, the acknowledgement of glanders as a contaminant in vaccines or serum is suggested.[41]

Back in Germany, FMD and bacterial diseases of horses were given attention as a matter of high-priority, and its spread was still hitting German livestock, horses, and meat. The Germans suspected an American attack, which they vowed its payback in the years to follow. *The New York Times* article "Cattle Disease in Germany. Foot and Mouth Affection Prevalent – Russia Held Responsible," hints at the Germans being quick to blame disease outbreaks on the Americans, saying, *"Had the livestock been imported from the United States, responsibility for the disease would probably have been laid to America. As it is Russian cattle are blamed."* [42]

As the scourge of FMD in Germany prompted the program by Fredrich Loeffler and Robert Frosch to find the cause of FMD in 1902 on the mainland, technical difficulties forced it to a more remote area, which led to the establishment of Germany's first agricultural facility on the isolated Island of Riems by Greifswald. This facility became known as Insel Riems. The Insel Riems facility coordinated activities with the University of Greifswald, named the Fredrich-Loeffler Institute, the first facility for the study of FMD and other diseases of animals, the production of vaccines, serum, and weaponized agents for biological warfare.[43]

The study of agricultural disease on Insel Riems would have certainly involved the tick-borne disease agents. Insects spread such diseases such as Cattle Tick Fever (Anaplasmosis), Trypanosomiasis, African Horse Sickness, among others. In fact, a later publication showed that in the early stages of FMD research on Riems, insects were studied for their ability to spread the virus.[44] A specific scientific publication from Insel Riems in 1938 studied the ability for ticks and other insects to spread FMD.[45] Later the Food and Agriculture Organization (FAO) of the U.N. listed ticks as a major hazard in the spread of FMD.[46]

This fact would have formed the basis of the German arthropod weapons program, and may have been used in the incidents of which John Loftus made another revelation from his sources – that Germans had sent typhus to Russia through prisoners of war in the years before the scourge hit Russia in World War I, which given their chemical weapons production a valuable context, since they used these chemicals as insecticides.[47] Soon after prisoners of war arrived in Russia, typhus broke out in refugee camps, possibly set up by Germany in Romania, sending waves of death and disease through the Russian empire.[48]

Already suspicious before the First World War, Russia's distrust of Western countries like Britain, Germany, and the United States, would come full circle following simultaneous outbreaks of typhus and later what became known as the "Spanish Influenza." However, to understand this correlation, we need to take a closer look to the events surrounding a little-known plot against the United States by Germans in secret acts of sabotage on the American home front before the War.

Endnotes

1   Even in primitive times, chemicals or plant alkaloids were employed for use against rival tribes or animals to hunt, such as poison arrows. Later in Roman times up to the medieval period, plant alkaloids and extracts of *Atropa belladonna* (deadly nightshade) or *Mandragora officianarum* (mandrake) were used to lace wine that could be given to the opposing armies. See: Ketchum, James S. *Chemical Warfare Secrets Almost Forgotten: a Personal Story of Medical Testing of Army Volunteers with Incapacitating Chemical Agents during the Cold War* (1955-1975). AuthorHouse, 2012, pp. 9-16.

2   Cochrane, Raymond C. "DTIC ADB228585: History of the Chemical Warfare Service in World War II. Biological Warfare Research in the United States, Volume 2 : Defense Technical Information Center." Internet Archive, Defense Technical Information Center (DTIC), 1 Nov. 1947, pp. 21 https://www.archive.org/details/DTIC_ADB228585/page/n21

3   Van Houweling, C. D. "Report of the Meetings on Foreign Animal Diseases Attended by State and Federal Regulatory Officials During February and March of 1955." *Report of the Meetings on Foreign Animal Diseases Attended by State and Federal Regulatory Officials During February and March of 1955*, USDA, 1957, pp. 03 Received from: https://archive.org/details/CAT10678550/page/3

4   *see*: Quigley, Carroll. *Tragedy and Hope: A History of the World in Our Time*. GSG & Associates, 2004. Pp.33-77

5   Volwiter, A. T. (Ed), 'William Trent's Journal at Fort Pitt, 1763', *Mississippi Valley Historical Review*, Vol. 11 (1924), pp. 390-413

6   Geissler, Erhard & John Ellis van Courtland Moon (Ed.). *Biological and Toxin Weapons: Research, Development and Use from the Middle Ages to 1945*. pp. 22.

7   Carus, W. Seth. *A Short History of Biological Warfare: from Pre-History to the 21st Century*. National Defense University Press, 2017, pp. 9-10

8   Fenn EA. "Biological warfare in eighteenth-century North America: beyond Jeffery Amherst." *J Am Hist*. 2000;86(4):1552-1580.

9   Loftus, John J., 2018 (personal communication). Additional researchers have also suggested the deliberate negligence to help Ireland during the famine, who was under British authority, see also: Anonymous Author. "An Argument That the Irish Famine Was Genocide." *The Irish Famine Was Genocide*, www.irishhistorylinks.net/History_Links/IrishFamineGenocide.html.

10   Van Houweling, C. D. "Report of the Meetings on Foreign Animal Diseases Attended by State and Federal Regulatory Officials During February and March of 1955." *Report of the Meetings on Foreign Animal Diseases Attended by State and Federal Regulatory Officials During February and March of 1955*, USDA, 1957, pp. 22 Received from: https://archive.org/details/CAT10678550/page/22

11   "Contagious Bovine Pleuropneumonia Eradication." *CSIROpedia*, 3 Dec. 2018, www.csiropedia.csiro.au/contagious-bovine-pleuropneumonia-eradication/

12   Loftus, J. Memorandum on biological warfare, 2018. (personal communication)

13   NATIONAL CAPITAL TOPICS NO TRACE OF FOOT AND MOUTH DISEASE IN THIS COUNTRY.; NO TRACE OF FOOT AND MOUTH DISEASE IN THIS COUNTRY. (1883, August 03). Retrieved September 04, 2020, from https://timesmachine.nytimes.com/timesmachine/1883/08/03/103613239.html?pageNumber=3

14   CATTLE IMPORTATIONS FROM ENGLAND. (1884, March 09). Retrieved September 04, 2020, from https://timesmachine.nytimes.com/timesmachine/1884/03/09/106274103.html?pageNumber=3

15   American Horses in Germany. (1895, May 06). Retrieved September 04, 2020, from https://timesmachine.nytimes.com/timesmachine/1895/05/06/102456345.html?pageNumber=6

16   AMERICAN HORSES IN GERMANY.; No Quarantine to be Imposed Yet -- The Fruit Correspondence. (1898, February 11). Retrieved September 04, 2020, from https://timesmachine.nytimes.com/timesmachine/1898/02/11/102548426.html?pageNumber=3

17   Germans Object to American Horses. (1900, March 15). Retrieved September 04, 2020, from https://timesmachine.nytimes.com/timesmachine/1900/03/15/102500928.html

18   BOERS INOCULATING HORSES?; Agents, Disguised as Cattlemen, Said to Have Caused Diseases in Animals Shipped from New Orleans. (1901, April 25). Retrieved September 04, 2020, from https://timesmachine.nytimes.com/timesmachine/1901/04/25/117962188.html?pageNumber=1

19   Doubts that Boers Inoculated Horses. (1901, April 29). Retrieved September 04, 2020, from https://timesmachine.nytimes.com/timesmachine/1901/04/29/117962798.html

20   DISEASED BRITISH MULES.; Pro-Boer Sympathizers Said to Have Inoculated Animals Shipped from New Orleans. (1902, June 22). Retrieved September 04, 2020, from https://timesmachine.nytimes.com/timesmachine/1902/06/22/101218316.html?pageNumber=2

21   AMERICAN BEEF BARRED FROM BRITISH ARMY; All but Home-Bred Product Excluded from Contracts. (1901, April 12). Retrieved September 04, 2020, from https://timesmachine.nytimes.com/timesmachine/1901/04/12/117960650.html

22   BOERS BRING SUIT IN NEW ORLEANS; Trying to Prevent Sailing of Mules for the British. (1901, April 3). Retrieved September 04, 2020, from https://timesmachine.nytimes.com/timesmachine/1901/04/03/117959389.html?pageNumber=6

23   HORSES DYING IN MISSISSIPPI.; Charbon Has Carried Off Practically All the Animals in Some Localities. (1901, July 6). Retrieved September 04, 2020, from https://timesmachine.nytimes.com/timesmachine/1901/07/06/117968044.html

24   AMERICAN HORSES SICK.; Those Purchased for Mexican Army De- velop a Peculiar Disease. (1901, August 4). Retrieved September 04, 2020, from https://timesmachine.nytimes.com/timesmachine/1901/08/04/102625830.html?pageNumber=3

25   ANIMALS FOR BRITISH ARMY.; 143,050 Horses and Mules Sent from New Orleans Since the War Began -- Valued at $13,483,052. (1901, December 20). Retrieved September 04, 2020, from https://timesmachine.nytimes.com/timesmachine/1901/12/20/101089913.html

26   BRITISH ARMY OFFICERS CHARGED WITH FRAUDS; Said to Have Bought Broken-Down Animals and Divided Profits. 15,779,000 FOR TRANSPORT House of Commons Votes That Amount After Bitter Debate -- Report on War Office Reorganization. (1901, June 07). Retrieved September 04, 2020, from https://timesmachine.nytimes.com/timesmachine/1901/06/07/101074225.html

27   HORSES HAVE THE GRIP; It Is Estimated that 10,000 Are Suffering from the Disease. In Several Hospitals 75 Per Cent. of the Horses Have It -- Work Animals the Principal Sufferers. (1901, June 22). Retrieved September 04, 2020, from https://timesmachine.nytimes.com/timesmachine/1901/06/22/101075593.html?pageNumber=3

28   White, E W. "Isolation in Influenza." British medical journal vol. 1,1941 (1898): 683-4. doi:10.1136/bmj.1.1941.683

29   Haddon, J. "Influenza and Pneumonia." British medical journal vol. 1,1520 (1890): 354-5. doi:10.1136/bmj.1.1520.354

30   Macpherson, L W. "Some Observations On The Epizootiology Of NewCastle Disease." Canadian journal of comparative medicine and veterinary science vol. 20,5 (1956): 155-68.

31   U. S. Department f Agriculture. (1902). Annual Report of the Bureau of Animal Industry for the Year 1902, Volume 19. Retrieved September 05, 2020, from https://play.google.com/books/reader?id=-P0EAQAAIAAJ

32   DISTRUST AMERICAN CATTLE.; Foreign Nations Afraid That Oriental Diseases Will Be Brought In from Philippines. (1903, July 5). Retrieved September 04, 2020, from https://timesmachine.nytimes.com/timesmachine/1903/07/05/108290770.html

33   Macpherson, L W. "Some Observations On The Epizootiology Of NewCastle Disease." Canadian journal of comparative medicine and veterinary science vol. 20,5 (1956): 155-68.

34   Whitmore, A, and C S Krishnaswami. "A Hitherto Undescribed Infective Disease in Rangoon." The Indian medical gazette vol. 47,7 (1912): 262-267.

35   SAFEGUARDING MEAT SUPPLY.; Prompt Work of Government Experts in Stamping

Ont Epidemic Among Cattle. (1903, October 27). Retrieved September 04, 2020, from https://timesmachine.nytimes.com/timesmachine/1903/10/27/102027748.html?pageNumber=8

36   Virology: Coronaviruses. Nature. 1968;220(5168):650. doi: 10.1038/220650b0. PMCID: PMC7086490.

37   Beach, J. R., and M. A. Stewart. *Diseases of Chickens*. University of California, 1942. pp. 39-41, 47-53

38   BEAUDETTE, F R. "Newcastle Disease in Poultry." *The Cornell Veterinarian*, U.S. National Library of Medicine, Vol. 36, No. 2, Apr. 1946, www.ncbi.nlm.nih.gov/pubmed/20990761 or https://babel.hathitrust.org/cgi/pt?id=uc1.b4179371&view=1up&seq=121

39   Macpherson, L. W. "Some Observations on the Epizootiology Of Newcastle Disease." Can J Comp Med Vet Sci., vol. 20, no. 5, May 1956, pp. 155–168., https://www.ncbi.nlm.nih.gov/pmc/articles/PMC1614269/pdf/vetsci00366-0007.pdf

40   Hunting, William. *Glanders: A Clinical Treatise*. H. & W. Brown, 1908., pp. 21, retrieved from: https://archive.org/details/b21463645/page/20

41   Ibid.

42   CATTLE DISEASE IN GERMANY; Foot and Mouth Affection Prevalent -- Russia Held Responsible. (1910, October 09). Retrieved September 05, 2020, from https://timesmachine.nytimes.com/timesmachine/1910/10/09/102048670.html?pageNumber=18

43   Schmiedebachm H. P. The Prussian State and microbiological research - Friedrich Loeffler and his approach to the "invisible" virus. *100 Years of Virology*. Springer-Verlag Wien. (1999) pp. 9-23.

44   Röhrer, H. 50 Jahre Forschung auf dem Riems. Archive für Experimentelle Veterinärmedizin. B. XIV, heft 5. (1960), pp.716-717 [translation by A. Finnegan 2020]

45   Hirschfelder, H. & J. Wolf. Die Bedeutung von Insekten und Zecken fur die Epidemiologie der Maul- und Klauenseuche [The Importance of Insects and Ticks for the Epidemiology of Foot-and-Mouth Disease]. Zschr. Hyg. Zool. 1938. 142-147

46   Food and Agriculture Organization (FAO). (1994). Foot-and-mouth disease: Sources of outbreaks and hazard categorization of modes of virus transmission. Fort Collins, CO: USDA, APHIS, VS, Centers for Epidemiology and Animal Health. Retrieved from: https://archive.org/details/CAT10871834/page/7/mode/1up

47   Loftus, John J. "Memorandum on Biological Weapons History." 2018

48   Holmes, Frederick. "Typhus on The Eastern Front." *Medicine in the First World War,* University of Kansas School of Medicine, www.kumc.edu/wwi/index-of-essays/typhus-on-the-eastern-front.html.

Chapter Two

SILENT WEAPONS FOR INFECTIOUS WARS:

THE COVERT OPERATIONS OF PLAGUE AND PESTILENCE AS A WEAPON OF WAR

A great war leaves the country with three armies – an army of cripples, an army of mourners, and an army of thieves.

– German Proverb

In the buildup to World War I, infectious wars were already playing out, though much of these factors would have been classified and still today are highly obscure in the eyes of the American public and the world at large. It can be concluded from the previous chapter that Britain was using dirty tricks to turn her ally against Germany, while turning Germany against her ally. This fomented the kick-off of events that led to an ongoing biological war that still maintains itself today. Several events leading up to and surrounding World War I will be looked at in more detail in this chapter.

THE GERMAN SABOTAGE PROGRAM OF 1914

In the years preceding the First Great War, a German sabotage campaign against America was set in motion on the order of the German Kaiser. It was carried out with the help of their agents in America under the supervision of certain men such as Ambassador Franz von Papen, and many additional military and intelligence operatives.[1] Some of these acts of sabotage used explosives to bomb and destroy munitions America was sending to Germany's enemies. Less-known, however, was a major bioterrorism campaign by Germany using germ weapons to sabotage horses used by the medical and military bases. In these attacks, the Germans used such germs as glanders and anthrax to infect the horses around the country.[2]

The plot was in large part successful, but within short-order, everything that could have gone wrong for the Germans, sure did. This was because British Intelligence was literally behind them every step of the way, as they broke the German code used in conveying messages via telegrams. Not to mention, British Intelligence did in fact penetrate the operation fully, as revealed in the personal diaries of a German general in communication with Dr. Helmut Klotz, in his memoir, *The Berlin Diaries: The Private Journals of a General in the German War Ministry Revealing the Secret Intrigue and Political Barralry of 1932-33*.[3]

The German sabotage against the United States described by Seth Carus in his paper "Bioterrorism and Biocrimes: The Illicit Use of Biological Agents since 1900," described one particularly interesting aspect of the German campaign. The effort involved a self-proclaimed German naval officer, Captain Erich von Steinmetz, who, according to reports, sneaks into America illegally dressed as a woman, to participate in the germ war against America. Following his later arrest, Steinmetz described to U.S. officials the details of his operation.[4]

However, according to British Secret Service agent, Henry Landau, in his memoir, *The Enemy Within: The Inside Story of German Sabotage in America*, Steinmetz brought his cultures of glanders boldly into to the Rockefeller Institute claiming he was a researcher and asked the staff to examine his cultures when the bacteria failed to take effect on the target animals.[5]

Other sources lend more insight to the story, and Steinmetz was certainly not on the same page or wavelength as his German compadres. The sloppy, oftentimes reckless nature of his participation, not to mention, outright rejection by other German agents supports the idea that he was employed by an interest outside of Germany.

The event was retold in Robert Koenig's work on German saboteur, Anton Dilger, in *The Fourth Horseman: One Man's Mission to Wage the Great War in America*, where Steinmetz certainly appears aloof among his German counterparts. For one, he shows up unexpectedly to German agent and explosives expert Walter Scheele's laboratory, with a battered suitcase that he claimed to have hand-carried all the way from Romania to New Jersey.

Instead of traveling through neutral Scandanavia to North America, as other German operatives like Anton Dilger and Arthur Zimmerman were ordered to do, Steinmetz adopted the name Steinberg, bought several dresses and, dressed as a woman, chose to travel through enemy territory by way of Russia with a suitcase full of germs, first through Siberia to Vlodivostock, then took a steamer-boat to San

Francisco, travelled across the United States to New Jersey, and finally, at Scheele's doorstep as an unexpected guest, rattling Scheele's nerves, obviously alarmed by this unusual tale. Furthermore, Steinmetz told Scheele of the luggage, a *"case of these germ cultures containing tetanus, some form of glanders or foot-and-mouth disease, and possibly the germ which they term 'dust germ' occasioning infantile paralysis or meningitis."*[6]

More unsettling to Scheele, he was not told of any of these germs to be used in his operation, that his line would be strictly explosives. Scheele studied chemistry at the University of Bonn and seemed to know enough about germs to know the difference between those used in the German affairs and those not used. Something was amiss, and the end result substantiates the idea that Steinmetz could have been a plant. After a heated argument, Scheele pummels Steinmetz and sends him on his way with the battered suitcase.[7]

Rising cases of meningitis were spreading before the 1918 Influenza pandemic. These certainly could have had nefarious origins in light of Steinmetz's likely possession of dust germs, as meningococcus has been termed dust germs because they are often found in dust and the bacteria does accompany infantile paralysis. Steinmetz can already be placed at the vicinity and nearby the Rockefeller Institute in these earlier times, leaving a very suspicious context. What Steinmetz was up to travelling through Russia to reach the United States is keenly suspicious. It would not be too out of line to suggest that Steinmetz was never actually a German agent, but rather a British or Russian double agent, sent in to penetrate the operation and give it an extra degree of severity.

Indeed, there is another work by University of Idaho Professor Emeritus Richard B. Spence, in his study of the 20th century occultist, Aleister Crowley, in *Secret Agent 666: Aleister Crowley, British Intelligence, and the Occult*, as Crowley's life at this time was rife with activity in the United States with German acquaintances, and some of the same names like Walter Scheele and Anton Dilger were mentioned. He describes a similar context, that British Intelligence had infiltrated the operation and were aiming to give it more bang for the buck, under one Admiral Sir Reginald "Blinker" Hall:

> Admiral Hall was anxious about the mounting threat in America and convinced that neutralizing it would require more than just counterpropaganda. He argued that the best way to combat German intrigues in the States was to expose them to the American public and government, who would abhor the destruction of property and fomenting of rebellion on their

soil. Following Hall's logic, preventing German outrages was not necessary or even desirable. Far better was to let them happen and then expose them. In fact, it might even be necessary to give the enemy a little help. The beastlier the Germans, the better.[8]

An interesting thing to note, is that in 1913, under British-controlled areas of Burma, there appeared a new variant of glanders, *Burkholderia pseudomallei*, known as melioidosis. The British could have been developing and testing new germ weapons, in parallel to early developments on influenza viruses, where the glanders variant (melioidosis) is seen for the first time in Rangoon, published as "An Account of a Glanders-like Disease Occurring in Rangoon."[9] Melioidosis was later identified as a biological weapons agent. Suspiciously, this occurs right before German intelligence started their sabotage campaign on American horses, heavily infiltrated by British Intelligence. This would have presented the British with an opportunity to further attack the United States as it had been doing since the formation of America.

What is notable in Steinmetz' activities, is that he can be placed at the Rockefeller Institute with meningococcus dust germs and this form of glanders and in the vicinity of the nearby medical horses, where he made attempts at infecting the horses, as mentioned by Landau.[10]

The German sabotage operation using germ weapons saw more notable success with Dr. Anton Dilger, an American physician who studied medicine in Germany before the First World War and was in a unique position to offer assistance to the Kaiser. Dilger's father was a German American Civil War general and highly-honored veteran, Hubert Dilger. Anton Dilger was travelling to Germany often to study medicine, when he offered his service to the Kaiser. This is said to have occurred following a traumatizing incident where a hospital was bombed and supposedly children were maimed and killed, which sparked Anton's need for retribution against the Americans.[11]

German Intelligence sent Anton Dilger back to America to set up a clandestine culture laboratory on the outskirts of Washington, D.C., just six miles from the White House.[12] Anton's brother, Carl Dilger, also joined him. Anton brought cultures of glanders and anthrax over from Germany to breed further at his secret American lab. They produced new variants for Hinsch, more suitable for the attack, who then passed them to the operatives carrying out the attacks on military horses.[13]

These activities, while having the effect of immobilizing the cavalries, had another, more sinister effect on human targets.[14] The horses would be used to make serum and vaccines.[15] While they could deliver a blow to the cavalries, they could deliver an even more destructive blow to humans all at the same time. This set a unique environment for what was later coined erroneously the "Spanish" Influenza of 1918.[16]

THE "SPANISH" INFLUENZA OF 1918

According to a PBS documentary, the initial start of the 1918 pandemic, seemingly began at Fort Riley in Kansas, in a camp called Camp Funston, and in Haskell County, likely from soldiers who were training at Camp Funston.[17] These soldiers were then thought to have carried the virus with them traveling through the country and into Europe before it spread worldwide. Eventually it spread globally, but it was coined the "Spanish Flu" because the American Press and many other countries censored the media from publishing anything about the new disease killing many soldiers under the threat of severe penalties.[18] Spain was the only one with a free press who reported on the disease and thus earned the name "Spanish Flu,"[19] even though it first appeared at Fort Riley and nearby Haskell County in Kansas.[20]

The aggressive 1918 Influenza surfaces just a month after the Rockefeller Institute finished up an experimental meningococcus vaccine program initiated in October and November of 1917, and soldiers lined up to test the new vaccine because of a rise in cases of bacterial meningitis.[21] The vaccine caused a significant number of severe reactions, and many could not finish the course of shots. Many reported flu-like symptoms indistinguishable from influenza. The following month, the first cases of the 1918 Influenza are recorded.[22]

But let's assume that the experimental meningococcus vaccines were not the source of the 1918 Influenza, it certainly would have enhanced it.[23] The germ sabotage to contaminate the military horses used for serums and vaccines produced by the Rockefeller Institute with destructive bacteria that cause fatal pneumonia would have given a perfect environment to aid and abet the influenza virus, which in turn enhances the fatal bacterial pneumonia.[24] The bacteria, however, would have to remain latent for long enough to not arouse suspicion of illness in the horses, and we will demonstrate one such bacteria shortly, but first lets cover details surrounding the virus itself.

According to John Loftus and what his sources have told him, the Russians and their very effective counterintelligence network placed a heavy emphasis on special weapons like germ weapons, because they thought the British developed the 1918 Influenza from an avian virus and used it as a weapon against them:

> Early warning of counter-revolutionary activities was only one of the benefits to the early Bolsheviks from the [counterintelligence network absorbed from the Russian Tsar's regime]. As a matter of high priority, their agents were also asked to obtain information about western plans to develop biological or chemical weapons that might be used against Russia in a counter-revolution. Emphasis was placed on "special weapons" developments in Great Britain and Germany as the largest threat to the USSR.
>
> It is no surprise that the Bolsheviks would place heavy emphasis on obtaining information about chemical and biological weapons. Russian losses during WWI were staggering: 65% of all the victims of chemical warfare attacks on both sides of the war were Russian. The Germans had attacked Russia with biological weapons such as Anthrax and Typhus, causing hundreds of thousands of deaths. Strange epidemics continued to plague Russia long after the war was over.
>
> Russian intelligence learned that British scientists had discovered and isolated the coronavirus[A] in their Porton Down laboratories as early as 1904. The Russians suspected (albeit without hard proof) that the British had then developed an avian virus that was the real source of the Spanish Flu epidemic of 1918 which killed many millions of Russians. [25]

Examining the possibility of the British developing the 1918 Influenza from an avian virus, there is some evidence that would corroborate it. Published research from 2019 has demonstrated the 1918 Influenza virus to be the combination of an avian influenza and human influenza A.[26] As for British activity, prior tactics described in the first chapter might give us some clues.

Indeed, the 1918 Influenza reached Australia from infected cases onboard ships coming from Britain and British-controlled Singapore.[27] There were also described cases of a unique fatal pneumonia similar to the fatal pneumonia seen in 1918 from a British Navy crew who docked in Philadelphia, killing them in a violent manner causing them to turn blue, apparently a few months before the start of the

---

A   This was an isolation of a coronavirus, but he is not referring specifically to the SARS-CoV-2 virus that caused COVID-19.

pandemic, but it had not spread.[28] This would reflect the same manner of spreading disease in the late 1700s with smallpox and again in the 1850s with pleuropneumonia where British vessels carried epidemics to the USA and Australia years apart.

The British were also heavily concentrating their scientific research on the combined infections of viral influenza and bacterial pneumonia,[29] and isolating human and avian influenza since the start of the 20th century.[30] This would have certainly appeared suspicious to the Russians, who had a very effective counterintelligence spy network since the Russian Tsar was in power.[31]

Next, although Fort Riley, Kansas was named as ground zero for the 1918 Influenza, other researchers have pointed out sporadic cases of a highly fatal disease mirroring the fatal pneumonia seen in 1918 erupted in British military camps as far back as 1916, causing what is termed *purulent bronchitis*, a bacterial and viral synergy, cited in paper, "The so-called Great Spanish Influenza Pandemic of 1918 may have originated in France in 1916."[32]

The following year, the same disease erupted in a British camp at the Aldershot barracks in England.[33] Other researchers suggested an origin in China and India, as there were similar outbreaks described there, but were not considered likely to be the origin.[34] The 1916 cases were also not considered as the start of the 1918 Influenza, but if Russian Intelligence was right and the British were developing such a biological weapon, it may have had several test-runs in the years leading up to 1918, and it would not be out of the question to test on their own military, something most militaries have an ugly history of doing.[35] Testing on army camps about to deploy to the frontlines of the war would have made it more conceivable. It is interesting to note that all regions just named were either British army camps or areas under British occupation, like those in China and India.

In 1889-1890, a Russian Influenza pandemic occurred which travelled worldwide but was mild and did not cause the devastation that the 1918 virus did, but it was thought that those exposed to this virus had a more severe and fatal reaction to the 1918 Influenza.[36] This fact may have aroused suspicion by Russian Intelligence.

Recall from the previous chapter, that in 1901, thousands of horses in New York became sick with the *grippe*, a term for influenza.[37] Epidemics of influenza were also raging in humans at this time.[38] This was also the same year that Boer agents were said to be inoculating horses in New Orleans to spread disease.[39] The Germans were at this time objecting to American horses due to disease.[40] Since so much activity described in the first chapter was occurring at this time, and if the past has taught us anything about British biological warfare, they were already shown how effective germs could be as an economic weapon. It is possible many unseen attempts and activities happened in the years leading up to the 1918 Influenza, but nothing conclusive can be said and they remain unseen for now.

Viral and Bacterial Synergy

Medical and Military horses were a unique target in the German sabotage campaign, since horses were used to produce serums and vaccines for human use, and this was the case for the experimental meningococcus vaccine conducted by the Rockefeller Institute at Fort Riley before the start of the 1918 Influenza, they used horse serum to make the vaccine.[41] Medical horses used to make serum and vaccines were often used and re-used to make multiple vaccines and serum for a diverse range of diseases and often used multiple live microbes,[42] and this could easily suppress the immune system of horses, especially meningococcus.

Meningococcus can suppress the immune system and activate additional infections,[43] sometimes referred to as *infectious catarrh*, which means "mixed infections."[44] Such combined infections can severely blunt the immune system rather than illicit a healthy response,[45] and the possibility of microbial contamination of the serums and vaccines is very high,[46] especially when using several strains of meningococcus bacteria in one vaccine or serum, which the Rockefeller vaccine did.[47] These multiple combined infections would complicate vaccination, leaving potentially permanent damage to the immune system, with a chronic, persistent infection to plague the afflicted.[48]

This compromised state would leave ripe conditions for a virus like influenza to rapidly mutate and shed for extended periods in the immunocompromised, and this was documented with the SARS-CoV-2,[49] and other published research documented long-term shedding of influenza virus in the immunocompromised.[50] In recent years, there were more than 20 mutations found in an immunocompromised patient with a SARS-CoV-2 infection.[51] Add this to the fact that many soldiers were packed in confined living quarters and ships during wartime. This would have been a perfect environment for a virus to evolve into a potent killer.

Melioidosis: The Vietnamese Timebomb

As for biological sabotage, the glanders variant melioidosis (*Burkholderia pseudomallei*) would have been a choice weapon against horses used for serums and vaccines. The advantage of this microbe is that there would be no apparent disease in these horses, as melioidosis has a much longer incubation period and was nicknamed the "Vietnamese time bomb" because it could often remain latent for months to years before erupting into an active infection.[52] This would mask the infection in horses being used for serum and vaccines. Melioidosis primarily causes pneumonia with a very high mortality rate and has been listed as a potential biological weapon.[53] British research on its cousin glanders understood that glanders commonly developed after influenza if the patient is infected with latent glanders."[54]

Recalling how Erich von Steinmetz, whose germs did not produce apparent disease in the horses nearby the Rockefeller Institute, was said to be in possession of "some form of glanders," indicating it was not the traditional glanders bacteria.[55] Certainly, the use of such germs against horses used in vaccines given to humans would have greatly enhanced any viral infection, especially epidemic influenza.[56] The horse serum and vaccines made from Rockefeller Institute horses were shipped and used worldwide in World War I.[57]

This would have produced a unique environment ripe for mutations of the 1918 Influenza virus in these hosts, allowing it to become the potent killer it became, destroying the immune system and activating the bacterial pneumonia that killed them. The 1918 Influenza virus was not the sole cause of death in the 1918 Influenza, as later samples of tissues taken from fatal cases of the pandemic revealed a bacterial pneumonia produced the fatal and violent death.[58] This would be expected with a virus that damages the immune system and activates bacterial pneumonia and Erich Traub will revisit this concept later in the book. In 1919, Louis Cruveilhier said, "If grippe condemns, the secondary infections execute."

BRITISH INFILTRATION OF GERMAN SABOTAGE

British Intelligence had fully infiltrated the German sabotage program, guiding it along every step of the way, while giving it more bang for the buck.[59] Earlier British published research on combined infections to create a viral and bacterial synergy demonstrated their foreknowledge of respiratory viruses like influenza activating additional bacterial infections like glanders and bacterial pneumonia.[60] Perhaps they only meant to enhance the German sabotage program to make it more costly and the situation spun out of control, providing ripe conditions for a full-scale pandemic as an unintended consequence.

On top of that, British Intelligence was certainly antagonistic in their role pinning the USA against the Germans.[61] According to John Loftus, his sources brought another revelation the reader may find hard to conceive, that at one time, U.S. Intelligence thought the British were an even bigger threat to American National Security than even Nazi Germany. However, in light of what I have laid out thus far, it is certainly understandable. It was this revelation that had me looking more deeply into British activities, and the evidence certainly supports it. Let's not forget what caused the formation of America to begin with.

Some of the German saboteurs may have been flipped to the British after getting caught and continued the campaign for British Intelligence.[62] This can be picked up throughout Robert Koenig's book on Anton Dilger. Interestingly enough, German spies are said to have eventually murdered Anton Dilger, their main saboteur, for what British Secret Service agent Henry Landau claimed as refusal to carry out orders in Spain.[63] He died in Spain under mysterious circumstances, and his brother Carl Dilger was certain that Anton Dilger was intentionally inoculated with Influenza germs as a weapon, in his case, a weapon of assassination.[64]

As British Intelligence "decoded" every cable the Germans were sending their saboteurs, they took the high ground in painting themselves as the saviors, expose Germany, point out the failures of U.S. Intelligence, and tarnish the reputation of both countries for the world at large, while further antagonizing the two against each other.[65] A perfect strategy for their strategic objectives in the build-up to World War I. With their antagonism in the shadows, Germany is exposed to the world with the Americans backing Britain. In biodefense advisor Seth Carus's working paper on biological warfare use in earlier times, German biological sabotage was employed heavily around the globe:

> The Germans conducted similar operations elsewhere, which the British discovered through reading decoded German cables. According to various reports, the Germans tried to introduce plague cultures into St. Petersburg in 1915, sent anthrax and glanders cultures to Romania in August 1916 to infect sheep being shipped to Russia, tried to infect Norwegian reindeer with glanders organisms in January 1917, infected 4,500 mules used by British forces in Mesopotamia during 1917 with glanders organisms, infected sheep, cattle, and horses being shipped from Argentina to Britain and to the Indian Army with glanders and anthrax during 1917 and 1918, and tried to infect

advancing Allied forces with glanders and cholera organisms during the German retreat in October 1918. The Germans also infected horses being shipped from Argentina to France and Italy. They believed the operation was so successful that it ended all such shipments. Another report suggests that the Germans attempted to introduce cholera organisms into Russia.[66]

While Germany certainly was responsible for many of these acts, we must ask, to what extent was British Intelligence helping them along and carrying out far more antagonistic acts of sabotage, giving them more bang for the buck, laying down the pretext for the United States to enter the war by her Majesty's side? In September of 1918, in Washington, D.C., a Lt. Col. Philip Doane, head of the Health and Sanitation Section of the Emergency Fleet Corporation, had already pointed blame to Germany for the pandemic:

> "It would be quite easy for one of these German agents to turn loose Spanish influenza germs in a theater or some other place where large numbers of persons are assembled. The Germans have started epidemics in Europe, and there is no reason why they should be particularly gentle with America."[67]

British Secret Service agents were also posing as German spies in Russia during WWI, where they involved the United States in German acts of sabotage in Russia. A declassified American Intelligence Report on a Soviet memorandum, "Prospective Uses of Bacterial Weapons in Future Wars," describes German sabotage operations using biological weapons and admits to how effective a weapon it actually was. In it describes how plague cultures were imported from the United States by British counterintelligence agent [Dorian] Blair to introduce plague-infected rats into the streets of Petrograd.[68]

This British Secret Service agent was Lt. Dorian Blair, who wrote a memoir called *Russian Hazard: The Adventures of a British Secret Service Agent in Russia* describing his involvement in the plan which also involved the Russian occultist Gregori Rasputin.[69] It was discussed in another publication later declassified by the CIA, "General Information on the Biological Weapon and Principles of Anti-Epidemic Defence of the Population," written by Soviet official I. N. Morgunov, revealing the deeper context of Blair's operation, appearing as a German agent, entangling the United States:

> In 1915, the German spy Gragersen imported a culture of plague bacillus from the United States into Russia. This cul-

ture was brought from Arkhangel'sk to Saratov, where it was to multiply and then be used in Petrograd. This diversionary act was not completed, because the German spy Bler[B] who had been put in charge of this operation was simultaneously working for Russian Intelligence.[70]

With all the information that has been laid out up to this point, the idea that Britain was formerly employing germ warfare against the United States, Australia, Ireland, and Russia is by no means unreasonable, in some cases, like smallpox, it is proven. Most sinister would be the overall achievement that unfolded with the 1918 Influenza in Europe that left many millions dead, with the virus serving as the dynamite to activate the bacterial pneumonia to deliver the death blow once the avian virus began to spread its wings.

This heavy toll on Russia from the multiple epidemics like typhus and influenza led them to begin concentrating on special weapons under their biowarfare program in attempt to defend and strike back to what they viewed as hostile acts by the Western world.[71] According to John Loftus citing his sources, they found a critical weakness to exploit – the American's failure to respond to or even denounce the earlier attacks by German and British sabotage:

> The communist leadership saw the American failure to react against these biological warfare attacks, or even denounce them in public, as a weakness that Russia could (and later did) exploit with their own use of biological warfare for clandestine attacks upon America. In 1921, Russia launched an all-out drive to develop offensive biological warfare systems as Russia's secret weapon against the West.[72]

As the First World War passed, typhus and the "Spanish" influenza devastated Russia causing bewildering death and destruction. Germany sent typhus to Russia, and this caused insect-borne disease to plague Russia with incapacitating diseases that would hex the Russian and later Soviet empire long after the fatal 1918 Influenza. It was in these epidemics that brought the attention to how much destruction could be waged with weaponized microbes and would set future models of attack using the different kinds of biological agents – those that kill, and those that *incapacitate*

B   *Bler* is Slavic phonetic spelling of the English name Blair, being Lt. Col. Dorian Blair, his involvement in which was confirmed in his memoir, Blair, Dorian (Lt. Col.), and C. H. Dand. *Russian Hazard the Adventures of a British Secret Service Agent in Russia*. Hale, 1937.

Endnotes

1   Landau, Henry. *The Enemy Within: The Inside Story of German Sabotage in America.* Putnam, 1937.

2   Ibid., pp. 47

3   Klotz, Helmut, ed. 1935. *The Berlin Diaries: The Private Journals of a General in the German War Ministry Revealing the Secret Intrigue and Political Barralry of 1932-33.* London: Jarrolds., pp. 68-71. Retrieved from: https://archive.org/details/in.ernet.dli.2015.536823/page/n75

4   Carus, W. Seth. *Bioterrorism and Biocrimes: the Illicit Use of Biological Agents since 1900.* Center for Counterproliferation Research, National Defense University, 2002., pp. 69

5   Landau, Henry. *The Enemy Within: The inside Story of German Sabotage in America.* Putnam, 1937., pp. 47

6   Koenig, Robert L. *The Fourth Horseman: One Man's Mission to Wage the Great War in America.* PublicAffairs, 2006., pp 90-91

7   Ibid., pp. 91

8   Spence, R. B. (2008). *Secret agent 666: Aleister Crowley, British intelligence and the occult.* Port Townsend, WA: Feral House., pp. 73-74

9   Whitmore A. An Account of a Glanders-like Disease occurring in Rangoon. *J Hyg (Lond).* 1913;13(1):1-34.1. doi:10.1017/s0022172400005234

10   Landau, Henry. *The Enemy Within: The inside Story of German Sabotage in America.* Putnam, 1937., pp. 47

11   Koenig, Robert L. *The Fourth Horseman: One Man's Mission to Wage the Great War in America.* Public Affairs, 2006.

12   Ibid.

13   Ibid.

14   Noted in report: Gates, F. L. "A Report On Antimeningitis Vaccination And Observations On Agglutinins In The Blood Of Chronic Meningococcus Carriers." *Journal of Experimental Medicine*, vol. 28, no. 4, 1918, pp. 460-461, doi:10.1084/jem.28.4.449.

15   Ibid.

16   Morens, David M., et al. "Predominant Role of Bacterial Pneumonia as a Cause of Death in Pandemic Influenza: Implications for Pandemic Influenza Preparedness." The Journal of Infectious Diseases, vol. 198, no. 7, 2008, pp. 962–970., doi:10.1086/591708.

17   Public Broadcasting Service. (n.d.). American Experience: Influenza Across America in 1918. PBS. Received from: https://www.pbs.org/wgbh/americanexperience/features/influenza-timeline/

18   Trine Day. (2023, August 11). TrineDay: *The Journey Podcast.* Episode 133. John Loftus: The sleeper agent, biological warfare, Allen Dulles, and his nazi-funding wall street clients. Spotify. https://open.spotify.com/episode/21avVmuIKqzZPjgcl9rVll

19   Little, B. (2020, May 26). As the 1918 flu emerged, cover-up and denial helped it spread. History.com. https://www.history.com/news/1918-pandemic-spanish-flu-censorship

20   Barry, J. M. (2004). *The Great Influenza.* Penguin.

21   Gates, F. L. "A Report On Antimeningitis Vaccination And Observations On Agglutinins In The Blood Of Chronic Meningococcus Carriers." *Journal of Experimental Medicine,* vol. 28, no. 4, 1918, pp. 449–474., doi:10.1084/jem.28.4.449.

22   Public Broadcasting Service. (n.d.). American Experience: Influenza Across America in 1918. PBS. Received from: https://www.pbs.org/wgbh/americanexperience/features/influenza-timeline/

23   Huisman, W et al. "Vaccine-induced enhancement of viral infections." Vaccine vol. 27,4 (2009): 505-12. doi:10.1016/j.vaccine.2008.10.087

24   *Nicolson, Garth L. and Gonzalo Ferreira de Mattos. "COVID-19 Coronavirus: Is Infec-*

tion along with Mycoplasma or Other Bacteria Linked to Progression to a Lethal Outcome?" International Journal of Physical Medicine and Rehabilitation 11 (2020): 282-302.

25   Loftus, John J. "Memorandum on Biological Weapons History." 2018.

26   He, Cheng-Qiang et al. "The matrix segment of the "Spanish flu" virus originated from intragenic recombination between avian and human influenza A viruses." Transboundary and emerging diseases vol. 66,5 (2019): 2188-2195. doi:10.1111/tbed.13282

27   Swinden, G. (2023, May 16). The Navy and the 1918-19 Influenza pandemic. JMVH, Vol.28 No. 3. https://jmvh.org/article/the-navy-and-the-1918-19-influenza-pandemic/

28   Barry, J. M. (2004). The Great Influenza. Penguin., pp. 2

29   Haddon, J. "Influenza and Pneumonia." *British medical journal* vol. 1,1520 (1890): 354-5. doi:10.1136/bmj.1.1520.354

30   White, E. W. "ISOLATION IN INFLUENZA." *Bmj*, vol. 1, no. 1941, 1898, pp. 683–684., doi:10.1136/bmj.1.1941.683.

31   Loftus, John J. "Memorandum on Biological Weapons History." 2018

32   Oxford, J S. "The so-called Great Spanish Influenza Pandemic of 1918 may have originated in France in 1916." *Philosophical transactions of the Royal Society of London. Series B, Biological sciences* vol. 356,1416 (2001): 1857-9. doi:10.1098/rstb.2001.1012

33   Abrahams, A., Hallows, N., Eyre, J. W. H., & French, H. (1917). PURULENT BRONCHITIS: ITS INFLUENZAL AND PNEUMOCOCCAL BACTERIOLOGY. The Lancet, 190(4906), 377–382. doi:10.1016/s0140-6736(01)52169-8 10.1016/s0140-6736(01)52169-8

34   Barry, John M. "The site of origin of the 1918 influenza pandemic and its public health implications." Journal of translational medicine vol. 2,1 3. 20 Jan. 2004, doi:10.1186/1479-5876-2-3

35   Human experimentation: An introduction to the ethical issues. Physicians Committee for Responsible Medicine. (n.d.). https://www.pcrm.org/ethical-science/human-experimentation-an-introduction-to-the-ethical-issues

36   Gagnon, Alain et al. "Age-specific mortality during the 1918 influenza pandemic: unravelling the mystery of high young adult mortality." PloS one vol. 8,8 e69586. 5 Aug. 2013, doi:10.1371/journal.pone.0069586

37   HORSES HAVE THE GRIP; It Is Estimated that 10,000 Are Suffering from the Disease. In Several Hospitals 75 Per Cent. of the Horses Have It -- Work Animals the Principal Sufferers. (1901, June 22). Retrieved September 04, 2020, from https://timesmachine.nytimes.com/timesmachine/1901/06/22/101075593.html?pageNumber=3

38   The New York Times. (1901d, January 14). 563,885 grip victims.; reports show the disease prevails in a broad belt from New York to the Rocky Mountains. The New York Times. https://timesmachine.nytimes.com/timesmachine/1901/01/14/118460360.html?pageNumber=1

39   BOERS INOCULATING HORSES?; Agents, Disguised as Cattlemen, Said to Have Caused Diseases in Animals Shipped from New Orleans. (1901, April 25). Retrieved September 04, 2020, from https://timesmachine.nytimes.com/timesmachine/1901/04/25/117962188.html?pageNumber=1

40   Germans Object to American Horses. (1900, March 15). Retrieved September 04, 2020, from https://timesmachine.nytimes.com/timesmachine/1900/03/15/102500928.html

41   Gates, F. L. "A Report On Antimeningitis Vaccination And Observations On Agglutinins In The Blood Of Chronic Meningococcus Carriers." *Journal of Experimental Medicine,* vol. 28, no. 4, 1918, pp. 449–474., doi:10.1084/jem.28.4.449.

42   "How New York City's Health Department Makes Serums and Vaccines for the United States Army," see Slide 7 Popular Science, December 1917 Courtesy Smithsonian Libraries, National Museum

43   Moore, P. S. "Respiratory Viruses and Mycoplasma as Cofactors for Epidemic Group A Meningococcal Meningitis." *JAMA: The Journal of the American Medical Association,* vol. 264,

no. 10, 1990, pp. 1271–1275., doi:10.1001/jama.264.10.1271.

44   Traub, E. & K. Beller. Stand und Aussichten der Erforschung des ansteckenden Katarrhs der Luftwege beim Pferd. [The Position and Outlook in Research on Infectious Respiratory Catarrh of the Horse]. Z. Veterinark, 53: 88-97. (1941). [Translated to English by A. Finnegan, 2019]

45   Awad, N F S et al. "Impact of single and mixed infections with Escherichia coli and Mycoplasma gallisepticum on Newcastle disease virus vaccine performance in broiler chickens: an in vivo perspective." *Journal of applied microbiology* vol. 127,2 (2019): 396-405. doi:10.1111/jam.14303

46   Armstrong, Shayn E et al. "The scope of mycoplasma contamination within the biopharmaceutical industry." *Biologicals : journal of the International Association of Biological Standardization* vol. 38,2 (2010): 211-3. doi:10.1016/j.biologicals.2010.03.002

47   Gates, F. L. "A Report On Antimeningitis Vaccination And Observations On Agglutinins In The Blood Of Chronic Meningococcus Carriers." *Journal of Experimental Medicine,* vol. 28, no. 4, 1918, pp. 460-461, doi:10.1084/jem.28.4.449

48   see: Naot, Yehudith. "Mycoplasmas as Immunomodulators." *Rapid Diagnosis of Mycoplasmas*, 1993, pp. 57–67., doi:10.1007/978-1-4615-2478-6_6.

49   Sonnleitner, Sissy Therese et al. "Cumulative SARS-CoV-2 mutations and corresponding changes in immunity in an immunocompromised patient indicate viral evolution within the host." *Nature communications* vol. 13,1 2560. 10 May. 2022, doi:10.1038/s41467-022-30163-4

50   Pinsky, Benjamin A et al. "Long-term shedding of influenza A virus in stool of immunocompromised child." *Emerging infectious diseases* vol. 16,7 (2010): 1165-7. doi:10.3201/eid1607.091248

51   Doucleff, M. (2021, February 05). Extraordinary patient offers surprising clues to origins of coronavirus variants. Retrieved February 20, 2021, from: https://www.npr.org/sections/goatsandsoda/2021/02/05/964447070/where-did-the-coronavirus-variants-come-from?

52   Dance, David Allan Brett. "Melioidosis and Glanders as Possible Biological Weapons." Bioterrorism and Infectious Agents: A New Dilemma for the 21st Century, 2009, pp. 99–145., doi:10.1007/978-1-4419-1266-4_4.

53   Ibid.

54   Hunting, William. *Glanders: A Clinical Treatise*. H. & W. Brown, 1908., pp. 21, retrieved from: https://archive.org/details/b21463645/page/20

55   Koenig, Robert L. *The Fourth Horseman: One Man's Mission to Wage the Great War in America*. Public Affairs, 2006.

56   Huisman, W et al. "Vaccine-induced enhancement of viral infections." *Vaccine* vol. 27,4 (2009): 505-12. doi:10.1016/j.vaccine.2008.10.087

57   Rockefeller Institute pamphlet PDF (1919), Retrieved from: https://digitalcommons.rockefeller.edu/cgi/viewcontent.cgi?article=1005&context=rockefeller-institute-descriptive-pamphlet

58   Morens, David M., et al. "Predominant Role of Bacterial Pneumonia as a Cause of Death in Pandemic Influenza: Implications for Pandemic Influenza Preparedness." The Journal of Infectious Diseases, vol. 198, no. 7, 2008, pp. 962–970.,

59   Klotz, Helmut, ed. 1935. The Berlin Diaries: *The Private Journals of a General in the German War Ministry Revealing the Secret Intrigue and Political Barralry of 1932-33*. London: Jarrolds., pp. 68-71. Retrieved from: https://archive.org/details/in.ernet.dli.2015.536823/page/n75

60   Haddon, J. "Influenza and Pneumonia." *British Medical Journal*, U.S. National Library of Medicine, 15 Feb. 1890, https://www.ncbi.nlm.nih.gov/pubmed/20752952

61   Landau, Henry. *The Enemy Within: The Inside Story of German Sabotage in America*.

Putnam, 1937.

62   This can be seen throughout Landau's account regarding the activities of the saboteurs and those setting up the operations.

63   Landau, Henry. *The Enemy Within: The inside Story of German Sabotage in America*. Putnam, 1937pp. 194

64   Koenig, Robert L. *The Fourth Horseman: One Man's Mission to Wage the Great War in America*. Public Affairs, 2006, pp. 272

65   Landau, Henry. *The Enemy Within: The inside Story of German Sabotage in America*. Putnam, 1937.

66   Carus, W. Seth. *Bioterrorism and Biocrimes: the Illicit Use of Biological Agents since 1900*. Center for Counterproliferation Research, National Defense University, 2002., pp. 70

67   "Placing Blame." PBS. American Experience: Influenza 1918, Public Broadcasting Service, www.pbs.org/wgbh/americanexperience/features/influenza-placing-blame/ Accessed 27 Aug. 2023.

68   Central Intelligence Agency (CIA) Intelligence Reports: PROSPECTIVE USES OF BACTERIOLOGICAL WARFARE IN FUTURE WARS. CIA-RDP80-00809A000600120022-4. Central Intelligence Agency (CIA), Reading Room, 2011. Retrieved from: https://www.cia.gov/readingroom/document/CIA-RDP80-00809A000600120022-4

69   Blair, Dorian (Lt. Col.), and C. H. Dand. *Russian Hazard the Adventures of a British Secret Service Agent in Russia*. Hale, 1937.

70   Central Intelligence Agency (CIA) Intelligence Reports: MEDICAL SERVICE IN MASS ATTACK USSR. "GENERAL INFORMATION ON THE BIOLOGICAL WEAPON AND PRINCIPLES OF ANTI-EPIDEMIC DEFENCE OF THE POPULATION." CIA-RDP81-01043R003800050002-9. Central Intelligence Agency (CIA), Reading Room, 2011. Retrieved from: https://www.cia.gov/readingroom/document/CIA-RDP81-01043R003800050002-9

71   Loftus, John J. "Memorandum on Biological Weapons History." 2018.

72   Ibid.

Chapter Three

RED PESTILENCE: THE SOVIET BIOLOGICAL WEAPONS PROGRAM

DEVELOPING THE MOST ADVANCED BIOLOGICAL WEAPONS PROGRAM IN EXISTENCE

... but his days were shortened by poison, perhaps the most incurable of poisons; the stings of remorse and despair, and the bitter remembrance of lost glory."
    – Edward Gibbon, *The Decline and Fall of the Roman Empire*

The Soviet Union, which is now the Russian Federation, began to concentrate and accelerate their biological warfare program early in the 20th century as a result of the devastating toll of the Spanish Flu and typhus epidemics that ravaged the Russian people from the days of World War I, eliciting suspicion that the pandemic was a deliberate act by the West.[1]

With a far-reaching, deeply embedded intelligence network positioning spies in the heart of each ally and enemy alike, the Soviet plan was a future of biological attack via stealth sabotage, vector warfare, espionage and psychological operations. Concerns about the British developing and using this capability had not been far-fetched. Therefore, intelligence gathering was not enough, the response was to push forward on a full-speed course to complete advancement in offensive biological weapons capability.[2]

LYSENKOISM: THE MARK OF THE SOVIET BEAST

Before we proceed to study the Soviet biological weapons program in operation from early times to present, we need to take a look at one of the minds who influenced and generated its framework, Trofim Lysenko, an agricultural biologist who promoted the concept that traits acquired in the lifetime are passed down generations.[3] While genetics are at the foundation of our biological makeup, Lysenko denied genetics. He mainly directed his ideas to the larger organisms like plant life and animals, and many of his ideas turned out to be wrong, although he was partially correct in some areas.

At any rate, intelligence reports show that there were other scientists like G. M. Bosh'yan who was developing and applying ideas of acquired characteristics to viruses and microbiology, which are much more malleable and adaptable, unlike the higher forms of life.[4] Under the Lysenko banner, intelligence reports show they were experimenting with many different methods and techniques which honed in on the malleability of viruses and microbes which could impart new qualities like that done by modern genetic engineering.[5]

These were primitive genetic engineering methods the Soviets were using, but the West scoffed at it because under the banner of Lysenko they deemed it pseudo-science.

Intelligence reports seem to indicate that some of these Soviet bioweaponeers were able to utilize conservative approaches with clever techniques for producing effective biological weapons, and under the banner of Lysenko it was well-hidden.[6] The Soviet Union believed in Lysenko's science, but it failed them. However, the biological weapons program succeeded onward under the banner of Lysenko, and it was never taken seriously by the West. The Soviet Union put the failures of Lysenko to good use hiding the biological weapons program under its banner. The Soviet bioweaponeers then gained the advantage over the West when they acquired both the Japanese Unit 731 and the German Insel Riems facilities at the end of World War II.[7, 8]

With the acquisition of Insel Riems at the end of World War II, the bulk of Erich Traub's most important work was hauled off to the U.S.S.R., giving them even more exceptional weapons than they ever could have dreamed of. Biological warfare was an alternative to the technological advancement of the West. If there was a way to take down Western civilization, who was far superior to the Soviet Union in technological terms, this was it – *biological warfare* – which did not need fancy lab equipment to do the trick, but clever methodologies with conservative approaches were always far superior.[9]

THE FIRST AND SECOND GENERATION OF SOVIET BIOWEAPONS

The Soviet program was divided into two parts or periods. The time from 1918-1972 was called the first generation, with 1973-1991 the second generation. Although Soviet bioweapons research had been conducted as far back as World War I, the first generation was officially underway in 1928 when a secret-decree, signed by Yakov Fishman, was issued by the Revolutionary Military Council as an assessment of the feasibility of creating biological agents for weapons of war.[10] This would sound much like the assessment given by Dr. George Merck to the War Research Service just 14 years later for the American offensive.[11]

The first generation of biological weapons development kicked off for the Soviet Union after realizing the devastation of the so-called "Spanish" Flu of 1918 and the typhus outbreaks in the days of World War I. With suspicions of the West intentionally spreading plagues, the Worker's and Peasant's Red Army (RKKA) Established the Military Chemical Agency in 1925, as a chemical warfare department that would eventually handle biological weapons research. To counter disease outbreaks, the Vaccine-Serum Laboratory was established. In 1933, the State Political Administration (OGPU) set up a laboratory in Suzdal called the Special Purpose Bureau to study highly infectious diseases. This bureau may have been some of the earlier areas where their ultra-secret working groups began to centralize on vaccine sabotage.

Later in the year the Special Purpose Bureau and the Vaccine-Serum Laboratory were combined and renamed several times.[12] It was through the Special Purpose Bureau that collaboration with Germany occurred to exchange information on chemical and biological agents and means of dispersal, once in 1921 and again in 1928 at Waffenprüf 9 chemical weapons artillery hanger in Tomka.[13, 14]

Communism under Soviet Russia was totalitarian through and through. Stalin had full control over the entire continent of the U.S.S.R. They lacked money and had nowhere near the technological advances of the West.[15] Yet, they made up for this in biological research and above all, spy networks.[16] Life in the trenches had the ability to pull more determination out of the human condition than any other lifestyle and Stalin directed this into creating the most advanced biological weapons program and unleashing it on the West.

In 1938, Joseph Stalin declared bacteriological war on the West with his lower generals disseminating a declaration of biological weapons capability, published in "Prospective Uses of Bacteriological Warfare in Future Wars," a memorandum for Soviet scientists and physicians turned bioweaponeers. In this memo, Stalin and his generals make it clear that bacteriological warfare research will be the weapon for future wars, admitting the *"use of pathogenic microbes for military purposes is all the more promising since the propagation of virulent bacterial cultures does not require large plants with extensive equipment, costly raw materials, and complex techniques."*[17]

In 1940, the RKKA Biotechnical Institute was moved and re-named several times up to WWII. Next, Fishman began preparing for a new laboratory called the Scientific Research Institute of Health.[18] As the Second World War broke out in 1942, three laboratories in the city of Moscow had been operating in an offensive capacity.[19]

Accompanying the expansion of biological warfare research facil-ities, three open-air testing sites had been established from before the second World War,[20] as well as Waffenprüf 9. German military units, along with Soviet units, trained here in the days of Soviet-German re-search cooperation. Germany was searching for a way to circumvent the Treaty of Versailles, which prohibited Germany from building and developing a military on their homeland, and their agreement with Russia would be solidified so that the two enemy nations would be working together in exchange for something the other did not have.[21]

For Germany, they needed to circumvent the Treaty of Versailles and build up their army where they were prohibited from doing in Germany. The Soviets, on the other hand, needed chemical weapons technology, especially to stomp out the insect-borne plagues that were ravaging the U.S.S.R. at the time.[22]

One testing site became well-known for its activities – *Vozrozh-deniye Island*, or *"Kingdom of Cockroaches"* – was an isolated island off the shores of the Aral Sea, better known as Rebirth Island. Here they field tested some of humanity's most hideous organisms such as plague, tularemia, anthrax, and many more.[23] The island had been set up early in the Soviet offensive, and unmarked graves belonging to Soviet scientists that died conducting experiments still exist to re-mind those setting foot on the island of its sinister past and the inevi-table cost of gambling with germ weapons. [24]

BIOPREPARAT: HIDDEN HAND OR SMOKESCREEN OF SOVIET GERMWARFARE?

The Soviet offensive took a very direct albeit hidden approach to the development of a full-scale biological weapons program. By 1973, at the start of the Second Generation of biological weapons de-velopment, the Soviet Union had established a new system for their program, known as Biopreparat. Biopreparat became the biological monster of the Soviet Union, with its tentacles reaching in all direc-tions over the vast Motherland. As each respective nation progressed their biological warfare initiative, they each had a place they could call home, the headquarters.

With the United States, it was Fort Detrick, with the British, it was Porton Down. With the Soviet Union, the Biopreparat headquarters in Stepnogorsk produced a massive stockpile of weaponized anthrax and various other biological weapons munitions. Biopreparat had several other unique factories and labs in which to research, produce, and weaponize biowarfare agents. Each facility focused on select agents.[25]

Other facilities included diverse research on biological agents, specializing in the production of bio-pesticides and various biological agents and bacteria such as tularemia. The State Research Center of Virology and Biotechnology, Vector, also called the Vector Institute, was a key facility that specialized in insect-borne diseases, respiratory viruses, and it was here that the later defector Ken Alibek weaponized smallpox and Marburg Virus, the sibling of Ebola Virus.

The Sverdlovsk bioweapons production facility was used to weaponize and produce anthrax. In 1979, an accident exposed the nearby villagers to anthrax and killed many people in the nearby villages, and this eventually aroused the suspicions of the West.[26]

A massive complex with many diverse facilities was set up in 1989 at Obolensk, just outside Moscow. This facility housed cultures of many pathogens of different classes. Operating like a closed city, each building was assigned to specific pathogen classes researching plague, tularemia, anthrax, glanders, melioidosis, bacterial toxins, among many more. This facility project, was known as BONFIRE, and worked on ways to genetically alter strains of disease to overcome treatments and vaccines, the success of which was optimal.[27]

The Soviet offensive was the most advanced biological weapons operation of any nation, especially after acquiring the German Insel Riems facility and all of the most important work of the Japanese program Unit 731. The Soviet Union took these weapons very seriously and concentrated all their forces in this area, while the West maintained an attitude of downplaying the potential of germ weapons as much as possible. We may not have ever known of or disrupted the Russian program, if not for key personnel defecting and exposing at least some of the operation. There were two main defectors, Vladimir Pasechnik and Ken Alibek (Kanatjan Alibekov).[28]

DEFECTOR #1: VLADIMIR PASECHNIK

Vladimir Pasechnik was the first to defect in the summer of 1989, after his superior, Ken Alibek, gave him permission to travel to Paris to close a deal with a French producer of chemical laboratory equipment. It was on this trip, he arranged the escape with British Intelligence, and made his escape shortly before he was scheduled to fly home. While in the Soviet Union, Pasechnik was given the opportunity to start a biotechnology institute with unlimited funding provided by the hands of the Soviet Ministry of Defense. The operation became the Institute of Ultra-Pure Biochemical Preparations, where Pasechnik would be weaponizing the plague bacteria, *Yersinia pestis,* among other agents.[29]

Vladimir Pasechnik had a high-degree of importance in hindering the development and secret nature of Biopreparat. It could be said that the exposure of the Biopreparat biological weapons program was a critical factor that helped to bring down the Soviet Union. Alibek's defection was less instrumental but much more publicized. However, Alibek's story was not exposing the more secret work discussed in this book, but it is likely that much of his revelations would have been disclosed but was prevented by Western Intelligence.

Reflecting on the circumstances before Pasechnik's defection, it became clear to Alibek that Pasechnik was not happy with the work he had undertaken. It was after his defection to Britain, where he expressed that his work in biological warfare operations placed a heavy strain on his moral conscience, causing him to plan an escape from the Soviet Union. What had once been a closely guarded secret would have been open to the world, but for reasons that will be explained shortly, the West refused to tell the world at large.

Pasechnik died of a stroke in 2001 while working for the British at Porton Down.[30] Naturally, one can't help but wonder whether it had been induced through a drug, poison, or exotic technology held by the Russians. His other biological weapons superiors had deeply resented Pasechnik's defection and vowed to get revenge on the former Soviet bioweaponeer, and even his children feared that someday his old employers might pay him a visit to "*deal with him.*"[31]

DEFECTOR #2: KEN ALIBEK (KANATJAN ALIBEKOV)

Ken Alibek, the second to defect from the Soviet empire, escaped just after the fall of the Soviet Union. After living in a country that appeared to be in shambles and collapsing and soon hoping to exit the business of bioweapons, he would learn with difficulty that such knowledge of the Soviet's deepest secrets and former operations would not part ways so easily. Soon he was allegedly being followed, stalked, and harassed to continue his work in the biological warfare program.

As a high-level Soviet officer, knowing where some of the biological bodies are buried, so to speak, the Russian empire was not willing to allow him to fade off into the sunset. Alibek had worked in numerous facilities over the years. He researched and successfully weaponized numerous agents like anthrax, tularemia, smallpox, among many others. He knew enough, but was it enough to compromise the program overall? This is a subject for further debate.

As a native of Kazakhstan, Alibek joined the military in his early years and planned to become a military psychiatrist, entering the Tomsk Medical Institute in 1973. His story would eventually be told in a revealing memoir written after his defection called *Biohazard: The Chilling True Story of the Largest Covert Biological Weapons Program in the World- Told from the Inside by the Man Who Ran It*. Alibek not only told of his tenure and participation in the program, but he gave us a deeper perspective into the Soviet Union's interest in biological warfare, confirming the analysis of my source, John Loftus, that the program begins far before World War II with the typhus epidemic:

> A year after taking power in 1917, the Bolshevik government plunged into savage conflict with anti-communist forces determined to bring down the fledgling workers' state. Red and White armies clashed from Siberia to the Crimean Peninsula, and by the time hostilities ended in 1921, as many as ten million people had lost their lives. The majority of the deaths did not result from injuries on the battlefield. They were caused by famine and disease.
>
> The casualties inflicted by a brutal epidemic of typhus from 1918 to 1921 made a deep impression on the commanders of the Red Army. Even if they knew nothing of the history of biological warfare, they could recognize that disease had served as a more potent weapon than bullets or artillery shells.[32]

As the German troops had invaded the Soviets in 1941, many had fallen ill with a sudden outbreak of tularemia. Alibek would later reveal that the outbreak was indeed the work of a Soviet attack using a weaponized strain of tularemia, but by 1941, the programs of all nations were well-underway.

In his memoir, Alibek cites work done at Vector on the development of effective biological weapons using neuroregulatory peptides to target the brain and mental health of its victims, in other words, neurotropic qualities of biological weapons that caused mental illness and psychiatric symptoms:

The Vector scientists had used a gene for beta-endorphin, a regulatory peptide, in their experiments. Beta-endorphin, capable in large amounts of producing psychological and neurological disorders and of suppressing certain immunological reactions, was one of the ingredients of the Bonfire program. It was synthesized by the Soviet Academy of Sciences.[33]

Alibek made another admission in his memoir about the neurotropic angles and their desire to engineer biological agents to target the mental health and well-being of its victims:[34]

> [...] I eventually discovered, developed psychotropic agents to induce altered mood and behavior in humans. Scientists worked with a number of biochemical substances including regulatory peptides, establishing a shadowy link with our Bonfire program. Another institute controlled by the Third Directorate, Medstatistika, gathered statistics related to biological research around the world. The pharmacology institute specialized in developing toxins to induce paralysis or death. All were connected in some manner to the Flute program, whose principal aim was to develop psychotropic and neurotropic biological agents for use by the KGB in special operations—including the "wet work" of political assassinations.[34]

After the collapse of the Soviet Union, Alibek made his escape to the United States in the middle of the night while coordinating with American Intelligence.[35] He was brought to America where he underwent weeks of interrogation and debriefing.[36] From that point on, he would consult with the Americans on the Soviet Union biological weapons program, and become a professor lecturing on bioterrorism and biowarfare, as well as co-founder of a biotechnology company with a former bioweaponeer from Fort Detrick.[37] However, it seemed that American Intelligence was not overly concerned with or believing Alibek's assessment on the level of advancement the Soviets actually had. He warned them of how advanced and serious their program became, but Western Intelligence didn't listen.

TRIPARTITE BLACKMAIL (USA-BRITAIN-RUSSIA)

In Alibek's memoir, there is a revealing section in particular that shows that following Pasechnik's defection, after he told the British and Americans about the Soviet Union's massive biological weapons program, both Britain and the United States kept it secret and decided not to tell the world about it.[38] The West said they would keep it secret in return for allowing them to travel to Russia and do an inspection of any group of selected facilities they wished to see.

The Soviets drew up an off-record agreement to be signed by the British and Americans, and the agreement was enacted between the three parties. Alibek was told that they decided to cover for the Soviet Union because it was thought that a public quarrel would endanger progress in other areas of arms control and perhaps weaken Mikhail Gorbachev. This is a vague statement but I will present a more likely possibility.

If the British and Americans threw the Soviet Union under the bus to the rest of the world and decried the Soviet Union's larges-cale bioweapons program, there would be a response from the Soviet Union. Events from the past would be brought out and exposed, like the reckless activities of the British and Americans, for example, the activities of German scientist Erich Traub and the open-air tests over populated areas with dubious germs that caused fatalities and illness in those exposed, which we will cover in later chapters. More information about the use of germ weapons in the Korean War might materialize. All sorts of other dirty secrets on the Americans and British could be exposed, since the Cambridge Five spies like Kim Philby and Donald Maclean had some of their most intimate secrets and gave them to the Soviet Union in the early 1950s.[39]

This could get very ugly. As an alternative route, each agreed to cover for the other and keep their biological warfare quarrels between themselves. This put in motion a dangerous game of perpetual blackmail and ensured the biological warfare activities of all involved could grow immensely in the years to come.

Endnotes

1   Loftus, John J. "Memorandum on Biological Weapons History." (personal communication) 2018

2   Ibid.

3   Graham, Loren. *Lysenko's Ghost: Epigenetics and Russia*. Harvard University Press, 2016.

4   Central Intelligence Agency (CIA) Intelligence Reports: INITIAL WORKS IN THE ADAPTATION OF MICROORGANISMS. CIA-RDP82-00039R000200100044-1. Central Intelligence Agency (CIA), Reading Room, 2012. Retrieved from: https://www.cia.gov/readingroom/document/CIA-RDP82-00039R000200100044-1

5   Central Intelligence Agency (CIA) Intelligence Reports: CONTROLLED MUTATION OF BACTERIA OF THE PASTEURELLA GROUP. CIA-RDP80-00809A000700250046-2. Central Intelligence Agency (CIA), Reading Room, 2011. Retrieved from: https://www.cia.gov/readingroom/document/CIA-RDP80-00809A000700250046-2

6   Central Intelligence Agency (CIA) Intelligence Reports: INITIAL WORKS IN THE ADAPTATION OF MICROORGANISMS. CIA-RDP82-00039R000200100044-1. Central Intelligence Agency (CIA), Reading Room, 2012. Retrieved from: https://www.cia.gov/library/readingroom/document/CIA-RDP82-00039R000200100044-1

7   Central Intelligence Agency (CIA) Intelligence Reports: MILITARY - BIOLOGICAL WARFARE. CIA-RDP80-00809A000600140080-8. Central Intelligence Agency (CIA), Reading Room. 2011. Retrieved from: https://www.cia.gov/library/readingroom/document/CIA-RDP80-00809A000600140080-8

8   Central Intelligence Agency (CIA) Intelligence Reports: The State Research Institute at Riems; Microbiological Research. CIA-RDP83-00415R000900020012-6. Central Intelligence Agency (CIA), Reading Room, 2011. Retrieved from: https://www.cia.gov/library/readingroom/document/CIA-RDP83-00415R000900020012-6

9   Erich Traub, one of the world's most talented in biological weapons and virology, accomplished many techniques that did not require fancy lab technologies.

10   Leitenberg, Milton, et al. *The Soviet Biological Weapons Program: a History*. Harvard University Press, 2012., pp. 16-51

11   War Bureau of Consultants Committee, and George W. Merck. 1945. Report to the Secretary of War by Mr. George W. Merck, Special Consultant for Biological Warfare. Report to the Secretary of War by Mr. George W. Merck, Special Consultant for Biological Warfare. National Acadamy of Science (NAS) Online Collections. Retrieved from: http://www.nasonline.org/about-nas/history/archives/collections/organized-collections/1945merckreport.pdf

12   Leitenberg, Milton, et al. *The Soviet Biological Weapons Program: a History*. Harvard University Press, 2012., pp. 16-51

13   Loftus, John J. "Memorandum on Biological Weapons History." (personal communication) 2018

14   Dâkov Ûrij Leontevič, and Bušueva Tatâna Semenovna. *The Red Army and the Wermacht: How the Soviets Militarized Germany, 1922-33, and Paved the Way for Fascism: from the Secret Archives of the Former Soviet Union*. Prometheus Books, 1995

15   Quigley, Carroll. *Tragedy and Hope: a History of the World in Our Time*. GSG & Associates, 2004.

16   Loftus, John J. "Memorandum on Biological Weapons History." (personal communication) 2018

17   Central Intelligence Agency (CIA) Intelligence Reports: PROSPECTIVE USES OF BACTERIOLOGICAL WARFARE IN FUTURE WARS. CIA-RDP80-00809A000600120022-4. Central Intelligence Agency (CIA), Reading Room, 2011. Retrieved from: https://www.cia.gov/readingroom/document/CIA-RDP80-00809A000600120022-4

18   Leitenberg, Milton, et al. *The Soviet Biological Weapons Program: a History*. Harvard University Press, 2012., pp. 16-51

19   Ibid.

20   Ibid.

21   Dâkov Ûrij Leontevič, and Bušueva Tatâna Semenovna. *The Red Army and the Wermacht: How the Soviets Militarized Germany, 1922-33, and Paved the Way for Fascism: from the Secret Archives of the Former Soviet Union*. Prometheus Books, 1995

22   Loftus, John J. "Memorandum on Biological Weapons History." (personal communication) 2018

23   Alibek, Ken, and Stephen Handelman. *Biohazard: the Chilling True Story of the Largest Covert Biological Weapons Program in the World, Told from the inside by the Man Who Ran It*. Dell Pub., 2000., pp. 15-28

24   Leitenberg, Milton, et al. *The Soviet Biological Weapons Program: a History*. Harvard University Press, 2012.

25   Ibid.

26   Ibid.

27   Alibek, Ken, and Stephen Handelman. *Biohazard: the Chilling True Story of the Largest Covert Biological Weapons Program in the World, Told from the inside by the Man Who Ran It*. Dell Pub., 2000.

28   Ibid.

29   Ibid.

30   Saxon, Wolfgang. 2001. "V. Pasechnik, 64, Is Dead; Germ Expert Who Defected." *The New York Times*. The New York Times. November 23, 2001. https://www.nytimes.com/2001/11/23/world/v-pasechnik-64-is-dead-germ-expert-who-defected.html

31   Bannerman, Lucy. 2018. "Sergei Skripal: Salisbury's Other Spy Lived in Fear of KGB Revenge." News | *The Times*. The Times. March 12, 2018. https://www.thetimes.co.uk/article/city-s-other-spy-lived-in-fear-of-kgb-revenge-fhkwhnvbp

32   Alibek, Ken, and Stephen Handelman. *Biohazard: The Chilling True Story of the Largest Covert Biological Weapons Program in the World, Told from the inside by the Man Who Ran It*. Dell Pub., 2000, pp. 32-33.

33   Ibid, pp. 261.

34   Ibid, pp. 171-172.

35   Ibid., pp. 250-256.

36   Ibid., pp. 257-268.

37   Ibid., pp. 290-292.

38   Ibid, pp. 151-152.

39   "Lost Briton Is Said to Admit Red Ties; Lords Hear Missing Diplomat's Recording of the Statement Is in Hands of F. B. I." *The New York Times*, The New York Times, 29 Oct. 1952, https://www.timesmachine.nytimes.com/timesmachine/1952/10/29/93586243.html

Chapter Four

Spy Rings and Sabotage

Day X and the Operational Phase of Soviet Biological Warfare

All men can see the tactics whereby I conquer, but what none can see is the strategy out of which victory is evolved.

— Sun Tzu, The Art of War

The key to a successful program of strategic weapons for the Soviet Union would be done through espionage and sabotage. We know that British Intelligence was highly compromised by Soviet double-agents like Kim Philby, Donald Maclean, Guy Burgess, of the Cambridge Five Spies.[1] It was the Soviet mole in MI6, Donald Maclean,[2] who cleared Germans like Erich Traub for the Operation Paperclip program in America, which was the secret government program that brought Nazi scientists to America to work for the U.S. Government after World War II, which was largely exposed in a book called *Secret Agenda: The United States Government, Nazi Scientists, and Project Paperclip, 1945 to 1990* by Linda Hunt in 1991.[3] Since British Intelligence was so highly compromised at that time, it would have been infinitely less challenging to flood the corporate sector, pharmaceutical giants, or the academic world and scientific communities in America.[4]

Their methodology would focus in several areas of attack: germ weapons of all kinds, especially vector warfare with ticks,[5] mosquitoes, fleas, and other insects.[6, 7] Even more diabolical was the sabotage of Western vaccines and serum. Aside from the already problematic nature of vaccines, these could be intentionally contaminated with stealth viruses and used to harm.[8] Early Soviet scientists were clearly mapping these methods out when they began to study how to overcome the so-called sterilization of vaccines and serum:

> In connection with this work, it was established that microorganisms exhibit a much higher resistance to powerful chemical

and physical influences than that which was ascribed to them hitherto. Thus, Bosh'yan was able to isolate living cultures from nutritive media which had been boiled and autoclaved repeatedly. Having this high resistance, microorganisms do not perish either in the host organism or outside of it as easily as had been assumed. Notwithstanding the prevalent view that a sterile vaccine contains only dead microorganisms, cultures of living microbes could be successfully grown from many formalinized vaccines and also some so-called chemical vaccines. [...] Numerous investigations of immune antitetanus serum which had been treated with phenol revealed that a culture of tetanus microbes could be invariably isolated from it. The initial live microbe culture could also be isolated from immune antianthrax serum and the active swine plague virus from the immune serum used against that disease. The identification of the microbes and viruses in question was quite certain. Microbe cultures were also obtained from many other sera used for medical and veterinary purposes.[9]

What was so desirable about the vaccine channel is that the line between a weapon and a vaccine can often be hard to distinguish when it comes to the strategic weapons, because the side effects can in many instances be just as bad as a weaponized disease. Likewise, a weaponized disease of the strategic class can unfold so slowly as to be denied a disease-causing agent under Western standards. We have not mastered the unpredictable and toxic nature of viruses and microbes, nor are our bodies designed to handle the stress of endless vaccinations and prophylactics to keep up with this war.

New weapons and stealth attacks of sabotage could resist antibiotics, contaminate Western vaccines, or use the antigens that cause the desired slow disease to unfold, because many of the antigens are too toxic and destructive long-term, especially when given on top of those who already had stealth infections passed from mother to child, already immunosuppressed from other stealth infections proliferating the population.[10]

SECTION K: BIOLOGICAL ESPIONAGE AND THE SUBVERSION OF WESTERN MEDICINE

A later defector of the KGB, Alexander Kouzminov, was another important Soviet official "in the know" about the Soviet biological weapons program, especially when it came to sabotage. In his memoir, *Biological Espionage: Special Operations of the Soviet and Russian Foreign Intelligence Services in the West,* there were deeper, covert plans in the Soviet/Russian Intelligence biological weapons program. It was Kouzminov's work at Directorate S (Special Operations), or Department 12 of the KGB First Chief Directorate and its successor, the Russian Foreign Intelligence Service (SVR), where he explains in detail the complex spy networks involving microbiology, science, and medicine:

> But as for us in Department 12, officially we assisted the government in carrying out the state agricultural and medical programmes by obtaining from overseas new fertilisers, modern medicines and biological products for medical, pharmacological and microbiological industries of the country'. But in fact we were supposed to obtain from the West the intelligence information which would help to produce and perfect Soviet (later Russian) biological weapons in many possible varieties. The list of the espionage targets [...] included Western government departments and state commissions, intelligence services, ministries of defense, agriculture, health, environment, civil defence and emergency, secret military medical and biological laboratories - in fact anything connected with research in the field of genetic engineering and the most dangerous human and animal pathogens. The department gathered intelligence information about plans for and means of protection against the potential application of biological weapons in target countries.
>
> Apart from that, we were also interested in which academic and, at first glance, unthreatening conventional research experiments with recombinant molecules and biological toxins could be applied to create new types of biological and toxic weapons. Our department was also interested in which laboratories, institutes, centres and private biotechnological companies were secretly involved in programmes to protect against bacteriological and toxin weapons. We had to investigate any possible security weaknesses associated with those organisations, and penetrate them.
>
> The other task of our department was to obtain new strains of modified pathogenic agents, samples of other novel biological materials from the West's secret military medical laboratories, and secretly deliver them to Russian clandestine lab-

oratories which developed and perfected their own offensive biological weapons...

People were another of Department 12's prime interests: professionals in biological and medical fields, especially those who were involved in experiments with recombinant molecules, toxins, and pathogens of dangerous human and animal diseases, which could be used for the development of a new generation of biological and toxin weapons. We were also interested in government and army personnel, and officials of intelligence services who had direct or indirect access to enemy biological weapons programs, as well as those who provided security for biological weapons laboratories and centres. Our goal was to recruit some of these people as special agents. We also recruited foreigners who could be used by the department as auxiliary agents. For example, those who could help to document and support the cover stories of our illegals, or even help with liaising them.

In the memorandum one continually met the phrases "The Instance," "Day X," and "direct actions." By "The Instance" was meant the Politburo of the Central Committee of the Communist Party of the Soviet Union. After disintegration of the Soviet Union, "The Instance" came to mean the "President of Russia and his Presidential Council," The formula "Day X" meant the beginning of a large-scale war against the West. "Direct actions" implied acts of biological sabotage and terrorism against the civilians, the army, and the economy of a potential enemy. "The potential strike targets" meant civil targets, including public drinking-water supplies, food stores, and processing plants; water-purification systems, vaccine, drug, and toxin repositories; and pharmaceutical and biotechnological plants.[11]

Many of Kouzminov's revelations corroborate the story put forward in this book. Later, we will explore the possibility of their methodology in operation, showing they were taking full advantage of not one but several weak points in American medical, science, intelligence, and biodefense. According to John Loftus, there were extensive and very effective counterintelligence spy networks known as the Russian Kolonii (RK) that the Tsar of Russia had employed, and the Bolsheviks who seized Russia assumed command of this network and it became the Soviet Kolonii (SK).[12]

While the United States had been so busy building the industrial revolution of technology and economy, the early Russians and later Soviet Union was busy continuing to penetrate Western society, corporate drug firms, medical and academic circles. It is likely they focused all their time, energy, and funding in these two areas - *intelligence* and *biological warfare*.[13]

I.V. Domaradskij, the Antiplague Institute, and the Plasmid Program

A third book on the Soviet biological weapons program from an insider was published by former molecular biologist and geneticist I.V. Domaradskij in *Biowarrior: Inside the Soviet Biological War Machine*. This was actually published before the works of Alibek and Kouzminov but was privately published without much publicity. In this memoir, he recounts his career working on several infectious diseases like cholera and weaponizing tularemia, plague, and pseudotuberculosis.

Domaradskij worked at Kirov, Rostov. Some of his work was also working on plasmids and proteins for weaponizing microbes under the cover of protein biosynthesis for applications in the production of agricultural feed for livestock. He gives a brief family history in which members of his family were arrested and disappeared in Stalin's great purge where many were either murdered or thrown in jail.

He then dives into his long career as a molecular biologist in which he decided to pursue after reading a copy of Theodore Rosebury's *Peace or Pestilence: Biological Warfare and How to Avoid It*.[14] Theodore Rosebury, by the way, was a prominent Camp Detrick scientist who was also a member of the communist front group the American Association of Scientific Workers.[15]

Domaradskij spent a great deal of time on "Problem No. 5," which had been code for the biological weapons program in the Soviet Union.[16] Domaradskij mentions the Biological and Toxin Weapons Convention (BTWC) treaty that replaced the 1925 Geneva Convention treaty, which allowed defensive research, whereas the Geneva Convention banned the testing and stockpiling of biological weapons entirely.

The Soviet Union signed the Biological and Toxin Weapons Convention (BTWC) treaty in 1972, and since this new treaty allowed defensive biological weapons research, it gave them a cover to greatly expand their offensive biological weapons program like never before by merely cloaking it as defensive work:

> As I said in the previous chapter, my move to Rostov coincided with the transformation of that institute, which at that point

69

began to emerge as the leading institute in the plague-control system on "Problem No. 5." My own deepening involvement-the gateway for me into the world of biological weapons- began here at Rostov with Problem No. 5. Since the early seventies, when the Biological and Toxin Weapons Convention was signed by the Soviet Union, the United States, and (as of January 1, 2001) 144 other nations, the emphasis of Problem No. 5 shifted. It began to serve as a "legend," or cover story, to hide the illegal and ultrasecret biological weapons program known as Problem "Ferment" (or Problem "F"). With the signing of the BTWC, biological defense was no longer a priority; under cover of the treaty, and unknown to the rest of the signatories, a greatly expanded and ambitious bioweapons program would rapidly take root in the USSR.

Developing such a program became the main task of a supersecret group, the Interagency Scientific and Technical Council for Molecular Biology and Genetics. Problem No. 5 became little more than a smokescreen for these hidden and dangerous activities. It was used both by the Ministry of Defense, and by a new organization, Biopreparat, the "civilian arm" of the biological weapons program.[17]

Domaradskij continued his assignments under Problem No. 5 and soon he would be working on plasmids under the guise of protein biosynthesis for agricultural foodstuffs at Glavmikrobioprom, noting that the *"entire Soviet biological weapons program went underground, and some kind of cover was needed to hide the fact that illicit research was going on. Biopreparat provided the bureaucratic cover."*[18]

Domaradskij discusses many of the endless quarrels in meetings he was to attend, and in particular he mentions informants to the KGB of scientists and academicians involved in the military program by reputable scientists with the West – V.M. Zhdanov, Yu. A. Ovchinnikov, and G.K. Skryabin:

> The organization of the Military Industrial Commission itself was far removed from science; its directors and staff were mainly officials, as well as military men. In order to devise future defense industry plans, therefore, the commission used our civilian scientists to gather information, which they used to recheck the data derived from intelligence.
>
> First, these civilian scientists gathered and analyzed all published data on molecular biology and genetics and presented a

summary of this data to the commission. Second, they visited
the most important conferences abroad and helped the commission analyze material submitted by the Main Intelligence
Service. Taking part as active informers were the famous scientists Yu. A. Ovchinnikov, G.K. Skryabin, and particularly,
V.M. Zhdanov, a noted virologist who had initially proposed
the worldwide eradication of smallpox and who had won the
high regard of many Western scientists. He was also responsible for many original ideas in virology. Zhdanov had traveled
abroad extensively and had often received foreign guests; this
sophisticated, worldly man was therefore a great asset to the
military. Every time any of these scientists took a trip abroad,
they had to present a report to the commission. Most probably, agreeing to gather such information was an indispensable
condition for any foreign travel.

[...]

All discussions with these scientists were held in secret in
the Military Industrial Commission and were not even disclosed to the heads of the academies (of science and of medicine) or the relevant departments. These discussions focused
on the necessity of matching Western results in the fields of
molecular biology and genetics in order to develop an effective, sophisticated bioweapons program; they also addressed
the creation of a special scientific and practical organization to
implement this program.[19]

Domaradskij reveals the extent of secrecy and compartmentaliza-
tion from even regular military and state officials, reinforcing the idea
that everything is disguised under covers like agricultural, medical
treatments, and vaccine production, and a weapon is never spoken of
as a weapon:

It was therefore interesting to see how Urakov solved his problems at party meetings. Since only a few party members were
admitted to any secret business (maybe thirty out of about five
hundred people attending), and since builders and laborers
were predominant among the Communists, everything was
said in figurative language, especially when discussing the results of any scientific work. Instead of "calling a spade a spade"
as Urakov would in our own meetings, at party sessions he
camouflaged our work by referring to our "newly developed
vaccines" or new "methods of treating dangerous diseases."[20]

LEV ZILBER, M. P. CHUMAKOV, AND SOVIET TICK RESEARCH

The Soviet program had an extensive amount of research concentrated in tick research,[21] for the stated purpose of research in biological weapons,[22] to vector encephalitis viruses and neurotropic animal viruses that resembled polio.[23] This was being mapped out in parallel with the study of animals and insects in the wild that spread human infection and study their stealth qualities and the ways in which they could be transmitted.[24] Once they assimilated the work of Insel Riems and Erich Traub at the end of WWII, they gained an exceptional understanding of the nature of dormant viruses and how to reawaken these viruses under physical stress from the toxic reaction of certain antigens or spike proteins.[25]

In 1937, the Soviet Union began testing new biological weapons on the Muslims and Mongolians in the Siberian and Southeastern Russian territories. Soviet academicians like M.P. Chumakov and Lev Zilber headed these expeditions and testing activities. John Loftus gives further insight from his sources:

> [...] in 1937 the epidemics started up again in the eastern and southern regions of the USSR. Stalin was testing these new-found strategies with clandestine attacks using biological weapons to weaken his restive Muslim and Mongolian populations. These laboratory-enhanced diseases were spread among the target civilian populations using insect vectors such as fleas and ticks that were native to the areas. [...] We may never learn the full extent to which the Soviets conducted bioweapons research through testing on human subjects. From the years leading up to WWII, all the way to its end, Soviet dictator Stalin prohibited all western doctors and epidemiologists from entering the Soviet Union. It was in this period that most likely made use of the free rein on the population within the communist empire. In the Muslim and Mongolian subsections of the Soviet Union, it is believed that tens of millions of lives may have been infected through insect-borne diseases such as ticks and mosquitoes, with around 2-3 million deaths.[26]

More people died in Stalin's experimental phase of the Soviet bacteriological warfare program than perhaps any other biological warfare program in existence. Many experimental phases were disguised as epidemiological surveys and tick studies disguised as academic research.[27, 28]

Later in this book, we will learn of how Western intelligence foolishly allowed American scientists to collaborate with Soviet bioweaponeers like V. M. Zhdanov, M. P. Chumakov, and former Red Army physicians to produce vaccines that would be deployed in the West.[29] Upon further investigation, we will begin to see a disturbing possibility in which the failures of Western Intelligence to put any resources to assess the Soviet biological weapons threat in the most critical days of the Cold War led to serious vulnerabilities which left American public health and biodefense incompetent against biological warfare and sabotage from the Soviet Union.[30]

With enough spies and saboteurs in the medical and academic fields and drug firms of the West, the Soviet Union could have a hidden channel for large-scale bioterrorism.[31] We will look at this in further depth in later chapters. However, it must be stressed that most of these weapons would be slow-acting and take a significant period of time to unfold and gain momentum, even many generations later for the weapon to achieve the desired effect – *tire and exhaust*.[32] Their strategy was always geared in the long-term sense like a patient waiting game. The result would exacerbate an ugly trio of chronic disease, mental illness, and *cancer*.

From the early expeditions to the Siberian regions, the Soviets were able to launch and develop their vector program, starting with tick encephalitis and the Ebola-like hemorrhagic fever viruses, as such, the hunt to mine and hybridize ticks, viruses, and microorganisms for use as weapons in ticks had begun.[33] Lev Zilber would be jailed at the height of the expedition for spreading the plagues, along with several of his men.[34] Chumakov had been one of Zilber's top scientists, yet it does not appear that he was among those jailed. Later activities indicate that Chumakov could have been high up in Soviet Intelligence.[35]

In either event, the tick program carried on, and later tick hybridization programs were initiated with *Ixodes* ticks.[36] In 1937, One of Stalin's generals made a declaration on bacteriological warfare to be used in future wars, and arthropods had been among the many means of delivery discussed.[37] According to a later declassified CIA report on the "Military Medical Academy Imeni Kirov," the expeditions by Chumakov and Zilber were focused on biological weapons through the use of ticks to vector their biological weapons:

b. Biological Warfare

[redacted] one high priority research project that was being conducted in this division as a result of a report from Siberia that the bite of a certain local species of forest tick (klesch) was found to rapidly cause encephalitis. This particular kind of encephalitis was named "vesene-letniy ensefalit" (spring-summer encephalitis) because the tick's bite results in the malady only during these two sessions of the year. As soon as word of this was received at the Academy, Evgenij Pavlovsky, the famed Soviet parasitologist, and a large staff of biologists immediately departed on an expedition to this remote section of Siberia to study this tick. The expedition returned some months later and expressed great enthusiasm over its findings and the possible application of this discovery to biological warfare. Reports such as the one from Siberia were numerous and came directly to the Academy.[38]

Another publication included in intelligence report "Possible Use of Chemical, Bacteriological, and Radiological Agents in a Future War" leaves its demands in a threatening tone saying that, should any country consider the use of chemical, biological, or nuclear weapons on the Soviet Union, they will retaliate tenfold back on the West.[39] Another report, titled "Soviet Guided Missile, Chemical, and Bacteriological Warfare in Hungary" mentions the use of rickettsia[A] and botulinum toxin against the West, admitting that it was with the help of Soviet spies in the U.S. who helped obtain the formula used by the West.[40]

There are dozens of old intelligence reports of Soviet activities focusing in the areas of transmission and vector studies with insects,[41] rodents,[42] the environmental factors of disease, suitable vectors for various rickettsia and spirochetes,[43] hybridization of ticks,[44] parasitology,[45] and various studies useful for a vector program.[46] In fact, the well-known bioweapons lab in the Siberian area, Vector, is the location for previous institutes where the tick and vector program had its footing with experimental outbreaks under Stalin studied by Lev Zilber, M. P. Chumakov, and their expedition team.[47] Many conferences were held for areas of research to study the natural foci of human infections in a given area.[48]

The Soviet Union scientists had an exceptional understanding of stealth, chronic infections, whereby the infected person will not show significant antibodies to confirm an infection, testing negative despite active infection. A December 1949 report, "Morphologic Characteristics of Acute Attacks in Chronic Brucellosis," lays out the process

---

A   **Rickettsia**: any of a various gram-negative, parasitic bacteria (order Rickettsiales and especially genus *Rickettsia*) that are transmitted by biting arthropods (such as lice or ticks) and cause a number of serious diseases (such as Rocky Mountain spotted fever and typhus)

showing the incompetence of antibody and blood testing to diagnose such stealth infections.[49]

In a July 1950 report "Preservation and Restoration of the Virulence of Leptospira" is clearly bioweapons research disguised as scientific research.[50] The spirochete *Leptospira* had later been researched in depth along with *Borrelia, Treponema, Spiroplasma,* and *Mycoplasma,* in the American program.[51] According to later Rocky Mountains Laboratory reports, *Leptospira* had been demonstrated to cause fungal infections in animals.[52]

In an October 1950 report "Health Campaign Continues: VD Decreases Mongol Population" discusses the health survey in the data gathering on the experimental epidemics unleashed by Stalin.[53] We know many of these could have been prevented because it was known in an even earlier report, "Tropical and Venereal Diseases in the Soviet Union," that show the successful control of these diseases were done by other measures and thus, in this case it was more or less left to spread.[54]

A March 1951 report, "Hybridization of Ixodes Ticks," demonstrates the mass propagation and cross-breeding of ticks for suitable vectors of disease in line with the work taking place at the Medical Military Academy Imeni Kirov, to produce new ticks that did not naturally exist, by cross-breeding them between compatible species to make newer species that could be more suitable reservoirs for disease agents in biological weapons.[55]

A September 1955 report "USSR Work on Hemorrhagic Nephroso-Nephritis" details Chumakov's work with tick-borne hemorrhagic fevers and its course of disease.[56] It states that these viruses could produce silent infections in animals, and it reveals that Chumakov was testing the virus on mentally ill patients. Chumakov would work extensively with both tick encephalitis virus, Crimean-Congo hemorrhagic fever, Omsk hemorrhagic fever, among others.[57] We will hear more about these viruses later in the book. These viral diseases were the early forms of Ebola and Marburg Virus and have direct connections to these earlier hemorrhagic fevers that appeared in these Siberian regions after testing bioweapons for Stalin.

In 1960, a translation of E.N. Pavlovskii's *Natural Foci of Human Infections* was published in English. This book, while seemingly unthreatening research on its face, was used to study the problems and tricks of the trade when it comes to utilization of ticks as natural "reservoirs" for the spread of weaponized disease to the enemy. Just as Domaradskij and others had disclosed, everything pertaining to research on biological weapons had to be hidden under the cloak of benign research.[58]

The communists had been aggressively researching animal neuro-virus diseases similar to human poliomyelitis since at least the early 1950's and certainly longer.[59] The Soviet Union's Day X against the West was in full swing at the start of the Cold War. This would be done with coordination from American scientists that were either helping the Soviet Union, or being played as pawns by them, as well as saboteurs from within the biological warfare program of the Americans during routine testing activities.[60] Let us now proceed to the story of German virologist Erich Traub, who's life work is at the center of this story, and the pioneer of the stealth, strategic biological weapons.

Endnotes

1   Newton, Verne W. *Cambridge Spies: the Untold Story of Maclean, Philby, and Burgess in America*. Madison Books, 1993

2   Philipps, Roland. *Spy Named Orphan: the Enigma of Donald Maclean*. VINTAGE, 2019.

3   Hunt, Linda. *Secret Agenda: The United States Government, Nazi Scientists, and Project Paperclip, 1945 to 1990*. St. Martins Press, 1991.

4   Kouzminov, Alexander. *Biological Espionage: Special Operations of the Soviet and Russian Foreign Intelligence Services in the West*. Manas Publications, 2006.

5   Central Intelligence Agency (CIA) Intelligence files: HYBRIDIZATION OF IXODES TICKS. CIA-RDP80-00809A000600380443-8. Central Intelligence Agency (CIA), Reading Room, 2011. Retrieved from: https://www.cia.gov/readingroom/document/CIA-RDP80-0080 9A000600380443-8

6   Pavlovskij Evgenij Nikanorovič. *Natural Foci of Human Infections*. Israel Program for Scientific Translations, 1963.

7   Central Intelligence Agency (CIA) Intelligence Reports: THE MILITARY MEDICAL ACADEMY IMENI KIROV. CIA-RDP82-00047R000400500002-8., pp. 02. Central Intelligence Agency (CIA), Reading Room, 2011. Retrieved from: https://www.cia.gov/readingroom/document/CIA-RDP82-00047R000400500002-8

8   Kouzminov, Alexander. *Biological Espionage: Special Operations of the Soviet and Russian Foreign Intelligence Services in the West*. Manas Publications, 2006., pp. 34-36

9   Central Intelligence Agency (CIA) Intelligence Reports: A NEW STAGE IN THE DEVELOPMENT OF MICROBIOLOGY AND IMMUNOLOGY. CIA-RDP80-00809A000600330601-7. Central Intelligence Agency (CIA), Reading Room, 2011. Retrieved from: https://www.cia.gov/readingroom/document/cia-rdp80-00809a000600330601-7

10   Cassisi, G, P Sarzi-Puttini, and M Cazzola. 2011. "Chronic Widespread Pain and Fibromyalgia: Could There Be Some Relationships with Infections and Vaccinations?" Clinical and Experimental Rheumatology. U.S. National Library of Medicine. 2011. https://www.ncbi.nlm.nih.gov/pubmed/22243559

11   Kouzminov, Alexander. *Biological Espionage: Special Operations of the Soviet and Russian Foreign Intelligence Services in the West*. Manas Publications, 2006., pp. 34-35

12   Loftus, John J. "Memorandum on Biological Weapons History." (personal communication) 2018

13   This would match the research done for this book with the claims revealed by Kouzminov seemed to sit in parallel. See: Kouzminov, Alexander. *Biological Espionage: Special Operations of the Soviet and Russian Foreign Intelligence Services in the West*. Manas Publications, 2006.

14   Domaradskiĭ Igor Valerianovich., and Wendy Orent. *Biowarrior: inside the Soviet/Russian Biological War Machine*. Prometheus, 2003.

15   FBI Investigation on Bacteriological warfare (2 of 5). n.d. Bacteriological Warfare in the United States. Internet Archive. Accessed July 30, 2019. Retrieved from: https://archive.org/stream/BacteriologicalWarfareInTheUnitedStates/fbi_bw2#page/n95/mode/1up

16   Domaradskiĭ Igor Valerianovich., and Wendy Orent. *Biowarrior: inside the Soviet/Russian Biological War Machine*. Prometheus, 2003..

17   Ibid., pp. 111-112

18   Ibid., pp. 117-118

19   Ibid., pp. 111-112

20   Ibid., pp. 117-118

21   Central Intelligence Agency (CIA) Intelligence files: HYBRIDIZATION OF IXODES TICKS. CIA-RDP80-00809A000600380443-8. Central Intelligence Agency (CIA), Reading Room, 2011. Retrieved from: https://www.cia.gov/library/readingroom/document/CIA-RDP80-00809A000600380443-

22   Central Intelligence Agency (CIA) Intelligence Reports: THE MILITARY MEDICAL ACADEMY IMENI KIROV. CIA-RDP82-00047R000400500002-8. Central Intelligence Agency (CIA), Reading Room, 2011. Retrieved from: https://www.cia.gov/library/readingroom/document/CIA-RDP82-00047R000400500002-8

23   Central Intelligence Agency (CIA) Intelligence Reports: ANIMAL NEUROVIRUS DISEASES SIMILAR TO HUMAN POLIOMYELITIS. CIA-RDP80-00809A000700170265-8 Central Intelligence Agency (CIA), Reading Room, 2011. Retrieved from: https://www.cia.gov/library/readingroom/document/CIA-RDP80-00809A000700170265-8

24   Pavlovskij Evgenij Nikanorovič. Natural Foci of Human Infections. Israel Program for Scientific Translations, 1963.

25   This was especially the case after the acquisition of Insel Riems, which composed all of Traub's work, as well as the morphology of the bacteriophage. See: Wittmann, W. (1999). 100 Years of Virology. The Legacy of Friedrich Loeffler - the Institute on the Isle of Riems, 28. doi:10.1007/978-3-7091-6425-9

26   Loftus, John J. "Memorandum on Biological Weapons History." 2018

27   Ibid.

28   Central Intelligence Agency (CIA) Intelligence files: HEALTH CAMPAIGN: VD DECREASES MONGOL POPULATION. CIA-RDP80-00809A000600350470-1. Central Intelligence Agency (CIA), Reading Room, 2011. Retrieved from: https://www.cia.gov/library/readingroom/document/CIA-RDP80-00809A000600350470-1

29   V. M. Zhdanov coordinated with Western countries on the smallpox vaccines, M. P. Chumakov worked alongside Albert B. Sabin on the polio vaccine, Red Army physician Wolf Szmuness emigrated to America and facilitated the Hepatitis B vaccine.

30   Zabrocka, K. (2013, May 22). Under the Microscope: Why US Intelligence underestimated the Soviet Biological Weapons Program. Retrieved February 19, 2021, from https://stacks.stanford.edu/file/druid:wk216hz5745/Zabrocka_Katarzyna_Thesis_Final.pdf

31   Kouzminov, Alexander. Biological Espionage: Special Operations of the Soviet and Russian Foreign Intelligence Services in the West. Manas Publications, 2006.

32   These would be classed as strategic weapons, and geared for long-term attacks.

33   Loftus, John J. "Memorandum on Biological Weapons History." (personal communication) 2018

34   Kisselev, Lev L., et al. "Lev Zilber, the Personality and the Scientist." Advances in Cancer Research, 1992, pp. 1–40., doi:10.1016/s0065-230x(08)60301-2.

35   This idea is based on the early tick expeditions, which Chumakov had a big role in, appears to have remained a free man, while his superior, Zilber, went off to prison. Later, Chumakov travels to the United States with his wife (see Swanson 2012), which was unheard of, to allow a husband and wife to travel outside of Russia. Typically, they would have made one stay behind, as collateral, to deter defections. Glavmikrobioprom bioweapons specialist, Domaradskij stated in his memoir that those who were able to travel abroad, it was accepted that being an informant was one of the conditions of travel (see Domaradskij 2003, pp. 142)

36   Central Intelligence Agency (CIA) Intelligence files: HYBRIDIZATION OF IXODES TICKS. CIA-RDP80-00809A000600380443-8. Central Intelligence Agency (CIA), Reading Room, 2011. Retrieved from: https://www.cia.gov/library/readingroom/document/CIA-RDP80-00809A000600380443-8.pdf

37   Central Intelligence Agency (CIA) Intelligence Reports: PROSPECTIVE USES OF BACTERIOLOGICAL WARFARE IN FUTURE WARS. CIA-RDP80-00809A000600120022-4. Central Intelligence Agency (CIA), Reading Room, 2011. Retrieved from: https://www.cia.gov/library/readingroom/document/CIA-RDP80-00809A000600120022-4

38   Central Intelligence Agency (CIA) Intelligence Reports: THE MILITARY MEDICAL ACADEMY IMENI KIROV. CIA-RDP82-00047R000400500002-8. Central Intelligence Agency (CIA), Reading Room, 2011. Retrieved from: https://www.cia.gov/library/readingroom/document/CIA-RDP82-00047R000400500002-8

39   Central Intelligence Agency (CIA) Intelligence Reports: POSSIBLE USE OF CHEMICAL, BACTERIOLOGICAL AND RADIOLOGICAL AGENTS IN A FUTURE WAR. CIA-RDP82-00046R000400030002-2 Central Intelligence Agency (CIA), Reading Room, 2011. Retrieved from: https://www.cia.gov/library/readingroom/document/CIA-RDP82-0004 6R000400030002-2

40   Central Intelligence Agency (CIA) Intelligence Reports: SOVIET GUIDED MIS-SILE, CHEMICAL, AND BACTERIOLOGICAL WARFARE WORK IN HUNGARY. CIA-RDP80-00809A000700090556-4. Central Intelligence Agency (CIA), Reading Room, 2011. Re-trieved from: https://www.cia.gov/library/readingroom/document/CIA-RDP80-0080 9A000700090556-4

41   Central Intelligence Agency (CIA) Intelligence Reports: RECENT USSR WORK ON IN-FECTIOUS DISEASES THAT HAVE NATURAL RESERVOIRS. CIA-RDP80-00809A000700200218-6. Central Intelligence Agency (CIA), Reading Room, 2011. Retrieved from: https://www.cia.gov/library/readingroom/document/CIA-RDP80-00809A000700200218-6

42   Central Intelligence Agency (CIA) Intelligence Reports: ROLE OF RODENTS AS RES-ERVOIRS OF EPIDEMIC INFECTIONS. CIA-RDP80-00809A000600270272-0 .Central Intelligence Agency (CIA), Reading Room, 2011. Retrieved from: https://www.cia.gov/library/reading-room/document/CIA-RDP80-00809A000600270272-0

43   Pavlovskij Evgenij Nikanorovič. *Natural Foci of Human Infections*. Israel Program for Scientific Translations, 1963.

44   Central Intelligence Agency (CIA) Intelligence files: HYBRIDIZATION OF IXODES TICKS. CIA-RDP80-00809A000600380443-8. Central Intelligence Agency (CIA), Reading Room, 2011. Retrieved from: https://www.cia.gov/library/readingroom/document/CIA-RDP80-0080 9A000600380443-8

45   Central Intelligence Agency (CIA) Intelligence Reports: SIXTH CONFERENCE ON PROBLEMS OF PARASITOLOGY, HELD AT THE ZOOLOGICAL INSTITUTE, ACADEMY OF SCIENCES USSR. CIA-RDP80-0. Central Intelligence Agency (CIA), Reading Room, 2011. Retrieved from: https://www.cia.gov/library/readingroom/document/CIA-RDP80-00809A000600400344-5

46   Pavlovskij Evgenij Nikanorovič. *Natural Foci of Human Infections*. Israel Program for Scientific Translations, 1963.

47   Kisselev, Lev L., et al. "Lev Zilber, the Personality and the Scientist." Advances in Cancer Research, 1992, pp. 1–40., doi:10.1016/s0065-230x(08)60301-2.

48   Central Intelligence Agency (CIA) Intelligence Reports: RECENT USSR WORK ON IN-FECTIOUS DISEASES THAT HAVE NATURAL RESERVOIRS. CIA-RDP80-00809A000700200218-6. Central Intelligence Agency (CIA), Reading Room, 2011. Retrieved from: https://www.cia.gov/library/readingroom/document/CIA-RDP80-00809A000700200218-6

49   Central Intelligence Agency (CIA) Intelligence Reports: MORPHOLOGIC CHARAC-TERISTICS OF ACUTE ATTACKS IN CHRONIC BRUCELLOSIS. CIA-RDP80-00809A000600270278-4 Central Intelligence Agency (CIA), Reading Room, 2011. Retrieved from: https://www.cia.gov/library/readingroom/document/CIA-RDP80-00809A000600270278-4

50   Central Intelligence Agency (CIA) Intelligence Reports: Central Intelligence Agen-cy (CIA), Reading Room, 2011. Retrieved from: PRESERVATION AND RESTORATION OF THE VIR-ULENCE OF LEPTOSPIRA. CIA-RDP80-00809A000600340591-8. Retrieved from: https://www.cia.gov/library/readingroom/document/CIA-RDP80-00809A000600340591-8

51   This can be seen in several documents available from the USDA along with pub-lished research. Much will be demonstrated in this book. Navy and USDA researchers can be found working with Borrelia anserina, USDA published about the use of Spiroplasma as an insecticide in mosquitoes. Treponema was studied in the Tuskegee syphilis study and by Rockefeller Institute's Hideyo Noguchi early on. The USDA and Plum Island published exten-sive research on Mycoplasma. Leptospira is also listed as a biological weapon in the American stockpile from Canadian Ministry of Defence document on Operation LAC.

52   Rocky Mountains Laboratory (RML), and Carl L. Larson. 1960. RML Annual Report: PHS-NIH Rocky Mountain Laboratory Calender Year 1960. RML Annual Report: PHS-NIH Rocky

Mountain Laboratory Calender Year 1960. Hamilton, MT: RML. https://contentdm.uvu.edu/digital/collection/Burgdorfer/id/18. See: pp. 05

53   Central Intelligence Agency (CIA) Intelligence files: HEALTH CAMPAIGN: VD DE-CREASES MONGOL POPULATION. CIA-RDP80-00809A000600350470-1. Central Intelligence Agency (CIA), Reading Room, 2011. Retrieved from: https://www.cia.gov/library/reading-room/document/CIA-RDP80-00809A000600350470-1

54   Central Intelligence Agency (CIA) Intelligence Reports: TROPICAL AND VENEREAL DISEASES IN THE SOVIET UNION. CIA-RDP82-00457R000500150003-1. Central Intelligence Agency (CIA), Reading Room, 2001. Retrieved from: https://www.cia.gov/library/reading-room/document/CIA-RDP82-00457R000500150003-1

55   Central Intelligence Agency (CIA) Intelligence files: HYBRIDIZATION OF IXO-DES TICKS. CIA-RDP80-00809A000600380443-8. Central Intelligence Agency (CIA), Read-ing Room, 2011. Retrieved from: https://www.cia.gov/library/readingroom/document/CIA-RDP80-00809A000600380443-8

56   Central Intelligence Agency (CIA) Intelligence Reports: USSR WORK ON HEMOR-RHAGIC NEPHROSO-NEPHRITIS. CIA-RDP80-00809A000700240068-9. Central Intelligence Agency (CIA), Reading Room, 2011. Retrieved from: https://www.cia.gov/library/reading-room/document/CIA-RDP80-00809A000700240068-9

57   Central Intelligence Agency (CIA) Intelligence Reports: SCIENTIFIC ABSTRACT A.Y. CHUMAKOV - M.P. CHUMAKOV. CIA-RDP86-00513R000509120004-0. Central Intelligence Agency (CIA), Reading Room, 2011., pp. 83-100. Retrieved from: https://www.cia.gov/library/readingroom/document/CIA-RDP86-00513R000509120004-0

58   Domaradskiĭ, I. V., and Wendy Orent. *Biowarrior: Inside the Soviet/Russian Biological War Machine*. Amherst, NY: Prometheus Books, 2003, pp. 111-112

59   Central Intelligence Agency (CIA) Intelligence Reports: ANIMAL NEUROVIRUS DISEASES SIMILAR TO HUMAN POLIOMYELITIS. CIA-RDP80-00809A000700170265-8 Central Intelligence Agency (CIA), Reading Room, 2011. Retrieved from: https://www.cia.gov/library/readingroom/document/CIA-RDP80-00809A000700170265-8

60   Kouzminov, Alexander. Biological Espionage: Special Operations of the Soviet and Russian Foreign Intelligence Services in the West. Manas Publications, 2006.

Chapter Five

THE BIRTH OF A BIOWEAPONEER

THE BEGINNINGS OF ERICH TRAUB,
SLEEPER OF GERM WEAPONS

Thereupon came the Evil Ahriman, who is all death, and he count-er-created the locust, which brings death unto cattle and plants.
– Vendidad (*Avesta* – The Sacred Books of Zoroastrianism, Book 3.)

D
r. Erich Traub, one of the world's most exceptional yet infa-mous pioneers in virology, immunology, and bioweaponeer-ing, was born on June 27, 1906, in Asperglen, a town in the county of Württemberg, Germany. Erich Traub was raised in a Lu-theran Christian family to parents Lydia Rommel and Michael Traub.[1]

In 1924, he graduated from high school in Stuttgart, and went on to study at the University of Tübingen, with major studies in mod-ern languages, becoming fluent in English and French. He traveled to England in 1926 acting as an interpreter for a German judge in a dog show through an English kennel club he belonged to and graduated his 2-year tenure in 1927.

In those two years he also acted as a secretary and translator for an American family in Switzerland, because of his ability to speak En-glish and German.[2] Early at this time, Traub also acted as an interpret-er for American virologist, Richard E. Shope while Shope was study-ing in Germany at the University of Giessen. Shope noticed Traub's interest and potential for working in virus research, and suggested he go to the United States to the Rockefeller Institute where Shope was to return.[3] Traub decided to take Shope's advice and went on to study veterinary medicine at the University of Munich, Berlin & Giessen.[4]

Upon graduation, Traub studied under Professor Dr. Oskar Sei-fried at Münich, and worked briefly under Professor Dr. Wilhelm Zwick in 1931, at the Institute for Veterinary Hygiene and Animal Diseases for the German Reich, University of Giessen.[5] His thesis focused on the hygiene of animal stables, published as "Hygienic Investigations of Animal Stalls with Special Consideration for Stable Air."[6]

Having worked under Seifried and Zwick gave Traub a unique opportunity to observe and study the hidden aspects of some of nature's most perplexing realms of animal disease, and he was truly one-of-a-kind among his contemporaries.[7] Traub's early mentors in Germany were known for their studies of a highly neurotropic[A] virus that caused mental illness called Borna Disease Virus (BDV).[8] Borna Disease had been increasingly establishing a presence in horses and other farm animals around the countryside of Württemberg and Stuttgart over many years.[9] Borna Disease Virus later became the model virus for studying severe, neurological problems and mental health disorders in the autistic spectrum.[10, 11] Seifried had already studied at the Rockefeller Institute, and Shope already knew him from his studies of hog cholera.

Soon Traub was accepted and given a Fellowship for studies in the United States at the Rockefeller Institute in July, 1932, as a "student" under the Immigration Act of 1924.[12] He left Germany on September 1, 1932 aboard the *S.S. Hamburg*,[13] a ship liner that would become known in later years as the ship used to smuggle Nazi spies in and out of America.[14]

THE ROCKEFELLER YEARS

Erich Traub began his tenure at the Rockefeller Institute to study animal diseases caused by viruses under Richard Shope and Dr. Carl TenBroeck,[15] who started very early with the Rockefeller Institute during its inception in the early years of the 20th century.[16] Beginning under Shope, Traub's first set of studies focused on the virus, pseudorabies,[17, 18] a swine herpesvirus unrelated to rabies producing a similar raging disease sometimes referred to as *mad itch*.[19] In June of 1933, Traub took a trip with Dr. Shope to Iowa to study the disease in swine and cattle, after an outbreak the summer before. Shope published the studies in several papers just several years later.[20, 21]

These studies were to assess the transmission of the disease in swine and ultimately to cattle, which was always fatal to the cattle. They looked at rats and arthropods like lice and possibly ticks for the transmission of pseudorabies, as rats had been in the stalls and the farmer had pulled a dead rat out of one of the stall's water trough, but the relationship was inconclusive.[22]

A   **Neurotropic:** the quality of a virus or pathogen, having an affinity for nervous tissue, attacking the Central Nervous System (CNS) and brain.

They found however, that the cows always contracted it when put in the same pen as the swine. Shope also found that when he infected rabbits with nasal droplets from an infected pig's nose, it quickly infected them, and rats experimentally infected with the nasal droplets from infected swine, also quickly developed the infection and died.[23]

He began to see a cycle of transmission whereby the rats were infected by the swine or cattle droppings. In turn, the pigs that eat rat carcasses develop the infection, then when an infected pig brushes its nose against a cow that has a cut or abrasion, they contract the disease, and thus, a cycle of transmission is established. Shope also found that, upon mixing the virus with swine blood, most of the samples from these various swine already had antibodies.[24] This likely gave Traub the idea that this was a common virus, perhaps a latent virus, that all swine contain. Traub was left with the impression that other animals might have a similar virus sleeping within them, too.[25]

At some point in the spring of 1933, Traub expressed a desire to make a trip back to Germany in the summer of that year, to marry his fiancé,[26, 27] Blanka Denner, but the Rockefeller Institute staff convinced him to hold off for one more year and advised him it would be best to make the trip the summer of the next year.[28] The staff were somewhat concerned about Traub's ability to return while the Reich had recently taken hold of Germany.

His tenure at the Rockefeller Institute, however, was not without some difficulty.[29] He seemed to be somewhat uneasy studying in the United States, away from his family and fiancé. In records kept at the Rockefeller archives, numerous letters back and forth between Institute staff have voiced concerns about Traub.[30]

Equally noted was Traub's praise and skill under Shope and Ten-Broeck's direction, in another letter just weeks later from Dr. TenBroeck to the Institute director, Simon Flexner, on May 19, 1933, indicating he was truly one of a kind:

> Dr. Traub is one of the most promising of the young men that we have here. He is an extremely hard worker, a great reader, and thinks for himself. This year, on his own initiative, he attempted and succeeded in cultivating the pseudorabies virus, without any preliminary training and without the elaborate facilities that some people feel necessary.[31]

The following summer, Traub arranged an opportunity to return home to see Blanka and his family. He married Blanka Denner on July 3, 1934, which he had planned two years prior while in the United

States.[32] Blanka joined her husband on his return to the United States and settled with him for the few years they had in America. The staff wanted him back in the United States at the end of that summer to attend some of the Institute's scheduled meetings.[33]

Once back, Traub became a member of the fraternity, Sigma Xi, Princeton chapter, and from 1934 to the following year, attended the German American Volksbund (*Amerika-deutscheur Volksbund*) at Camp Siegfried,[34] a summer camp on Long island that attempted to promote and normalize Nazi ideologies and urgently tried to sway favor for Germany during the buildup to war. According to his colleagues and associates in the United States, he never talked about politics or spoke of Hitler or the Reich, and it was always strictly about science, which he was very passionate about.[35]

According to declassified FBI files on Traub, he spoke to a small number of his colleagues and professors about the *German American Volksbund*, claiming that for a short while he joined and went to rallies for the sake of Blanka, who felt isolated and without any German friends in America. She felt as though she had to always defend herself and Germany, and this was supposedly to help her cope with life in America. But she was not very happy in the United States, and having a social life was apparently difficult for her. It was Blanka, according to FBI interviews of his colleagues, that was so enthusiastic for the Nazi party and supportive of Adolph Hitler.[36]

In 1935, his third year at the Institute, Traub had discovered the virus of Lymphocytic Choriomeningitis (LCM) while injecting the brains of mice with a foreign protein suspended in a broth. Traub discovered that this foreign protein would elucidate a chronic, debilitating condition from the septic shock resulting from the injections. Within short order, an epidemic was spreading in the mouse colony from Traub's experiments. A virus was isolated, and it was the LCM virus that had been isolated by other virologists the year before in Maryland. The virus causes both fatal and chronic diseases. In the fatal form, it was similar to poliomyelitis, while the chronic form resembles Lyme disease. [37]

The virus was also pathogenic to humans and infected several of the animal keepers at the Institute.[38] It was unknowingly present in sleeping form before he injected the foreign protein into the mice brains and awakened it into an active viral infection because of the physical trauma induced by the stress or septic shock it produced. His discovery of LCM virus set the majority of his life's work in immunology, virology, and of course, bioweaponeering.[39]

Just five days after Traub published his breakthrough publication on LCM virus, Blanka gave birth to their first child, Walter Hellmuth

Traub, on March 27, 1935, at the Princeton Hospital in Princeton, NJ. Traub's firstborn was now a U.S. citizen.[40]

Traub would receive international praise for his clever work on the LCM virus,[41] and he would also be recognized for his studies of pseudorabies and Eastern Equine Encephalitis virus (EEE) transmitted by mosquitoes and carried by birds. EEE is a virus related to West Nile Virus that affects horses as well as humans. Encephalitis is swelling of the brain and can be fatal, like that seen in rabies.

In April of 1935, Traub briefly returned to study the ability of pseudorabies to infect the cells of immunized guinea pigs. The idea was to add the virus to an already immunized animal, in which case would neutralize the virus since it had already been immunized and thus, antibodies to fight it. Not so, he found. Traub observed, that the virus was not neutralized, and once inside the cells of immunized animals, the immunity was not necessarily present, and the virus would continue to multiply at a much slower rate.[42]

Traub then returned to LCM virus to further study the results of the earlier outbreak. These results were published in "An Epidemic in a Mouse Colony Due to the Virus of Lymphocytic Choriomeningitis," estimating that about fifty percent of the mice were infected, although present in a mild form. He also found that, although milder in form, the infection rate was much higher than in typical fatal disease,[43] and this gave him additional clues in maximizing infection rates when making effective biological weapons for the Reich.

Following Traub's studies of pseudorabies and his breakthrough studies of LCM virus, Dr. Carl TenBroeck and several students, including Erich Traub, discovered a more virulent form of Western Equine Encephalomyelitis Virus (WEE) on the east coast, respectively naming it Eastern Equine Encephalomyelitis Virus (EEE). The results of his first experiment with EEE virus, "Protective Vaccination of Horses with Modified Equine Encephalomyelitis Virus" was published in May 1935.[44]

First, Traub ran the virus through many serial passages in pigeons until it could no longer be attenuated any further, and isolated infectious material from the brains of these pigeons.[45] He then injected it into lambs, then took the infective material from the brains of these lambs and injected it into horses, and some of the horses also developed encephalitis and died.[46] He found that the infective material from the brains of these horses was highly virulent for guinea-pigs and yet it was not the same as the EEE he injected,[47] as it produced a modified, new agent, possibly the same virus isolated by the Rockefeller Foundation staff in Africa the following year, which became known as West Nile Virus.[48]

That July, Traub published additional studies with TenBroeck on the vector, pathogenicity, and transmission of EEE in "Epidemiology of Equine Encephalomyelitis Virus in the Eastern United States."[49] According to the Rockefeller Institute's official history, by 1936, Traub had already been making great strides in modifying the virus as well as understanding the complex, environmental host-vector relationships of the virus.[50]

Traub's studies of EEE with TenBroeck gave Traub, from a very early time, a more relevant context in which he could later supervise studies that included insect-vectored tests conducted on and around Plum Island, then known as Fort Terry, owned by the Army Chemical Corps.[51]

Traub had been working diligently on these viruses that would become the basis of his life work – potent viruses that he could either elucidate from within the body or transmit through various ways, such as mosquitoes, mites, or other insects.[52] These viruses would cause slow, debilitating conditions that progressed over the lifespan of the individual or animal, passing through generations, becoming more silent yet destructive to the central nervous system with each passing generation.

In early 1936, Traub returned to his studies of LCM virus, publishing "Persistence of Lymphocytic Choriomeningitis Virus in Immune Animals and its Relation to Immunity," noting that many would continue to harbor and shed the virus despite any symptoms.[53]

It is this 1936 paper which became the basis for what later became known as *immune tolerance*,[54] a damaged immune system that will tolerate pathogens and toxic material it should otherwise fend off. It stops fending off harmful pathogens, tolerating them instead, and in turn, such pathogens invade the body and central nervous system, causing devious effects without visible symptoms or antibodies, and this is an important part of the reason why many of those sick with chronic diseases like Lyme disease and chronic fatigue syndrome cannot get diagnosed as sick by the public health system and its medical practitioners.

It is clear from the records that the Rockefeller Institute staff valued Traub's tenure, perhaps even more than he. They saw Traub as their most valuable player, an exceptionally skilled virologist. Numerous letters have cited their interest in keeping him at the Institute, even hinting at moving around issues of immigration law.[55] But Traub clearly had some conflict remaining in the United States, likely because of Blanka's unhappiness and feelings of isolation from Germany.[56] Late in 1936, Traub requested to be excused from participation in the Institute activities for the period of one year, and to return in 1937.[57]

Traub's file shows that during his time back in Germany he visited several German laboratories, though specifics on this are not mentioned. It is most likely that he visited Insel Riems, because in 1937 a researcher from Insel Riems published a paper studying Foot-and-Mouth Disease Virus (FMD) in the central nervous systems of small animals and mice in which the test mice were acquired from the Rockefeller Institute in Princeton, NJ, which would have come from Traub.[58]

Upon his return, Traub continued his work on LCM producing modified variants of the virus passing the virus through guinea pigs and mice. He continued studying the strange new phenomenon, later to be baptized *immune tolerance,* describing it in a 1939 paper as "perfect parasitism" of the body by the virus.[59] Traub clearly began to see the immunological relationships between the virus and the animals infected, as well as virulence. He also noted in the infected animals that there was exceptionally slow antiviral activity of the immune system in fighting off the infection, with hardly the level of antibodies one would expect. This virus also passed from mother to newborn and started to cause cancer in the mice, which was not published in his American studies, but he mentioned it in later German papers recalling his American studies.[60, 61]

It is also of interest to note that during his time studying LCM virus in mice, multiple infections were produced, which had been the phenomenon known as "infectious catarrh," or "mixed infections," similar to those seen in the Spanish Flu of 1918. It was here that strains of mycoplasma were isolated, a bacteria similar to meningococcus but lacks a cell wall. Traub supervised and assisted a researcher under him, John B. Nelson, to further study these microbes which Traub's LCM studies had produced in the mice, and these were published in three papers by Nelson in 1937.[62, 63, 64]

In addition to the mycoplasma, Traub also gained some experience with the bacteria *Listeria monocytogenes,* a bacteria that causes food poisoning (listeriosis) in humans. This experience Traub only briefly mentions in passing in later papers Traub published under the Reich in 1942.[65]

Soon Traub was appointed associate of the Rockefeller staff, along with his colleague Albert B. Sabin, appearing in an article from *The New York Times* on June 29, 1937, "Promoted at Institute: Rockefeller Medical Research Staff Members Are Shifted."[66] His value to the Institute was clear to the staff, watching Traub concentrate in his meticulous studies and original ideas in which other students had yet to understand. They felt however, he was overworking himself, and desperately needed a break, perhaps a vacation, addressed in a letter from Dr. TenBroeck to newly appointed Institute director, Herbert Gasser, dated December 16, 1938.[67] Among his colleagues, he was well-respected, spoken of in the highest terms and earned a very good reputation as a virologist and bacteriologist.[68]

Traub's promotion, however, would be short-lived. Within a year, following the mounting tensions between Germany and the rest of the world, Traub decided to return to his native Germany to enter into professorship at the University of Giessen, with the coming outbreak of World War II just a few years out, Traub packed up and returned to the homeland.[69]

Endnotes

1   National Archives. Joint-Intelligence Objectives Agency file on Erich Traub (RG 330). NARS. Joint Intelligence Objectives Agency (JIOA), JIOA Administrative Records. (1949-54).

2   Ibid.

3   National Archives. RG 65 Erich Traub, (Declassified FBI Investigations on the Loyalties of Erich Traub). Federal Bureau of Investigation (FBI): NARA., Doc. # QO1-458431291

4   Dinter, Z. Persönaliches, Begegnungen mit Erich Traub.[Personal Encounters with Erich Traub] Berl. Munch. Tier. Woch. 96. 70-72. (1984)

5   Traub, Erich. "Information for Desired Staff Appointment." Received by The Rockefeller Institute for Medical Research, 66th Street and York Avenue, 25 Mar. 1932, New York, NY

6   Traub, E. Hygienische Untersuchungen in Tierställen unter besonderer Berücksichtigung der Stalluft. [Hygienic Investigations of Animal Stables with Special Consideration for Stable Air.] Zeitschrift für Infektionskrankheiten. Haus. Vol. 45, No. 1. 1-35. (1932). [Translated to English by A. Finnegan, 2019].

7   Dinter, Z. Persönaliches, Begegnungen mit Erich Traub. Berl. Munch. Tier. Woch. 96. 70-72. (1984)

8   Zwick, W., Seifried, O., & J. Witte. Weitere Untersuchungen über die seuchenhafte gehirn-Rückenmarksentzündung der Pferde (Bornasche Krankheit). Z. Inf. Krkh. Haustiere. 32, 150, (1927)

9   Reichard, R. E., & Uskavitch, R. (1975). Borna disease: A literature review. Beltsville, MD: Agricultural Research Service, U.S. Dept. of Agriculture, Northeast Region.

10   Bode, L, R Ferszt, and G Czech. 1993. "Borna Disease Virus Infection and Affective Disorders in Man." Archives of Virology. Supplementum. U.S. National Library of Medicine. 1993. https://www.ncbi.nlm.nih.gov/pubmed/8219801

11   Carbone, K M et al. "Borna disease virus (BDV)-induced model of autism: application to vaccine safety test design." *Molecular psychiatry* vol. 7 Suppl 2 (2002): S36-7. doi:10.1038/sj.mp.4001174

12   Flinn, W. E. (1934, February 5). Letter to the American Consul at Stuttgart from Assistant Business Manager of The Rockefeller Institute for Medical Research [Letter to American Consul at Stuttgart]. U.S.A., New York, New York.

13   Flinn, Waldo R. Letter to Department of Immigration. 1932. "Letter to the Commissioner General of Immigration," September 9, 1932.

14   Loftus, J. personal communication

15   National Archives. Joint-Intelligence Objectives Agency file on Erich Traub (RG 330). NARS. Joint Intelligence Objectives Agency (JIOA), JIOA Administrative Records. (1949-54).

16   Corner, G. W. (1965). *A history of the Rockefeller Institute: 1901-1953: Origins and growth.* New York: The Rockefeller Institute Press.

17   Traub, Erich. Letter to Waldo R. Flinn. 1933. "Letter to Waldo R. Flinn," June 12, 1933.

18   Shope, R. E. (1935). Experiments on The Epidemiology Of Pseudorabies: I. Mode Of Transmission Of The Disease In Swine And Their Possible Role In Its Spread To Cattle. Journal of Experimental Medicine, 62(1), 85-99. doi:10.1084/jem.62.1.85

19   "Pseudorabies (PRV)." n.d. USDA APHIS | Pseudorabies (PRV). USDA APHIS | Pseudorabies (PRV). Accessed August 1, 2019. https://www.aphis.usda.gov/aphis/ourfocus/animalhealth/nvap/NVAP-Reference-Guide/Control-and-Eradication/Pseudorabies

20   Shope, R. E. (1935). Experiments on The Epidemiology Of Pseudorabies: I. Mode Of Transmission Of The Disease In Swine And Their Possible Role In Its Spread To Cattle. *Journal of Experimental Medicine*, 62(1), 85-99. doi:10.1084/jem.62.1.85

21   Shope, R. E. (1935). Experiments on The Epidemiology Of Pseudorabies: II. Prevalence Of The Disease Among Middle Western Swine And The Possible Role Of Rats In Herd-To-Herd Infections. *Journal of Experimental Medicine*, 62(1), 101-117. doi:10.1084/jem.62.1.101

22   Shope, R. E. (1935). Experiments on The Epidemiology Of Pseudorabies: II. Prevalence Of The Disease Among Middle Western Swine And The Possible Role Of Rats In Herd-To-Herd Infections. *Journal of Experimental Medicine*, 62(1), 101-117. doi:10.1084/jem.62.1.101

23   Shope, R. E. (1935). Experiments on The Epidemiology Of Pseudorabies: I. Mode Of Transmission Of The Disease In Swine And Their Possible Role In Its Spread To Cattle. *Journal of Experimental Medicine*, 62(1), 85-99. doi:10.1084/jem.62.1.85

24   See Shope 1935a, Shope 1935b

25   Traub, E. Cultivation of Pseudorabies Virus. *Journal of Experimental Medicine*, 58(6), 663-681. (1934). doi:10.1084/jem.58.6.663.

26   TenBroeck, C., Dr. (1933, May 6). [Letter to Mr. Waldo R. Flinn]. U.S.A., New York, New York.

27   Flinn, Waldo R. Letter to Department of Immigration. 1934. "Letter to Dana Hodgdon, Chief, Visa Division," January 22, 1934.

28   TenBroeck, C., Dr. (1933, May 6). [Letter to Mr. Waldo R. Flinn]. U.S.A., New York, New York.

29   TenBroeck, C., Dr. (1934, March 24). [Letter to Mr. Waldo R. Flinn]. U.S.A., New York, New York.

30   TenBroeck, C., Dr. (1933, May 6). [Letter to Mr. Waldo R. Flinn]. U.S.A., New York, New York.

31   TenBroeck, C., Dr. (1933, May 19). Correspondence [Letter to Dr. Simon Flexner]. U.S.A., New York, New York.

32   Traub, Erich, (1933, August 26). [Letter to Mr. Waldo R. Flinn]. U.S.A., New York, New York.

33   TenBroeck, C., Dr. (1934, January 30). [Letter to Mr. Waldo R. Flinn]. U.S.A., New York, New York.

34   National Archives. Joint-Intelligence Objectives Agency file on Erich Traub (RG 330). NARS. Joint Intelligence Objectives Agency (JIOA), JIOA Administrative Records. (1949-54).

35   National Archives. RG 65 Erich Traub, (Declassified FBI Investigations on the Loyalties of Erich Traub). Federal Bureau of Investigation (FBI): NARA., Doc. # QO1-458431291

36   Ibid.

37   Traub, E. A Filterable Virus Recovered from White Mice. Science, 81. (2099), 298-299. doi:10.1126/science.81.2099.298. (1935).

38   Corner, G. W. (1965). *A history of the Rockefeller Institute: 1901-1953: Origins and growth.* New York: The Rockefeller Institute Press., pp. 408-409

39   National Archives, Joint Intelligence Objectives Agency (JIOA), JIOA Administrative Records. (1949-54). Joint-Intelligence Objectives Agency file on Erich Traub (RG 330). NARS.

40   National Archives. Joint-Intelligence Objectives Agency file on Erich Traub (RG 330). NARS. Joint Intelligence Objectives Agency (JIOA), JIOA Administrative Records. (1949-54).

41   Traub, E. LCM Virus Research, Retrospect and Prospects. Lymphocytic Choriomeningitis Virus and Other Arenaviruses, 3-10. doi:10.1007/978-3-642-65681-1_1. (1973)

42   Traub, E. Multiplication In Vitro Of Pseudorabies Virus in The Testicle Tissue of Immunized Guinea Pigs. *Journal of Experimental Medicine*, 61(6), 833-838. doi:10.1084/jem.61.6.833. (1935).

43   Traub, E. An Epidemic in A Mouse Colony Due to The Virus of Acute Lymphocytic Choriomeningitis. *Journal of Experimental Medicine*, 63(4), 533-546. doi:10.1084/jem.63.4.533. (1936).

44   Traub, E., & Broeck, C. T. (1935). Protective Vaccination of Horses with Modified Equine Encephalomyelitis Virus. *Science*, 81(2110), 572-572. doi:10.1126/science.81.2110.572

45   Ibid.

46   Ibid.

47   Ibid.

48   Smithburn, K. C., T. P. Hughes, A. W. Burke, and J. H. Paul. 1940. "A Neurotropic Virus Isolated from the Blood of a Native of Uganda 1." *The American Journal of Tropical Medicine and Hygiene* s1-20 (4): 471–92. https://doi.org/10.4269/ajtmh.1940.s1-20.471.

49   TenBroeck, C., et al. (1935). Epidemiology Of Equine Encephalomyelitis In The Eastern United States. *Journal of Experimental Medicine*, 62(5), 677-685. doi:10.1084/jem.62.5.677

50   Corner, G. W. (1965). *A history of the Rockefeller Institute: 1901-1953: Origins and growth*. New York: The Rockefeller Institute Press, pp. 312-313

51   National Archives. Joint-Intelligence Objectives Agency file on Erich Traub (RG 330). NARS. Joint Intelligence Objectives Agency (JIOA), JIOA Administrative Records. (1949-54).

52   Traub, E. & F. Kesting. Ueber die Ausscheidung des E.E.E.-Virus und das gelegentliche Vorkommen von Kontaktinfektionen bestimmter Art bei Mausen. [Secretion of the EEE-virus and occasional incidence of certain contact infections in mice]. Zbl. bakt. Abt. I. Orig. 166 (6). 462-475. (1956).

53   Traub, E. Persistence of Lymphocytic Choriomeningitis Virus in Immune Animals and Its Relation To Immunity. Journal of Experimental Medicine, 63(6), 847-861. doi:10.1084/jem.63.6.847. (1936).

54   Dinter, Z. Persönaliches, Begegnungen mit Erich Traub.[Personal Encounters with Erich Traub] Berl. Munch. Tier. Woch. 96. 70-72. (1984)

55   Flinn, Waldo R. (1934, January 29). ["Letter to Dr. Carl TenBroeck."] Rockefeller Institute. New York, NY

56   National Archives. RG 65 Erich Traub, (Declassified FBI Investigations on the Loyalties of Erich Traub). Federal Bureau of Investigation (FBI): NARA., Doc. # QO1-458431291

57   Traub, E. Correspondence [Letter to Mr. A. D. Robinson]. U.S.A., Princeton, New Jersey. (1936, June 30).

58   Nagel, H C. Untersuchungen uber das Verhalten des Maul und Klauenseuche-Virus im Zentralnervensystem kleiner Versuchstiere. Dtsche. Tier. Woch. 45: 624-625. (1937)

59   Traub, E. Epidemiology of Lymphocytic Choriomeningitis In A Mouse Stock Observed for Four Years. *Journal of Experimental Medicine*, 69(6), 801-817. doi:10.1084/jem.69.6.801. (1939).

60   Traub, E. Epidemiology of Lymphocytic Choriomeningitis In A Mouse Stock Observed for Four Years. *Journal of Experimental Medicine*, 69(6), 801-817. doi:10.1084/jem.69.6.801. (1939).

61   Traub, E. Ueber den Einfluß der latenten Choriomeningitis-Infektion auf die Entstehung der Lymphomatose bei weißen Mause [On the Influence of Latent Choriomeningitis Infection on the Development of Lymphomatosis in White Mice]. Zentrl. Bakt. I. Orig. 147 (16). 1-25. (1941). [Translated to English by A. Finnegan, 2019]

62   Nelson JB. INFECTIOUS CATARRH OF MICE : I. A NATURAL OUTBREAK OF THE DISEASE. J Exp Med. 1937 May 31;65(6):833-41. doi: 10.1084/jem.65.6.833. PMID: 19870637; PMCID: PMC2133528.

63   Nelson JB. INFECTIOUS CATARRH OF MICE : II. THE DETECTION AND ISOLATION OF COCCOBACILLIFORM BODIES. J Exp Med. 1937 May 31;65(6):843-9. doi: 10.1084/jem.65.6.843. PMID: 19870638; PMCID: PMC2133524.

64   Nelson JB. INFECTIOUS CATARRH OF MICE : III. THE ETIOLOGICAL SIGNIFICANCE OF THE COCCOBACILLIFORM BODIES. J Exp Med. 1937 May 31;65(6):851-60. doi: 10.1084/ jem.65.6.851. PMID: 19870639; PMCID: PMC2133521.

65   Traub, E. Ueber eine mit Listerella-ähnlichen Bakterien vergesellschaftete Menin-go-Encephalomyelitis der Kaninchen. [About a Meningo-Encephalomyelitis of Rabbits Asso-ciated with Listerella-like Bacteria]. Zntrl. Bakt. I. Orig. 149 (1). 38-49. (1942). [Translated to English by A. Finnegan, 2019]

66   Promoted at Institute: Rockefeller Medical Research Staff Members Are Shifted. (1937, June 29). New York Times. Retrieved February 28, 2018, from https://timesmachine. nytimes.com/timesmachine/1937/06/29/118978767.html?pageNumber=10

67   TenBroeck, C., Dr. (1936, December 16). Correspondence [Letter to Dr. Herbert S. Gasser]. Rockefeller Institute for Medical Research, New York, New York.

68   National Archives. RG 65 Erich Traub, (Declassified FBI Investigations on the Loyal-ties of Erich Traub). Federal Bureau of Investigation (FBI): NARA., Doc. # QO1-458431291

69   Traub, E. . Correspondence [Letter to Dr. Carl TenBroeck]. Rockefeller Institute for Medical Research, Princeton, New Jersey. (1938, April 7)

Chapter Six

BUILDING THE BIOWEAPONS PART I

ERICH TRAUB LEARNS THE ESOTERIC ART OF GERM WEAPONS WITH KARL BELLER

Nature has the deep cunning which hides itself under the appearance of openness, so that simple people think they can see through her quite well, and all the while she is secretly preparing a refutation of their confident prophecies

– George Eliot, *The Mill on the Floss*

From the time of Erich Traub's return to Germany, he was accepted into the University of Giessen to study in virology, bacteriology, and veterinary medicine under Professor Dr. Karl Beller. Dr. Beller's history and acquisition of Traub at the Institute was summarized by Klaus Munk in a later textbook on the history of German virology, with Beller taking the lead position of veterinary research after Professor Wilhelm Zwick retired.[1]

At this time, Traub wrote a post-doctoral thesis, "Active Immunity and Active Immunization Against Viral Diseases," an in-depth paper on the nature of immunity, including forms that were only meant to prevent losses and did not stop disease or give true immunity. He spoke at length about the different kinds of immunization approaches and gave both criticism and praise for the different methods, as well as explaining the various approaches other researchers took in their attempts at explaining the science of immunity.[2]

It is also interesting to note that in his thesis paper, Traub mentions diseases of blood sucking insects being able to reactivate vaccine viruses, that is, a live virus vaccine, it can potentially regain virulence when a mosquito bite transmits African Horse Sickness to the vaccine recipient, as African Horse Sickness contains antigens that can be suppressive to the immune system, reactivating the vaccine virus and the ability to spread. This would be much like he had done with foreign protein in his mice to awaken the sleeping LCM virus to start up an epidemic from scratch. He says:

> The [vaccine] virus circulates in the blood of the horses during the fever period, which may be a drawback in that [African] horse sickness is most likely transmitted by blood-sucking insects [and since] it is not guaranteed that the vaccine virus in the [animal] cannot [regain its virulence] back into the original agent. However, this risk should be lessened by the fact that the vaccinations are carried out in a season in which blood-sucking insects do not occur or only in small numbers.[3]

Traub also continued studies on Eastern Equine Encephalitis (EEE) which he started while he was at the Rockefeller Institute. When he continued this work at Giessen, he began running the virus in serial passages through different animals, such as the horse, rabbits, guinea-pigs, mice, and pigeons. He was able to create modifications of the virus, for instance, increase the neurotropic qualities by running it through mice.[4] This also gave him more complex experience adapting the virus to various animals they did not infect before, which then could be used to convey weapons to enemy targets through the use of animals, like we had established in the early chapters.

As an assistant professor under Beller at Giessen, Traub had a few students under him, such as Dr. Werner Schäfer, who went to Africa in 1939, and returned by the start of the war to later join Traub at Insel Riems.[5] He and Traub would also publish a paper that year on the virus of LCM in mouse blood.[6]

It was at this time Schäfer retrieved a strain of avian spirochetes, *Borrelia anserina*, then known as *Spirochaeta gallinarum*, which was given to him by Rockefeller-funded psychologist, Franz Jahnel. This was the spirochete from birds that was weaponized by Traub and would become in later years, *Borrelia burgdorferi*, the agent responsible for Lyme Disease, later supported by evidence in a 1989 publication, "Shared flagellar epitopes of *Borrelia burgdorferi* and *Borrelia anserina*."[7] Schäfer began growing the spirochetes in chick embryos, acknowledging their need, for a cheap way to maintain the spirochete and to have a fully virulent strain for research and teaching purposes. The results were published in "The Maintenance of *Spirochaeta gallinarum* by Passages in Fowl Embryos:"

> Since we have to have a fully virulent *Spirochaeta gallinarum* strain in our institute for research and teaching purposes, we

have tried to replace the expensive chicken passages with a complete, simple and cheap breeding procedure.[8]

That same year, Traub contributed two chapters to a German book on animal disease, *Handbook of Virus Diseases: with particular attention to their experimental research*, edited by Eugen Gildemeister, Otto Waldmann, and Eugen Haagen.[9] Traub's contribution was an entire chapter on LCM, "Choriomeningitis of Mice,"[10] as well as a chapter with Karl Beller on fowl plague (avian influenza) and similar avian diseases, in "Fowl Plague and Related Virus Diseases of Birds."[11]

In this chapter, it is clear where Traub's experience with avian spirochetosis (*Borrelia anserina*) comes into play – as the *differential diagnosis* to fowl plague – which means it is a disease that mirrors fowl plague and only an expert can tell them apart.[12] Schäfer's bacteriological work under Traub and Beller produced another paper on pseudotuberculosis, a bacteria of chickens, another disease that mirrored both avian spirochetosis and fowl plague.[13] Combining and mixing the qualities of these different agents together served as an excellent way to confuse diagnosis with new biological weapons never seen before.

Dr. Karl Beller published several additional chapters in the *Handbook for Virus Diseases* in 1939 while Traub was his assistant Professor. There was a chapter, "Heartwater and other animal rickettsioses." It is here that Erich Traub gained his important research on ticks and tick-borne disease.

Heartwater is a *rickettsia*, a bacteria related to ehrlichiosis[A], another rickettsia that mainly affects cattle and ruminants. He describes the disease agents *Rickettsia ruminantium* (now called *Cowdria ruminantium*) and *Rickettsia canis* (now called *Ehrlichia canis*), both of which are closely related to the agent of human monocytic ehrlichiosis (*Ehrlichia chaffeensis*) which is now a major tick-borne disease and co-infection of Lyme disease in the United States and abroad.[14] He also describes the complex illness in dogs that result from a mix of infections like *Babesia, Ehrlichia, Bartonella*, and *Leishmaniasis*, present in some hard-bodied ticks that do not feed on humans.

Beller describes their ability to cause the same *immune tolerance* that Traub found in his mice with LCM virus at the Rockefeller Institute. Also, it is interesting to note that Beller's studies of *Rickettsia ruminantium* demonstrate that although the chief host of the tick that transmits this rickettsia is cattle, they attach themselves to all warm-blooded animals and also to humans.[15]

A   **Ehrlichiosis** : Infection with parasitic rickettsia of the genus *Ehrlichia*, especially *E. sennetsu*, that are transmitted by ticks and produce manifestations in humans similar to those of Rocky Mountain spotted fever, including rash, muscle pain, and fever.

Beller makes another major admission in this chapter by noting the ability for relapsing fever spirochetes (*Borrelia*) to be transmitted occasionally by the brown dog tick, a hard-bodied tick. All the way up to 1983 when Lyme disease was discovered by Willy Burgdorfer, he and the American scientists had maintained that spirochetes could not be transmitted by hard-bodied ticks, yet Traub's mentor is saying just that back in 1939. Even though this tick does not affect humans, it gave Traub the foreknowledge that it was possible to transmit spirochetes using hard-bodied ticks.

All Traub had to do was get these infectious agents into hard-bodied ticks that were a real nuisance to humans, such as the *Amblyomma* or the *Ixodes* ticks, and he would have insects to naturally spread his serpentine weapons that could induce the same immune tolerance he would spend his life studying.

Traub mentions extensive experiments on horses with blood parasites in a 1941 paper, linking him to direct experience with disease agents like *Babesia*.[16] Adding a weaponized avian relapsing fever spirochete (*Borrelia anserina*) to the mix would cause a complex mix of infections that would not only be very confusing to physicians and diagnosis, but also very resistant to treatment.

MILITARY SERVICE AND VETERINARY AFFAIRS

According to records at the German Federal Archives from the University of Giessen, the German Research Foundation (*Deutschen Forschungsgemeinschaft*) was funding Erich Traub's work and paid for him to continue his Rockefeller studies on EEE and LCM virus. Traub published a follow-up paper on Eastern Equine Encephalitis in guinea pigs for the production of serum.

Traub once again admits in here that vaccine viruses can be spread by blood-sucking insects when the vaccine virus is circulating the blood:

> Since [the] horse disease is probably transmitted by blood-sucking insects that take the pathogen from the blood, it must be required [that the] virus to be used as a vaccine [...] does not appear in the blood at all, or only in such small quantities, that the mosquitoes cannot get infected.[17]

At this time, Traub published several studies on diseases of swine looking at the similarities and differences between swine polio (Teschen disease), pseudorabies, and the virus of swine fever.[18] He also published a study of an attempted vaccine for swine polio, but the results had clear implications for biological weapons work hidden under the cover of vaccine studies.[19]

These studies were soon interrupted by the outbreak of war and Traub was drafted for military service. He sent a letter to the German Research Foundation in February of 1940, concluding his work with the grant he was given by them.[20] He was sent to the front lines in France, but was too valuable to end up a casualty of war, so they pulled him from the front lines to continue important bioweapons work as a veterinarian.

In April of 1940, Traub, Beller, and another colleague published a study of Bovine Papular Stomatitis, a poxvirus similar to smallpox, in "Studies on Bovine Papular Stomatitis," a viral infection that looked much like Foot-and-Mouth Disease but is a member of the poxvirus family. They began experiments trying to adapt it to different animals to change its properties.[21]

It was in this study, they mixed the virus in broth containing strains of *Serratia marcescens* (*Bacillus prodigiosus*), a so-called "harmless" bacterium to cattle and was used in later simulant tests in America. The filters used hold back the bacteria as the mixture passes through the filter and any virus will pass through it, but the bacteria will be held back. In this case however, the virus had transferred genetic material to the bacteria giving it pathogenic properties and changing its qualities.[22] In other words, he weaponized the simulant bacteria *Serratia marcescens*.[23]

For his German patriotism, Erich Traub would become a member of the NSKK (Motor Transportation Corp), the NSV (Welfare Association), the NS (Student Fraternity), and the *Reichsluftschutzbund* (Air Raid Protection), which he claimed was a requirement for him to join the academic institutions.[24]

Through the years 1940-1942, Traub made some important studies for the military in several epidemics in veterinary horses for the Reich, occurring in Germany and France. He would spend this time researching and giving lectures on Equine Infectious Anemia Virus (EIA), infectious respiratory catarrh ("mixed infections"), Streptococci, equine encephalitis, lymphocytic choriomeningitis (LCM), *Listeria monocytogenes* (listeriosis) in Angora rabbits, swine polio (Teschen Disease), Newcastle Disease Virus (NDV), avian influenza (fowl plague) of birds, with some other studies of infectious diseases of humans.[25]

In 1941, Traub published a very important study on LCM virus – its ability to cause cancer.[26] This had deep implications for his weapons work, as it is, that not only was the virus able to cause chronic neurodegenerative disease, but it also likewise promoted cancer:

> Taking into account the tropism[B] of the choriomeningitis virus, it is concluded from the test results and the observations described in the text [described] that the latent, long-lasting viral infection promotes the development of the Lymphomatosis. [...]. The effect of the virus is considered to be a chronic stimulus to the cells of the lymphoid tissue. It is thus similar to the effect of carcinogenic chemicals in experimentally generated mouse cancer.[27]

Moreover, he noted the ability for the virus to transmit through generations, becoming, *"more and more of a completely silent infection, so that even a connoisseur of the epidemic could no longer [visibly] distinguish between infected and healthy mice."*[28]

INFECTIOUS CATARRH – "MIXED INFECTIONS"

When Traub was serving the German military in the areas of France, he worked on a series of studies on *infectious catarrh* involving an epidemic in horses owned by a veterinary company in France near the Pyrenees, but soon German military horses also became sick.[29]

It was suggested by other veterinarians that the disease may have been equine infectious anemia, the HIV of horses, and since they could not rule it out, several studies of infectious anemia were made by Traub and Beller, who ruled it out, because the quick onset and highly contagious nature of the epidemic spoke against the infectious anemia virus, which spreads at a much slower rate and these horses lacked evidence to indicate it.[30]

Traub and Beller also conducted some experiments with blood parasites, likely a *Babesia* of horses, to also rule that out from the diagnosis. Eventually the diagnosis was confirmed to be infectious catarrh, a mixed infection first triggered by a viral infection that blunted the immune system and brought on a mix of infections with *Mycoplasma* and *Streptococci*, explaining the epidemic.[31] This mirrored his earlier studies of LCM virus, when he awakened the virus from dormancy and produced a mix of bacterial and viral infections at the same time. Another interesting thing to note, is that Beller had also published a paper about the synergy that occurs between bacteria and

---

B   Tropism – *i.e.* destructive effect

virus, in this instance, between the bacteria *Mycobacterium bovis* used as the BCG tuberculosis vaccine and the ability of Foot-and-Mouth Disease Virus to enable the bacteria to regain virulence.[32] These veterinary studies show that Traub and Beller understood very well the mechanics behind the 1918 Influenza, where the virus activates a mix of infections devastate the body after an initial viral infection.[33]

Professor Beller and Dr. Traub published follow-up papers to explain the disease, in "The Position and Outlook in Research on Infectious Respiratory Catarrh of the Horse," which describes a disease process similar to the Spanish Influenza of 1918, whereby a virus throws the immune system into disarray and kicks on a secondary bacterial pneumonia, like *Streptococcus*, found in great numbers in the diseased horses:

> [...] we have reason to believe that these streptococci are not the primary cause of the disease, that they do not have any essential pathogenicity for the horse, but that [they are] pathogens of a secondary infection on the grounds of [an initial] viral disease, which are responsible for the various modifications of the [typical disease] and their chronic course with the numerous relapses [of the disease] condition.[34]

Traub concluded this with a long final report on the *Streptococci* of the horse, explaining the complicated disease it presents to veterinarians and doctors. These mixed infections occurred because the immune system was suppressed and thus brought on multiple additional infections.[35] When making a biological weapon, it was wise to produce an agent that could bring on symptoms of many diseases simultaneously, confusing the doctors and thus, unable to assess the proper treatment.

SWINE POLIO (PORCINE ENCEPHALOMYELITIS)

Erich Traub spent some time on the virus termed swine polio that causes paralysis in pigs and conducted a lengthy study on vaccines for the disease.[36] This work shows considerable potential for *dual-use* capability, that is, serving as either vaccine or a weapon. This is more or less the case for all of Traub's vaccine research but in this paper in particular, it demonstrates he was creating more stealth qualities in vaccinated animals who were still killed by the virus after vaccination but the inflammatory signs within the central nervous system were completely absent.

Pseudorabies (Swine Herpesvirus – Aujeszky's Disease)

In 1941, Traub was conducting experiments with pseudorabies virus, and noted its ability to infect while remaining clear from the blood, therefore being infected but a blood test would be negative.[37] This was an important quality for his stealth weapons in later years. It is interesting to note, Traub reveals in this paper that Richard E. Shope had sent him the virus while he was in Germany.

Swine Fever (Hog Cholera)

While Traub was conducting research on pseudorabies and swine polio, he also spent some time conducting experiments with the virus of hog cholera, which is known as classical swine fever, as opposed to African Swine Fever, which would be researched at Plum Island in later years.[38]

Borna Disease Virus

In Traub's experiments with swine polio, he mentions that he was conducting experiments with Borna Disease Virus,[39] the highly neurotropic virus that he began his career studying under Professor Wilhelm Zwick. This virus would later be used as the animal model to study various kinds of psychiatric abnormalities and was also demonstrated in cases of human psychiatric disorders.[40] It has broad spectrum pathogenicity, meaning it can infect a broad range of animals, and even human infections have been known to occur.

Equine Infectious Anemia (EIA): The HIV of Horses

In this same period of time, during the years 1941-1942, Traub worked with Beller to study the immunology and transmission of Equine Infectious Anemia (EIA). EIA is a retrovirus and *lentivirus*, the same family as HIV and it is considered the HIV of horses.[41] The Immunity experiments were not published publicly until 1951, indicating they may have been classified until that time.[42] In their experiments on EIA, they attempted to treat the horses with Salvarsan and Neosalvarsan, which had been the antibiotic of choice, against spirochetes, but occasionally used for other diseases.[43]

Earlier in those studies, Traub and Werner Schäfer conducted studies on antibodies for the disease.[44] The virus was highly suppressive to the immune system, and the publication stated that neither immunity tests nor antibody tests were successful. The only antibodies found were not against the virus, but some other substance, and most of the antigen they isolated from the spleen of infected horses, did not react or have antibodies even though they were infected.[45]

These immunity tests on EIA spoke about the immune tolerant state that often occurs in blood parasites, which include the common Lyme disease co-infection babesiosis:

> In human and animal protozoal diseases, after the survival of the [initial period of disease, the disease remains] existing [in a balanced] state between parasite and [host], in which the [host] is usually resistant to a new infection [due to it already being chronically infected, but] [d]ue to damaging influences on the body, this state of equilibrium can change in favor of the parasite.[46]

Transmission experiments with equine infectious anemia spoke about insects to spread the disease, such as horse-flies, beetles, and mosquitoes, which had been studied since the start of World War I, but their experiments were conducted by infecting the horse by contact with infected urine.[47] We will hear more about this virus later in the book.

LISTERIA MONOCYTOGENES (LISTERIOSIS)

In 1942 Traub was confronted with yet another mystery disease, after the *Luftwaffe* repeatedly delivered diseased and dead Angora rabbits from a rabbit farm. The rabbits had economic value, but also medical and experimental research value. They were particularly concerned because the rabbits were used to make vaccines, which could pass disease to both humans and veterinary animals. Vaccine material, again, becomes a target for bioterrorism in wartime activities.[48]

These studies were confusing like the infectious catarrh was in horses, and the conclusion was difficult to arrive at, but strains of *Listeria* germs could be isolated from the brainstem. He also found co-infecting fungus called *Encephalitizoon caniculi*.

The results of this study were inconclusive, but he found similarities to his work with infectious catarrh, with rickettsia and tick-borne diseases while under Beller at Giessen, and not to mention, his work on LCM virus. The only common denominator for these diseases of rabbits was his isolation of *Listeria* germs in most cases.[49]

Outbreak of Avian Influenza and Newcastle Disease Virus (NDV)

The year 1942 saw multiple outbreaks that occurred on chicken farms in Germany at the time, and Traub began research to study the virus and identify factors around it.[50] In a follow-up publication, he was assessing whether these were variants of avian influenza, or a separate virus. He concluded it to be a variant of avian influenza, known as Newcastle Disease Virus (NDV).[51]

This would set the course for the following years, when he gained considerable experience working with the disease in chickens, which can also infect humans.[52] One of Traub's observations, in assessing the origin of the epidemic, spoke to the fact that the disease was only known to occur in Britain, and according to some of his colleagues, this virus was recognized as a war-time disease, and although no saboteurs had been caught, the possibility was there, along with the use of migratory birds to spread the disease:

> Such has not been found on our continent until now, [but] only in England (Newcastle Disease). It is therefore a case in which one could suspect [a naturally occurring] development of the virus in the chicken [from this country], if one would not have to reckon with completely uncontrollable and difficult factors of detection, (i.e. with an introduction of the virus by migratory birds or even with hostile action).[53]

Endnotes

1   Munk K.: Virologie in Deutschland. Die Entwicklung eines Fachgebietes. Basel, Karger, 1995, pp 4-49 (DOI:10.1159/000423810) [Translated by A. Finnegan 2019]

2   Traub, E. Uber Immunität und aktive Immunisierung gegen Viruskrankheiten [About Immunity and Active Immunization Against Viral Diseases.] Zeit. Infek. Krank. Hyg. Haus. Vol. 45 (1). 169-213. (1939). [Translated by A. Finnegan 2019]

3   Ibid. pp. 192-193

4   Traub, E. Experimentelle Untersuchungen über einen durch Taubenpassage veränderten Virusstamm der amerikanischen Pferdeenzephalomyelitis. [Experimental Investigations on a strain of american equine encephalomyelitis modified by pigeon passages]. Zbl. Baki, 143: 7-22. (1938) [Translated by A. Finnegan 2019]

5   Maier, E. (2017, January). Flashback... Virus Research: A Foul Enemy in Fowl. Max Planck Research, 78-79.

6   Traub, E. & W. Schäfer. Serologische Untersuchungen über die Immunität der Mäuse gegen lymphozytische Choriomeningitis. [Serologic investigations on the immunity of mice against lymphocytic choriomeningitis.] Zntrl. Bakt. I. Orig. 144 (6): 331-345. (1939). [Translated by A. Finnegan 2019]

7   Walker, R., Greene, R., Nicholson, W., & Levine, J. (1989). Shared flagellar epitopes of Borrelia burgdorferi and Borrelia anserina. Veterinary Microbiology, 19(4), 361-371. doi:10.1016/0378-1135(89)90101-6

8   Schäfer, W. (1939). Fortführung von Spirochaeta gallinarum-Stämmen von Eipassagen. [The Maintenance of Spirochaeta gallinarum by Passage in Fowl Embryos.] Vet. Bull., 11, 220. [translated by A. Finnegan 2019]

9   Gildemeister, Eugen, et al. Handbuch Der Viruskrankheiten Mit Besonderer berücksichtigung Ihrer Experimentellen Erforschung. G. Fischer, 1939. [Translated by A. Finnegan 2019]

10   Traub, E. Choriomeningitis der Maus. Handbuch Der Viruskrankheiten Mit Besonderer berücksichtigung Ihrer Experimentellen Erforschung. G. Fischer, 1939., Bd. 2, pp. 355-364 [Translated by A. Finnegan 2019]

11   Traub, E. & K. Beller. Geflügelpest und ahnliche Viruskrankheiten der Vögel. [Fowl Pest and Related Viral Diseases of Birds]. Handbuch der Viruskrankheiten, herausgegeben von Gildemeister, Haagen u. Waldmann. Bd. 1, Ch. 7. 590–606. Jena: Gustav Fischer (1939)., pp. 597 [Translated by A. Finnegan 2019]

12   Ibid.

13   Schäfer, W. Das Vorkommen des B. pseudotuberculosis rod. oder eines ihm ähnlichen Erregers bei Hühnerküken. [The occurrence of B. pseudotuberculosis rod. or a related pathogen in young chickens]. Tierärztl. Rdsch. No. 4, 72-73. (1939)

14   Springer YP, Johnson PTJ. Large-scale health disparities associated with Lyme disease and human monocytic ehrlichiosis in the United States, 2007-2013. PLoS One. 2018 Sep 27;13(9):e0204609. doi: 10.1371/journal.pone.0204609. PMID: 30261027; PMCID: PMC6160131.

15   Beller, K. Herzwasser und sonstige tierische Rickettsiosen. Handbuch Der Viruskrankheiten Mit Besonderer berücksichtigung Ihrer Experimentellen Erforschung. G. Fischer, 1939., Bd. 2, pp. 606-623

16   Traub, E. Ansteckender Katarrh der Luftwege im Pferdebestande einer Veterinärkompanie. [Infectious Respiratory Catarrh in the Horses of a Veterinary Company] Dtsch. tierarztl. Wschr, 49: 439-444. (1941). [Translated to English by A. Finnegan, 2019]

17   Traub, E. Experimentelle Untersuchungen über einen durch Taubenpassage

veränderten Virusstamm der amerikanischen Pferdeenzephalomyelitis. [Experimental Investigations on a strain of american equine encephalomyelitis modified by pigeon passages]. Zbl. Baki, 143: 7-22. (1938) [Translated to English by A. Finnegan, 2019]

18   Traub, E. Die ansteckende Schweinelähme im Vergleich mit der Pseudowut und Schweinepest. [Contagious Porcine Encephalomyelitis Compared with Aujeszky's Disease and Swine Fever.]. Tierärz. Rund. No. 10. 122-123. (1941). [Translated to English by A. Finnegan, 2019]

19   Traub, E. Aktive Immunisierung gegen die ansteckende Schweinelähme mit Adsorbatimpstoffen. [Active Immunization against Porcine Encephalomyelitis by Adsorbate Vaccines]. Arch, wiss. prakt. Tierheuk. 77. 52-66. (1941). [Translated to English by A. Finnegan, 2019]

20   Traub, Erich. [Letter to the Deutschen Forschungsgemeinschaft, February 24, 1940]

21   Traub, E., et al. Untersuchungen über die Stomatitis papulosa des Rinde. [Studies on bovine papular stomatitis] Zeit. Infek. Krank. Hyg. Haus. 56 (2): 85-103. (1940). [Translated to English by A. Finnegan, 2019]

22   Traub, E., et al. Untersuchungen über die Stomatitis papulosa des Rinde. [Studies on bovine papular stomatitis] Zeit. Infek. Krank. Hyg. Haus. 56 (2): 85-103. (1940). [Translated to English by A. Finnegan, 2019]

23   Ibid.

24   National Archives. RG 65 Erich Traub, (Declassified FBI Investigations on the Loyalties of Erich Traub). Federal Bureau of Investigation (FBI): NARA., Doc. # QO1-458431291

25   Joint Intelligence Objectives Agency (JIOA), JIOA Administrative Records. (1949-54). Joint-Intelligence Objectives Agency file on Erich Traub (RG 330). NARS.

26   Traub, E. Ueber den Einfluß der latenten Choriomeningitis-Infektion auf die Entstehung der Lymphomatose bei weißen Mause [On the Influence of Latent Choriomeningitis Infection on the Development of Lymphomatosis in White Mice]. Zentrl. Bakt. I. Orig. 147 (16). 1-25. (1941). [Translated to English by A. Finnegan, 2019]

27   Ibid.

28   Traub, E. Ueber den Einfluß der latenten Choriomeningitis-Infektion auf die Entstehung der Lymphomatose bei weißen Mause [On the Influence of Latent Choriomeningitis Infection on the Development of Lymphomatosis in White Mice]. Zentrl. Bakt. I. Orig. 147 (16). 1-25. (1941). [Translated to English by A. Finnegan, 2019]

29   Traub, E. Ansteckender Katarrh der Luftwege im Pferdebestande einer Veterinärkompanie. [Infectious Respiratory Catarrh in the Horses of a Veterinary Company] Dtsch. tierarztl. Wschr, 49: 439-444. (1941). [Translated to English by A. Finnegan, 2019]

30   Ibid.

31   ibid.

32   Beller, K. Wiedererlanguag der Virulenz von BCG-Kulturen durch Meerschweinchenpassagen, zugleich ein Beitrag zur Syntropie zwischen Tuberkulose und Maul- und Klauenseuche. [Recovery of the virulence of BCG cultures through guinea pig passages, at the same time a contribution to the syntropia between tuberculosis and foot and mouth disease]. Zeitschr. f. Infekt. d. Haustiere. 59: 25-31. (1942)

33   Morens, David M., et al. "Predominant Role of Bacterial Pneumonia as a Cause of Death in Pandemic Influenza: Implications for Pandemic Influenza Preparedness." The Journal of Infectious Diseases, vol. 198, no. 7, 2008, pp. 962–970., doi:10.1086/591708.

34   Traub, E. & K. Beller. Stand und Aussichten der Erforschung des ansteckenden Katarrhs der Luftwege beim Pferd. [The Position and Outlook in Research on Infectious Re-

spiratory Catarrh of the Horse]. Z. Veterinark, 53: 88-97. (1941). [Translated to English by A. Finnegan, 2019]

35   Traub, E. & E. Gratzl. Zum Vorkommen von hämolytischen Streptokokken bei den kattarhalisch-entz ündlichen Erkrankungen der Luftwege des Pferdes. [Occurrence of Hemolytic Streptococci in Catarrhal Respiratory Diseases of Horses]. Archiv fur wiss. und prakt. Tier. 77. 347-377. (1942) [Translated to English by A. Finnegan, 2019]

36   Traub, E. Aktive Immunisierung gegen die ansteckende Schweinelähme mit Adsorbatimpstoffen. [Active Immunization against Porcine Encephalomyelitis by Adsorbate Vaccines]. Arch, wiss. prakt. Tierheuk. 77. 52-66. (1941). [Translated to English by A. Finnegan, 2019]

37   Traub, E. Die ansteckende Schweinelähme im Vergleich mit der Pseudowut und Schweinepest. [Contagious Porcine Encephalomyelitis Compared with Aujeszky's Disease and Swine Fever.]. Tierärz. Rund. No. 10. 122-123. (1941). [Translated to English by A. Finnegan, 2019]

38   Traub, E. Die ansteckende Schweinelähme im Vergleich mit der Pseudowut und Schweinepest. [Contagious Porcine Encephalomyelitis Compared with Aujeszky's Disease and Swine Fever.]. Tierärz. Rund. No. 10. 122-123. (1941). [Translated to English by A. Finnegan, 2019]

39   Traub, E. Aktive Immunisierung gegen die ansteckende Schweinelähme mit Adsorbatimpstoffen. [Active Immunization against Porcine Encephalomyelitis by Adsorbate Vaccines]. Arch, wiss. prakt. Tierheuk. 77. 52-66. (1941). [Translated to English by A. Finnegan, 2019]

40   Bode, L, R Ferszt, and G Czech. 1993. "Borna Disease Virus Infection and Affective Disorders in Man." Archives of Virology. Supplementum. U.S. National Library of Medicine. 1993. https://www.ncbi.nlm.nih.gov/pubmed/8219801

41   Stephens, R., Casey, J., & Rice, N. (1986). Equine infectious anemia virus gag and pol genes: relatedness to visna and AIDS virus. Science, 231(4738), 589–594. doi:10.1126/science.3003905

42   Traub, E. & K. Beller. Untersuchungen uber die ansteckende Blutarmut der Pferde. Immunitatsversuche. [Immunization experiments in equine infectious anaemia]. Monatshefte fur Praktische Tierheilkunde; 3:193-206. (1942, 1951). [Translated to English by A. Finnegan (2019)]

43   Traub, E. & K. Beller. Untersuchungen uber die ansteckende Blutarmut der Pferde. Immunitatsversuche. [Immunization experiments in equine infectious anaemia]. Monatshefte fur Praktische Tierheilkunde; 3:193-206. (1942, 1951). [Translated to English by A. Finnegan (2019)]

44   Traub, E., et al. Komplementbindungversuche bei der ansteckenden Blutarmut der Pferde. [Complement-binding experiments on Infectious anemia of the horse]. Berl. Munch. Tierarztl Wochenschr. 134-135. (1941). [Translated to English by A. Finnegan, 2019]

45   Traub, E. & K. Beller. Untersuchungen uber die ansteckende Blutarmut der Pferde. Immunitatsversuche. [Immunization experiments in equine infectious anaemia]. Monatshefte fur Praktische Tierheilkunde; 3:193-206. (1942, 1951). [Translated to English by A. Finnegan (2019)]

46   Traub, E. & K. Beller. Untersuchungen uber die ansteckende Blutarmut der Pferde. Immunitatsversuche. [Immunization experiments in equine infectious anaemia]. Monatshefte fur Praktische Tierheilkunde; 3:193-206. (1942, 1951). [Translated to English by A. Finnegan (2019)]

47   Traub, E. & K. Beller. Untersuchungen uber die ansteckende Blutarmut der Pferde. II. Ubertragungsversuche. [Research on equine infectious anemia. II. Transmission experiments.] Archiv fur wiss. und prakt. Tier. 77:411-422. (1942)

48   Traub, E. Ueber eine mit Listerella- ähnlichen Bakterien vergesellschaftete Menin-go-Encephalomyelitis der Kaninchen. [About a Meningo-Encephalomyelitis of Rabbits Asso-ciated with Listerella-like Bacteria]. Zntrl. Bakt. I. Orig. 149 (1). 38-49. (1942). [Translated to English by A. Finnegan, 2019]

49   Ibid.

50   Traub, E., Eine atypische Form der Geflügelpest in Hessen-Nassau. [The Atypical Form of Fowl Pest in Hessen-Nassau] Tierarztl Rundschau : 42-45. (1942a)

51   Traub, E., Immunbiologischer Vergleich von Geflügelpest-Virusstämmen aus Schlesien und Nassau. [Immunobiological comparison of avian influenza virus strains from Silesia and Nassau.] Tierärztlichen Rundschau 48, 1-3. (1942b).

52   Traub, E. Weitere Mitteilungen uber die aktive Immunisierung mit Adsorbatimp-stoffen gegen die atypische Geflügelpest. [Further news about active immunization with ad-sorbate vaccines against atypical avian influenza]. Z. Infekt. krankh. Haustiere 60, 367-379. (1944).

53   Traub, E., Eine atypische Form der Geflügelpest in Hessen-Nassau. [The Atypical Form of Fowl Pest in Hessen-Nassau] Tierarztl Rundschau : 42-45. (1942a) [Translated to En-glish by A. Finnegan, 2019]

Chapter Seven

BUILDING THE BIOWEAPONS PT. II

ERICH TRAUB AND THE INSEL RIEMS INSTITUTE OF ULTRA-SECRET BIOWEAPONS

I looked, and behold, an ashen horse; and he who sat on it had the name Death; and Hades was following with him. Authority was given to them over a fourth of the earth, to kill with sword and with famine and with pestilence and by the wild beasts of the earth

– Jeremiah 27:8

In the later part of 1942, Traub was recruited to direct the research at Insel Riems on matters of biological warfare,[1] leading a position in charge of the department of microbiology, later becoming head of the research laboratories and vice-president of the Institute under Dr. Otto Waldmann.[2] Beller coordinated to some degree with Insel Riems from the University of Giessen, and Traub was the most valuable player for Insel Riems to acquire.

Traub began his time at Riems with further research into the Newcastle Disease Virus, and Behringwerke AG, the IG Farben subsidiary, asked for Traub to study inoculations and vaccines against avian influenza.[3] Waldmann gave permission for Behringwerke AG to produce the vaccine against avian influenza, but said it would not be possible to produce the vaccine at Insel Riems in the long-term.[4]

It was at Insel Riems that Traub became an expert in Foot-and-Mouth Disease Virus (FMD).[5] Traub would also study Newcastle Disease, swine erysipelas, brucellosis,[6] and conducted experiments on a human influenza adsorbate vaccine and weaponized agents for use in war.[7]

ERICH TRAUB TRANSFORMS THE RIEMS INSTITUTE

Traub's first order of business on Insel Riems was to work on the antigens of Foot-and-Mouth Disease Virus. He worked on this project with Insel Riems biochemist, Gottfried Pyl.[8] They extracted the antigens with an ultracentrifuge[A] and separated them for other uses, such as weaponizing other disease agents.

Open-air tests with variants of FMD and weaponized agents modified by these FMD antigens were later initiated and hidden under defensive FMD research, giving any onlookers or foreign eyes an impression it was limited to preventing FMD. First, tests were made with the virus in droplets of water that could be dispersed as a mist but improved it by making the virus in a powdered, dry form, a process called *lyophilization*.[9]

Traub and his pathologist Heinz Röhrer ran them through different animals in serial passages to establish different *tropisms*,[10] at the same time, creating methodologies to distinguish the different strains that brought test results back rapidly cutting the time for results down from weeks to hours.[11] Serums were made in various production facilities, including a slaughterhouse and chicken farm.[12] Insel Riems was set up to produce massive amounts of serum and vaccines,[13, 14] but the true nature of Insel Riems was concentrated on the development of highly effective and esoteric biological weapons as Germany's aide-de-camp. [15]

The reader may recall from earlier chapters that in 1937, Insel Riems researcher Heinz-Christoph Nagel produced a neurotropic Foot-and-Mouth Disease virus by repeatedly passing the virus through mice, which were sent to him from the Rockefeller Institute by Traub.[16] The mouse colonies at that time were infected with LCM virus, and likely had a role in the FMD experiments. This may have been the method for weaponizing other viruses and germs, which gave it a marked neurotropism. It allowed the agent to take to new hosts via cell fusion, and a similar effect was noted much later by one of Traub's Iranian counterparts in 1974."[17]

Otto Waldmann, the leading veterinary scientist and member of the National Socialist Workers' Party (NSDAP), sat as president of Insel Riems. Waldmann was recognized as a leading authority on FMD, and created an original vaccine/serum for FMD, but it was not sufficient.[18] Waldmann was not as involved in the research as Traub was. Dr. Traub took second-in-command at Riems, but it was he who led and directed the entire phase of research on Insel Riems.[19]

One interesting fact about Otto Waldmann, was that Waldmann was scientifically expelled from the German University of Veterinary

---

A   **Ultracentrifuge**: A high-velocity centrifuge used in the separation of colloidal or submicroscopic particles. **Centrifuge**: A centrifugal machine; specifically, a form of centrifugal machine employed to separate the solid particles suspended in a fluid, such as the blood or urine.

Medicine in Berlin in 1919 for his participation in early communist activities known as the Spartacist Uprising.[20] Even still, he assisted in fighting a major FMD outbreak back in 1911-12 and based on that merit he was qualified and joined the faculty at the University of Greifswald and the Friedrich-Loeffler Institute, the parent institute of Riems.[21] Waldmann eventually gained control of Riems and by the Second World War his old past may have been forgotten.

One of the more notable scientists stationed at Riems included Heinz Röhrer, director of pathology, who, along with Traub, worked on neurotropic variants of FMD, as "mouse polio."[22, 23] Röhrer was a National Socialist since 1931, active in the party but kept to the scientific research, appointed to the University of Greifswald as a lecturer and specialist in equine and bovine diseases.[24] Röhrer's skill was useful in the adaptation, in a similar fashion as Traub, and critical to the execution of biological weapons activity on the island. Röhrer also worked at the ASID serum plant in Dessau, an important station for producing serums in coordination with Insel Riems work.[25] It was here that they were producing serum for the *Leptospira* spirochete which causes Weil's Disease (leptospirosis), and they were also producing a serum for multiple sclerosis, which is likely to have been for the *Borrelia* spirochetes in his weaponization of the Lyme disease spirochete.[26]

Director of the chemical department was chief chemist, Gottfried Pyl, formerly a biochemist at IG Farben,[27] Pyl worked out chemical analysis, production of synthesized amino acids, diagnostics, extraction, and synthesis of chemical additives such as aluminum hydroxide and formalin for adsorbate vaccines, with his assistant chemist K. O. Hobohm, he and Pyl would purify and synthesize preparations of chemicals, antigen, and pathogenic components from FMD and other agents.[28, 29]

Hubert Möhlmann, headed the production department and developed vaccine and serum material, which could serve as *dual use* – meaning offensive or defensive work.[30] Möhlmann was appointed to the scientific council as a professor in 1943.[31]

Werner Schäfer, Traub's protegé back at the University of Giessen, was a valuable researcher who spent time on Riems with Traub. He was born in 1912, started out life as a carpenter, yet decided at some point to enter into veterinary school and study animal disease. After entering the University under Beller and Traub, he went to Africa in 1939 to work on a number of animal diseases with biological warfare significance.[32]

Schäfer's bioagents were constructed together with Traub, and these were intended not just for animals, but also human use, indicating a clear dual-use purpose.[33, 34] Schäfer would move on to the Kaiser-Wilhelm Institute, later called the Max Planck Institute, as well as future collaboration with the United States on the Special Virus Cancer Program (SVCP) working on leukemia viruses and other animal viruses with significance in cancer research.[35, 36]

Another notable scientist on Insel Riems, Helmut Ruska, who's brother Ernst developed the electron microscope and set up a department at the facility specifically for its use.[37] Helmut's brother went on to achieve international fame for his invention, and Helmut Ruska spent numerous years in the United States after the War.[38]

Gerhard Schramm, known for his work on the Tobacco Mosaic Virus (TMV), also spent some time on Riems in collaboration with Traub and Schäfer working on human influenza,[39] and Newcastle Disease.[40] Schramm ran the ultracentrifuge and advised the scientists at Riems on plant pathogens with potential for biological warfare.[41]

In a literary work on the official history of Insel Riems, "Research on the Island of Riems from 1933 to 1945 Under Special Consideration of Nazi Forced labor," by Jans U. Lichte, of the Institute for the History of Medicine, described the history and activities on Insel Riems. After the Nazis came to power, Waldmann had the black and white Nazi Party (NSDAP) flag hoisted up on Riems to declare loyalty to Adolf Hitler and Nazi Germany, to continue the research, regardless of whether or not they agreed with his position. During the war, despite his alleged advocation against weaponizing numerous, highly contagious diseases like rinderpest, a highly contagious and destructive virus of cattle, and FMD, Riems began to specialize in biological warfare relating to animal disease, with equal implications for human targets.[42]

In 1942 and 1943, they initiated successful field experiments that took place in Eastern Europe, and they continued to pour resources into furthering their hidden arsenal.[43] What other agents those field experiments contained was largely kept secret within the Reich and in Russia. During this time, Traub began to assess the spread of FMD by the aerogenic route. He found however, that the virus did not spread well in animal stalls by the airborne route, and published work on this in later years.[44] This may have been the point at which ticks and other insects were considered and used. Field studies with rinderpest were also noted. According to this history, forced human labor was indeed used in some capacity on Insel Riems.[45]

Earlier in the war, leaflets thought to contain FMD or other agents were allegedly dropped from British and Allied planes. Numerous outbreaks of FMD occurred simultaneously, but no conclusive evidence could establish the link to the leaflets. It was claimed that the fear of mounting threats to Germany was used increasingly as justification for further research & development in biological warfare. There may be a fair level of truth in this assumption, as evidenced by Traub's reports on the avian influenza and Newcastle Disease spreading through Germany.[46]

While leading the Riems institute, Traub had a few young ladies under him, Miss Johanna Frank and Anne-Lise Bürger, working as assistant lab technicians.[47] His main technician, Anne-Lise Bürger, was born in Stuttgart, Germany in 1922, attending high school and moving on to a two-year medical school for technical assistants, passing her final exam with the "best grade," continuing to become assistant medical technician at the University of Giessen from 1941-1942, and went on to Insel Riems as a lab technician for Dr. Erich Traub.[48]

In 1943, numerous experiments were being conducted on human subjects across Germany involving typhus, malaria, spotted fever, epidemic hepatitis, and influenza. Nuremberg documents detail numerous experiments that were carried out by Traub's old Rockefeller colleague, Eugen Haagen, under contract for Behringwerke, at the Buchenwald and Dachau concentration camps.[49]

Some new faces at Riems in 1943 arrived as guest researchers from the Axis-allied Spain and even from Yugoslavia, scientists like Fausto Manso-Rodriguez and Zvonimir Dinter,[50] both of whom worked with Traub. Serum production was equally underway on various bacterium and rickettsia, as his assistant, Anne Bürger, had particular skills in cultivation of a range of highly infectious diseases, according to later reports.[51]

Several research projects conducted by Werner Schäfer under Traub's leadership around this time were carried out on further experiments with swine paralysis (Teschen disease) to study further effects on the virus content in the central nervous system.[52] Schäfer also conducted studies of the interference effect of FMD virus in experimental infections, where the virus may contain enzymes that destroy immune receptors making re-infection with other viruses difficult, and what it meant in relation to immunity.[53] Schäfer then looked into the virus content of blood and organs in guinea pigs infected with the FMD virus, noting its ability to take to the lining of the tissues that make up the central nervous system.[54]

In a much later edition of the *Berlin and Munich Veterinary Weekly*, an article written by Dr. Zvonimir Dinter, who frequently penned memories through expressive writing,[55] wrote an experience based on his memories of working together with Erich Traub on Riems, in "Personal Encounters with Erich Traub,"[B] and using fictional accounts to make analogies to the real experience, it gives a better idea of the mysterious personality of Dr. Traub, and the atmosphere or work conditions at Insel Riems:

On Riems 1943. It is autumn 1943 and 8 o'clock in the morning on Riems. When I came from the guest house to the microbiological department of the institute, TRAUB'S hardworking technical assistant, ANNE-LIESE BÜRGER, was already in full swing. Always in boots with a short skirt, she hurried down the corridor this time, past me. She called out to me that "the boss was already there." Her call was not necessary because the boss, TRAUB, always seemed to be "already there." He, too, was already in full swing; from the writing room to the laboratory and back, always at a quick pace. I see him in front of me as if it had been yesterday: the slim, medium-sized figure in the snow-white smock; the face with reddish mottled cheeks; one hand taking out of his smock pocket grains (wheat?) that he was gnawing at, and between the fingers of the other hand the "eternal" cigarette.

When TRAUB saw me approaching, he turned to me with his characteristic sidelong glance and a slightly ironic smile: "The Americans are much more intense; that's why they create things." I got the hint. It was an indirect criticism of my always late arrival (although the waiter in the Riems Casino served breakfast early). A little later we were all in the large laboratory. By "all" I mean TRAUB, two [technical assistants], as well as my Spanish colleague MANSO and me (both of us as visiting researchers). From time to time our colleague MÖHLMANN would join us. Everyone had their own workstation and racks with rows of tubes. We pipetted like a competition. It went on like this day in, day out. It was the final test phase of TRAUB's method to determine variants ("subtypes") of the foot and mouth disease virus - especially the virus in tongue vesicles - by means of complement fixation, a method that has been used worldwide since then.

Personally, I didn't like the "eternal" pipetting at all. I stayed with it for about an hour, but then "slipped away" under the pretext that I had to "go to my mice" and atypical avian influenza to work out differences, and I examined, among other things, the different behavior of these viruses after intracranial inoculation on mice. So I went to the stable. There I put the glass containers with the mice and a loaded vaccination syringe in front of me and looked out, took one look across the window into the laboratory, where the intensive pipetting was going on. If TRAUB had come by, I would have started vaccinating the mice.

... No wonder that later, at an internal graduation ceremony for work on variants of the FMD-Virus, TRAUB said in his short address: "I would also like to mention our guest researchers, of whom Mr. MANSO is diligent, Mr. DINTER on the other hand..." Traub's sincerity was disarming; because he ended the sentence with "was lazy." I didn't blame him; he was right.

New Year 1944. Despite wartime, everything was available on Riems that was necessary for a living - except cigarettes and schnapps. That is why colleague MANSO went to Berlin in the old year to buy cigarettes. Before that, he asked me to show the boss his titrations of the foot-and-mouth disease virus on guinea pigs for the New Year. On the morning of the New Year 1944, we, TRAUB and I, met in the stable room. TRAUB took no account of the fact that it was New Year's Day: "Holidays were conceived for lazybones" - he instructed me. The presentation went on in silence - up to the virus dilution of 10^{-6}. At this dilution, TRAUB suddenly roared. His cheeks became redder than usual. After all animals of the 10^{-5} dilution were negative, the one animal of the 10^{-5} dilution was "illogically" positive. A "sloppiness" must have occurred while pipetting. He took the animal out of my hand to take a closer look. But no sooner had I heard TRAUB's rising anger than the positive animal flew away from him through the air to me. How good it was that I was once a goalkeeper: I caught it in time. But TRAUB went out of the stable cursing (I only heard so much of his cursing that it referred to "Spaniards" as a nation). Later, when I was sitting in my writing room, there was a knock on the door. It was TRAUB. He kindly invited me to coffee and cake in the afternoon. The guinea pig incident seemed already completely forgotten.

Traub, "who started the whole thing." The TRAUB'S lived in a villa on Riems. When I entered the villa it was already twilight. You could hear the monotonous splashing of the Baltic Sea. It was a mood in which memories are easily awakened.

After the coffee and cake, TRAUB told me, when I asked, how he came to the USA.

RICHARD E. SHOPE, the famous virologist from the Rockefeller Institute, spent his time in the early 1930s, among other things, at Giessen. Zwick's work on Borna disease attracted the researchers to Giessen... TRAUB, who had already mastered English as a student, was assigned to SHOPE as a language translator. SHOPE soon saw TRAUB'S interest and talent for virus research and invited him to the Rockefeller Institute. Shope was right in his assumption. Much later (1959) he told me himself. [56]

By 1944, Traub published several more papers on avian influenza, Newcastle Disease, and Foot-and-Mouth Disease. He published a follow-up to his earlier work on atypical avian influenza, or Newcastle disease.[57] He also published further papers with guest researcher Fausto Manso-Rodriguez, published research about the antibody responses to different variants of FMD,[58] as well as working with Dinter on FMD which did not get published until 1946.[59] Traub was teaching these guest researchers his earlier work about the different antigens of FMD. This work had clear implications for offensive research for the weaponization of FMD. He would teach them how to use the antigens to weaponize other pathogens and adapt them to infect new animals for the spread against a target country.

Also that year, Insel Riems gained a valuable addition to their facility, through their electron microscope department under Helmut Ruska, a scientist with Siemens & Halske AG.[60] During his time at Riems, Ruska had been publishing work on mycoplasma and bacteriophages, in which they had been assessing the ability of *potentiation* of virus, or causing it to revert back to active form, by lyophilization and irradiation.[61, 62] The mycoplasma was first being studied from mice, which Traub had encountered at the Rockefeller Institute with John B. Nelson.[63]

This year also saw Erich Traub, Werner Schäfer, Gerhard Schramm, and Hugo Miehler, in concentrated studies on avian influenza,[64] also under contract with Behringwerke AG, with additional construction of human influenza vaccines.[65] This work continued throughout the war and would be worked on further following the war's end. These studies also show clear implications for weapons work, with Traub concentrating and purifying antigens and virus.[66, 67]

Declassified records from the CIA indicate that human tests may have occurred at Riems, to assess the pathogenicity of avian influenza to human targets.[68, 69] Since Riems was an isolated facility offshore from Germany, it would have been used for experiments with such highly contagious agents like influenza, avian influenza, and Newcastle Disease Virus, diseases considered too risky for trials on the mainland. Considering that Traub and Schäfer had been constructing an influenza vaccine for human use, contracted through Behringwerke AG the same year as Haagen's tests on influenza at Buchenwald, is probably not a coincidence.[70]

Additionally, many animal pathogens with potential for human pathogenicity were studied under the guise of veterinary problems, cleverly disguised from prying enemy eyes. The facility was well equipped to produce large amounts of biological weapons material, while serum and vaccine production was underway, and worked with several other large corporations such as ASID and Behringwerke AG. At that time, Traub had been working with several corporations and universities, establishing a name for himself within the German science community and among the pharmaceutical conglomerates.[71]

In Dr. Kurt Blöme's talks with Heinrich Himmler, commander of the SS-Waffen (Schutzstaffel) regarding biological warfare, it was decided to secure strains of rinderpest, but securing it was not so easy. The obstacle was due to established laws across Europe forbidding them from storing the virus due to its highly contagious nature that could wipe out Europe's livestock, which gave them great difficulty in finding strains, and eventually, Himmler decided to send Traub on a trip to Turkey to secure cultures of rinderpest and he made the long journey there and back.[72]

Nearing the end of the war, Himmler, had been pushing for more aggressive biological warfare development with his medical and agricultural authorities, Kurt Blöme, Walter Schrieber, and Otto Waldman. Dr. Blöme set up in Poland at the SS Military Medical Academy at Posen to run experiments on plague and similar agents under the guise of medical cancer research, while Dr. Schrieber headed vaccine departments,[73] and Dr. Waldmann ran the agricultural and animal disease division for the Department of the Interior on the Isle of Riems.[74]

Although Schrieber and Waldmann may have produced vaccines and protective measures for Germans and their livestock at some capacity, these served equally as covers for more compartmentalized biological weapons programs. There was discussion between Himmler and Blöme suggesting the use of insects to spread diseases to enemy forces, and Blöme also proposed the use of insects for effective delivery of crop-destroying potato beetles along with the weaponized animal and human diseases such as typhus-infected lice to be tested on prisoners at Buchenwald and Dachau.[75]

Experimental vaccines for typhus, malaria, epidemic hepatitis, spotted fever, dysentery, and influenza were tested on camp inmates during the War, resulting in the deaths of hundreds upon thousands.[76,77] Entomological warfare studies using malaria-infected mosquitoes were carried out at Buchenwald concentration camp under contract with Behringwerke AG, and carried out by scientists like Klaus Schilling, Gerhard Rose, Eugen Haagen, among others.[78] The Reich also had a sepsis program (phlegmon),[79] to which LCM and swine erysipelas would have been a candidate for, since both are established human pathogens and cause septicemic reactions.[80]

Dr. Werner Schäfer also worked on rinderpest with Traub at Riems. It was claimed that the rinderpest may have been non-infectious when they finally got it back to Riems. However, other sources claim they succeeded in growing and fully weaponizing it. In later Counter Intelligence Corps (CIC) interviews with Dr. Blöme after the war, he told them that indeed, it had been a success.[81]

An academic publication out of Germany, based on the activities of the University of Greifswald under National Socialism, presented some long-lost testimony of the biological weapons activity at the Insel Riems Institute. In 1945, while Traub and the rest of Insel Riems staff were busy working on special problems of biological warfare significance, they began to shape their neurotropic-modified FMD for tests over Lake Peipus near Byelorussia, by putting reindeer on a raft in the middle of the lake and spraying the animals with the weaponized pathogens, causing an 80% infection rate.[82]

By August of 1945, according to Traub, *"The Riems Institute was able to produce up to 200,000 liters of vaccine a year. The serum production amounted to 200,000-300,000 liters per year."*[83] Around this time, however, Germany was losing the war, and according to reports, Riems would fall under the occupied zone of Russia.[84]

As the Soviet Union began to occupy East Germany, FBI files indicated that Traub was in an alleged conflict with Waldmann, because he wanted to move all the laboratory equipment and research out of Riems and over to West Germany, where it could be under control of Western countries, while Waldmann, apparently nervous that if they attempted to flee, thought there would be serious repercussions if they weren't successful, and decided to stay put.[85] "A less redacted intelligence report on the situation released to this author shows that Traub and three others had three ships arranged to pick them up and move the equipment but Waldmann threatened to shoot anyone attempting to leave the island."[86] Waldmann would later escape and left them behind to head for Argentina with Swiss assistance, late in 1945 towards the end of the war.[87]

Insel Riems was soon captured by the Russian Army, who descended upon Riems at night, and the staff showed up to work only to find their labs locked and chained off, and Russian soldiers quickly taking them as political prisoners.[88] The Russians disassembled the entire research laboratory and hauled all of Traub's most important work to Russia and there upon one of the laboratory walls someone had made the statement clear, "Research is finished."[89]

Endnotes

1   Eberle, Henrik. "Ein Wertvolles Instrument": Die Universität Greifswald Im Nationalsozialismus. Bohlau Verlag, 2015. [pp. 538-541]

2   Lichte, J. U. (1983). Die Forschung auf der Insel Riems von 1933 bis 1945 unter besonderer Berücksichtigung der NS-Zwangsarbeiter (Inaugural Dissertation). Nordenham, Germany: The Medical Faculty of the Ernst-Moritz-Arndt University of Greifswald.

3   Behringwerke AG, [Letter from Albert Demnitz to the Reich Minister in Berlin on the possibility for production of vaccine by Traub against the pathogen of fowl plague]. June 18, 1943.

4   Waldmann, O. [Letter to Reichs minister in Berlin regarding Traub's vaccine against fowl plague by Behringwerke]. August 02, 1943

5   Wittmann, W. (1999). *100 Years of Virology. The Legacy of Friedrich Loeffler - the Institute on the Isle of Riems*, 28. doi:10.1007/978-3-7091-6425-9

6   National Archives. Joint-Intelligence Objectives Agency file on Erich Traub (RG 330). NARS. Joint Intelligence Objectives Agency (JIOA), JIOA Administrative Records. (1949-54).

7   Behringwerke AG. (1943, June 18). Behringwerke [Letter to The Reich Ministery of the Interior]. Insel Riems Institute, Isle of Riems, Germany.

8   Traub, E. & G. Pyl. Untersuchungen über das komplementbindende Antigen bei Maul-und Klauenseuche. [Studies on the complement-binding antigen in foot-and-mouth disease] Z. Immun. Forsch.104, 158-165. (1943).

9   Eberle, Henrik. "Ein Wertvolles Instrument": Die Universität Greifswald Im Nationalsozialismus. Bohlau Verlag, 2015. [pp. 538-541]

10   Röhrer, Heinz. "Die Histopathologie Des Zentralnervensystems Bei Der Spinalen Mäuselähmung (Poliomyelitis Murium)." Virchows Archiv Für Pathologische Anatomie Und Physiologie Und Für Klinische Medizin, vol. 312, no. 1-3, 1944, pp. 740–755., doi:10.1007/bf02655974.

11   Traub, E. & F. M. Rodriguez. Uber die Herstellung komplementbindender Meerschweinchensera fur die Typendiagnose bei Maul- und Klauenseuche. [On the Complement-Fixation test of Guinea-pig sera for the typing of Foot-and-Mouth Disease.] Zbl. Bakt. I. Orig. 151, 380-388. (1944).

12   Central Intelligence Agency (CIA) Intelligence Reports: 1. PRODUCTION OF FOOT-AND-MOUTH DISEASE VACCINE AT THE FRIEDRICH LOEFFLER INSTITUTE RIEMS ISLAND 2. SECOND VIRUS PRODUCING STATION. CIA-RDP80-00810A007800710008-3. Central Intelligence Agency (CIA), Reading Room, 2011. Retrieved from: https://www.cia.gov/library/readingroom/document/CIA-RDP80-00810A007800710008-3

13   Central Intelligence Agency (CIA) Intelligence Reports: Installations of the Serum-Werk VEB Dessau (Formerly ASID), East Germany 1953 (CIA Information Report). Central Intelligence Agency (CIA), Reading Room, 2011. Retrieved from: https://www.cia.gov/library/readingroom/document/cia-rdp82-00457r016300350010-6.

14   Central Intelligence Agency (CIA) Intelligence Reports: The State Research Institute at Riems; Microbiological Research. CIA-RDP83-00415R000900020012-6. Central Intelligence Agency (CIA), Reading Room, 2011. Retrieved from: https://www.cia.gov/library/readingroom/document/CIA-RDP83-00415R000900020012-6

15   Eberle, Henrik. "Ein Wertvolles Instrument": Die Universität Greifswald Im Nationalsozialismus. Bohlau Verlag, 2015. [pp. 538-541]

16   Nagel, H C. Untersuchungen uber das Verhalten des Maul und Klauenseuche-Virus im Zentralnervensystem kleiner Versuchstiere. Dtsche. Tier. Woch. 45: 624-625. (1937)

17   Irvin, A., Brown, C., Kanhai, G. K., Stagg, D., & Rowe, L. W. (1974). Cell fusion, using sendai virus, to effect inter-species transfer of a cell-associated parasite (Theileria parva). International Journal for Parasitology, 4(5), 519-521. doi:10.1016/0020-7519(74)90070-8

18   Waldmann, O., Dr. (1938). Report on Preparation of the Vaccine of Riems for Foot-and-Mouth Disease. In Report on Preparation of the Vaccine of Riems for Foot-and- Mouth Disease, presented at the Thirteenth International Veterinary Congress at Zurich-Interlaken, Switzerland, 21-27 August 1938 (Vol. XVII, No. 2, pp. 282-283). Zurich-Interlaken, Switzerland: Office International des Epizooties, Bulletin I.

19   Central Intelligence Agency (CIA) Intelligence Reports: The State Research Institute at Riems; Microbiological Research. CIA-RDP83-00415R000900020012-6. Central Intelligence Agency (CIA), Reading Room, 2011. Retrieved from: https://www.cia.gov/library/readingroom/document/CIA-RDP83-00415R000900020012-6

20   Eberle, Henrik. "Ein Wertvolles Instrument": Die Universität Greifswald Im Nationalsozialismus. Bohlau Verlag, 2015. [pp. 538-541]

21   Ibid.

22   Röhrer, Heinz. "Die Histopathologie Des Zentralnervensystems Bei Der Spinalen Mäuselähmung (Poliomyelitis Murium)." Virchows Archiv Für Pathologische Anatomie Und Physiologie Und Für Klinische Medizin, vol. 312, no. 1-3, 1944, pp. 740–755., doi:10.1007/bf02655974.

23   Central Intelligence Agency (CIA) Intelligence Reports: The State Research Institute at Riems; Microbiological Research. CIA-RDP83-00415R000900020012-6. Central Intelligence Agency (CIA), Reading Room, 2011. Retrieved from: https://www.cia.gov/library/readingroom/document/CIA-RDP83-00415R000900020012-6

24   Eberle, Henrik. "Ein Wertvolles Instrument": Die Universität Greifswald Im Nationalsozialismus. Bohlau Verlag, 2015. [pp. 538-541]

25   Röhrer, H. 50 Jahre Forschung auf dem Riems. [50 years of research on the Riems]. Arch. Exp. Vet. Med. 14: 713-763. (1960).

26   Central Intelligence Agency (CIA) Intelligence Reports: BACTERIOLOGICAL ESTABLISHMENTS IN THE SOVIET ZONE OF GERMANY. CIA-RDP83-00415R002400170002-4. Central Intelligence Agency (CIA), Reading Room, 2006. Retrieved from: https://www.cia.gov/library/readingroom/document/CIA-RDP83-00415R002400170002-4

27   Central Intelligence Agency (CIA) Intelligence Reports: THE BACTERIOLOGICAL RESEARCH INSTITUTE ON THE ISLAND OF RIEMS. CIA-RDP83-00415R002200020014-9. Central Intelligence Agency (CIA), Reading Room, 2011. Retrieved from: https://www.cia.gov/library/readingroom/document/CIA-RDP83-00415R002200020014-9.

28   Traub, E. & G. Pyl. Untersuchungen über das komplementbindende Antigen bei Maul-und Klauenseuche. [Studies on the complement-binding antigen in foot-and-mouth disease] Z. Immun. Forsch.104, 158-165. (1943). [Translated to English by A. Finnegan (2019)]

29   Pyl, G. K. O. Hobohm. Zur Kenntnis der Zusatze nichtbiologischer Herkunft in der Riemser Maul- und Klauenseuche-Vakzine. [For knowledge of the additives of non-biological origin in the Riems foot-and-mouth disease vaccine]. Berl. Munch. Tierarztl. Wschr.; Feb. 18th. 58:56-58. (1944).

30   Central Intelligence Agency (CIA) Intelligence Reports: The State Research Institute at Riems; Microbiological Research. CIA-RDP83-00415R000900020012-6. Central Intelligence Agency (CIA), Reading Room, 2011. Retrieved from: https://www.cia.gov/library/readingroom/document/CIA-RDP83-00415R000900020012-6

31   Central Intelligence Agency (CIA) Intelligence Reports: SOVIET SCIENTISTS AND SCIENTIFIC ORGANIZATIONS (132). CIA-RDP85T00875R000300010008-6. Central Intelligence Agency (CIA), Reading Room, 2003. Retrieved from: https://www.cia.gov/library/readingroom/document/CIA-RDP85T00875R000300010008-6

32   Maier, E. (2017, January). *Flashback... Virus Research: A Foul Enemy in Fowl*. Max Planck Research, 78-79.

33   Behringwerke AG. (1943, June 18). Behringwerke [Letter to The Reich Ministery of the Interior]. Insel Riems Institute, Isle of Riems, Germany.

34   Traub, E. & W. Schäfer. Immunisierung von Mausen gegen Influenza mit Adsor-batimpstoffen von Viruskonzentraten. [Immunization of Mice Against Influenza with Concen-trated Virus Adsorbate Vaccines]. Monatshefte fur Veterinmedizine. 1. 369-373 (1946)

35   Schäfer, Werner, and E. Seifert. 2004. "Production of a Potent Complement-Fixing Murine Leukemia Virus-Anti-Serum from the Rabbit and Its Reactions with Various Types of Tissue Culture Cells."Virology. Academic Press. June 4, 2004. https://www.sciencedirect.com/science/article/abs/pii/0042682268902730

36   Schäfer, W. (1963). Structure of Some Animal Viruses and Significance of their Components. Bacteriological Review, 27.

37   Lichte, J. U. (1983). Die Forschung auf der Insel Riems von 1933 bis 1945 unter besonderer Berücksichtigung der NS-Zwangsarbeiter (Inaugural Dissertation). Nordenham, Germany: The Medical Faculty of the Ernst-Moritz-Arndt University of Greifswald., pp. 53

38   Wittmann, W. (1999). *100 Years of Virology. The Legacy of Friedrich Loeffler - the Insti-tute on the Isle of Riems*, 28. doi:10.1007/978-3-7091-6425-9

39   Traub, E. & W. Schäfer. Immunisierung von Mausen gegen Influenza mit Adsor-batimpstoffen von Viruskonzentraten. [Immunization of Mice Against Influenza with Concen-trated Virus Adsorbate Vaccines]. Monatshefte fur Veterinmedizine. 1. 369-373 (1946).

40   Traub, E., Schäfer, W. & Schramm, G., Untersuchen uber das Virus der Atypischen Geflugelpest. [Studies of the Virus of Atypical Fowl Plague]. Z. Naturforsch B. 157-167 (1949).

41   Deichmann, Ute. 1996. Biologists under Hitler. Cambridge, MA: Harvard University Press., pp. 99-102, 210-213, 298-99, 313-317, 421-38

42   Lichte, J. U. (1983). Die Forschung auf der Insel Riems von 1933 bis 1945 unter besonderer Berücksichtigung der NS-Zwangsarbeiter (Inaugural Dissertation). Nordenham, Germany: The Medical Faculty of the Ernst-Moritz-Arndt University of Greifswald.

43   Eberle, Henrik. "Ein Wertvolles Instrument": Die Universität Greifswald Im Nation-alsozialismus. Bohlau Verlag, 2015. [pp. 538-541]

44   E Traub, G Wittmann. Experimenteller Beitrag zur Klärung der Frage der Verbre-itung des Maul-und Klauenseuche-Virus durch die Luft. [Experimental Contribution to Elu-cidating the Question of Airborne Transmission of the Foot and Mouth Disease Virus]. Berl. Münch. Tier. Woch. (1957).

45   Lichte, J. U. (1983). Die Forschung auf der Insel Riems von 1933 bis 1945 unter besonderer Berücksichtigung der NS-Zwangsarbeiter (Inaugural Dissertation). Nordenham, Germany: The Medical Faculty of the Ernst-Moritz-Arndt University of Greifswald.

46   Ibid.

47   Traub, E., Schneider, B., Zuchtung des Virus der Maul- und Klauenseuche im bebru-teten Huhnerei. [Breeding of the Virus of Foot-and-Mouth Disease Virus in Chicken Embryos]. Z Naturforsch B. May-Jun; 3 (5-6):178-87. (1948)

48   National Archives, Joint Intelligence Objectives Agency, J.I.O.A. Administrative Re-cords. (1950). Memorandum on Anne Bürger, C. F. Berrens, Naval Medical Research Institute, to Chief of Naval Operations, 27 November 1950, Navy Escape Clause (RG 330). NARS.

49   Haagen, E. (n.d.). Letter and report to the director of general medicine at the Reich Research Council concerning research [influenza, typhus, and epidemic jaundice]. Retrieved from http://nuremberg.law.harvard.edu/documents/1173-letter-and-report-to-the-direc-tor?q=influenza#p.3 doi:Evidence Code: NO-138 HLSL/Item No.: 1172

50   Dinter, Z. Persönaliches, Begegnungen mit Erich Traub. Berl. Munch. Tier. Woch. 96. 70-72. (1984)

51   National Archives, Joint Intelligence Objectives Agency, J.I.O.A. Administrative Records. (1950). Memorandum on Anne Bürger, C. F. Berrens, Naval Medical Research Institute, to Chief of Naval Operations, 27 November 1950, Navy Escape Clause (RG 330). NARS.

52   Schäfer, W. Über den Virusgehalt des Zentralnervensystems von Ferkeln nach intracerebraler Infektion mit Schweinelähmevirus. [About the virus content in the central nervous system after intracerebral infection with swine paralysis]. Berl. u. Münch. Tierärztl. Wschr. No. 2, Aug 1946.

53   Schäfer, W. Über einen Blockierungseffekt bei der künstlichen Maul- und Klauenseuche-Infektion der Meerschweinchen und seine Beziehungen zur Immunität. [About the blocking effect of the artificial Foot-and-Mouth Disease infection and its relation to immunity]. Berl. u. Münch. Tierärztl. Wschr. No. 6, Dec. 1946.

54   Schäfer, W. Untersuchungen über den Virusgehalt des Blutes und der Organe bei der Maul- und Klauenseucheinfektion von Meerschweinchen.[Studies on the virus content of blood and organs from the foot-and-mouth disease infection in guinea pigs]. Monatshefte für Veterinärmedizin. 6-10, 1946.

55   Rockborn, G., B. Liess, P.-P. Pastoret, S. Edwards, and A. San Gabriel. 1992. "Zvonimir Dinter—In Memoriam." *Veterinary Microbiology* 33 (1-4): 3–4. https://doi.org/10.1016/0378-1135(92)90029-

56   Dinter, Z. Persönaliches, Begegnungen mit Erich Traub. [personal memories of Erich Traub]. Berl. Munch. Tier. Woch. 96. 70-72. (1984)

57   Traub, E. Weitere Mitteilungen uber die aktive Immunisierung mit Adsorbatimpfstoffen gegen die atypische Geflügelpest. [Further news about active immunization with adsorbate vaccines against atypical avian influenza]. Z. Infekt. krankh. Haustiere 60, 367-379. (1944).

58   Traub, E. & F. M. Rodriguez. Uber die Herstellung komplementbindender Meerschweinchensera fur die Typendiagnose bei Maul- und Klauenseuche. [On the Complement-Fixation test of Guinea-pig sera for the typing of Foot-and-Mouth Disease.] Zbl. Bakt. I. Orig. 151, 380-388. (1944).

59   Traub, E & Z. Dinter. Uber den Einfluß der Virulenz und der Antigenstruktur von Maul- und Klauenseuche-Virusstämmen auf das Immunisierungvermögen der daraus bereiteten Vaccinen [The Influence of Virulence and Antigenic Structure of Foot-and-Mouth Disease Virus on the Immunogenicity of Vaccines Prepared from Them]. Monatshefte fur Veterinmedizine. 6. 91-96. (1946). [Translated to English by A. Finnegan (2019)]

60   Lichte, J. U. (2011). Die Forschung auf der Insel Riems von 1933 bis 1945 unter besonderer Berücksichtigung der NS-Zwangsarbeiter (Inaugural Dissertation). Nordenham, Germany: The Medical Faculty of the Ernst-Moritz-Arndt University of Greifswald.

61   Ruska, H. Über die Elementarkörper des Virus der Bronchopneumonie der Maus. [On the Elementary Bordies of Bronchopneumonia of Mice]. Klinische Wochenschrift 23 (1944), S. 121-122

62   Ruska, H. Zur Frage der Potenzierung von Bakteriophagenlösungen durch Zerschäumen. [On the question of potentiation of bacteriophage solutions by foaming] Kolloid-Zeitschrift 110 (1948), S. 175-177 [research conducted in 1944-45, not published until 1948]

63   Nelson, J B. "INFECTIOUS CATARRH OF MICE : I. A NATURAL OUTBREAK OF THE DISEASE." *The Journal of experimental medicine* vol. 65,6 (1937): 833-41. doi:10.1084/jem.65.6.833

64   Traub, E., Schäfer, W. & Schramm, G., Untersuchen uber das Virus der Atypischen Geflugelpest. [Studies of the Virus of Atypical Fowl Plague]. Z. Naturforsch B. 157-167 (1949).

65   Traub, E. & W. Schäfer. Immunisierung von Mausen gegen Influenza mit Adsor-batimpstoffen von Viruskonzentraten. [Immunization of Mice Against Influenza with Concentrated Virus Adsorbate Vaccines]. Monatshefte fur Veterinmedizine. 1. 369-373 (1946).

66   Traub, E.; Miehler, H. Konzentration und Reinigung von Geflugelpest-Virusstammen. [Concentration and purification of avian influenza virus]. Monatsh Vet Med. 35-38. (1946).

67   Traub, E. & W. Schäfer. Immunisierung von Mausen gegen Influenza mit Adsor-batimpstoffen von Viruskonzentraten. [Immunization of Mice Against Influenza with Concentrated Virus Adsorbate Vaccines]. Monatshefte fur Veterinmedizine. 1. 369-373 (1946).

68   Central Intelligence Agency (CIA) Intelligence Reports: THE BACTERIOLOGICAL RESEARCH INSTITUTE ON THE ISLAND OF RIEMS. CIA-RDP83-00415R002200020014-9. Central Intelligence Agency (CIA), Reading Room, 2011. Retrieved from: https://www.cia.gov/library/readingroom/document/CIA-RDP83-00415R002200020014-9

69   Traub, E. Vaccine Production at Riems [Letter to The Reich Ministery of the Interior]. Insel Riems Institute, Isle of Riems, Germany. (1945, August 11).

70   Behringwerke AG. (1943, June 18). Behringwerke [Letter to The Reich Ministery of the Interior]. Insel Riems Institute, Isle of Riems, Germany.

71   Central Intelligence Agency (CIA) Intelligence Reports: The State Research Institute at Riems; Microbiological Research. CIA-RDP83-00415R000900020012-6. Central Intelligence Agency (CIA), Reading Room, 2011. Retrieved from: https://www.cia.gov/library/readingroom/document/CIA-RDP83-00415R000900020012-6

72   National Archives. Joint intelligence Objectives Agency (JIOA), JIOA Administrative Records. (n.d.). Interview of ALSOS Scientists: Dr. Kurt Blöme (RG 330 INSCOM dossier XE001248). NARS.

73   Hunt, Linda. Secret Agenda the United States Government, Nazi Scientists, 1945 to 1990. St. Martins Pr, 1991.

74   Lichte, J. U. (1983). Die Forschung auf der Insel Riems von 1933 bis 1945 unter besonderer Berücksichtigung der NS-Zwangsarbeiter (Inaugural Dissertation). Nordenham, Germany: The Medical Faculty of the Ernst-Moritz-Arndt University of Greifswald.

75   National Archives. Joint intelligence Objectives Agency (JIOA), JIOA Administrative Records. (n.d.). Interview of ALSOS Scientists: Dr. Kurt Blöme (RG 330 INSCOM dossier XE001248). NARS.

76   Haagen, E. (n.d.). Letter and report to the director of general medicine at the Reich Research Council concerning research [influenza, typhus, and epidemic jaundice]. Retrieved from   http://nuremberg.law.harvard.edu/documents/1173-letter-and-report-to-the-director?q=influenza#p.3 doi:Evidence Code: NO-138 HLSL/Item No.: 1172

77   Hunt, Linda. Secret Agenda the United States Government, Nazi Scientists, 1945 to 1990. St. Martins Pr, 1991.

78   Kliewe, H., Dr. (n.d.). Memorandum concerning a plan to establish a medical research institute near Posen, including experiments with biological weapons, plague vaccines, and poisons, with related documents. Retrieved from http://nuremberg.law.harvard.edu/documents/5638-memorandum-concerning-a-plan?q=Memorandum concerning a plan to establish a medical research institute near Posen, including experiments with biological weapons, plague vaccines, and poisons, with related documents#p.1. Evidence Code: NO-1309/HLSL Item No.: 5638

79   Grawitz, Ernst. n.d. "Report to Himmler Concerning the Phlegmon Experiments at Dachau." Nuremberg Trials Project. Harvard Law School Library. Accessed August 1, 2019. http://nuremberg.law.harvard.edu/documents/4141-report-to-himmler-concerning#p.1

80   Traub worked with both, and later contracted under Behringwerke AG to produce an erysipelas vaccine, before his return to the United States. See Traub 1947, Traub 1948.

81   National Archives. Joint intelligence Objectives Agency (JIOA), JIOA Administrative Records. (n.d.). Interview of ALSOS Scientists: Dr. Kurt Blöme (RG 330 INSCOM dossier XE001248). NARS.

82   Eberle, Henrik. "Ein Wertvolles Instrument": Die Universität Greifswald Im Nationalsozialismus. Bohlau Verlag, 2015. [pp. 538-541]

83   Central Intelligence Agency (CIA) Intelligence Reports: The State Research Institute at Riems; Microbiological Research. CIA-RDP83-00415R000900020012-6. Central Intelligence Agency (CIA), Reading Room, 2011. Retrieved from: https://www.cia.gov/library/readingroom/docs/CIA-RDP83-00415R000900020012-6

84   Central Intelligence Agency (CIA) Intelligence Reports: THE BACTERIOLOGICAL RESEARCH INSTITUTE ON THE ISLAND OF RIEMS. CIA-RDP83-00415R002200020014-9. Central Intelligence Agency (CIA), Reading Room, 2011. Retrieved from: https://www.cia.gov/library/readingroom/document/CIA-RDP83-00415R002200020014-9

85   National Archives. RG 65 Erich Traub, (Declassified FBI Investigations on the Loyalties of Erich Traub). Federal Bureau of Investigation (FBI): NARA., Doc. # QO1-458431291

86   Central Intelligence Agency (CIA). The Bacteriological Research Institute on the Island of Riems. C03157285. 2023.

87   Lichte, J. U. (1983). Die Forschung auf der Insel Riems von 1933 bis 1945 unter besonderer Berücksichtigung der NS-Zwangsarbeiter (Inaugural Dissertation). Nordenham, Germany: The Medical Faculty of the Ernst-Moritz-Arndt University of Greifswald.

88   Central Intelligence Agency (CIA) Intelligence Reports: The State Research Institute at Riems; Microbiological Research. CIA-RDP83-00415R000900020012-6. Central Intelligence Agency (CIA), Reading Room, 2011. Retrieved from: https://www.cia.gov/library/readingroom/document/CIA-RDP83-00415R000900020012-6.pdf

89   Wittmann, W. (1999). 100 Years of Virology. The Legacy of Friedrich Loeffler - the Institute on the Isle of Riems, 28. doi:10.1007/978-3-7091-6425-9, pp. 28

Chapter Eight

THE SOVIET SLEEPER AGENTS

THE RUSSIAN OCCUPATION OF INSEL RIEMS AND THE ACQUISITION OF ERICH TRAUB

Beware the beast Man, for he is the Devil's pawn. Alone among God's primates, he kills for sport or lust or greed. Yea, he will murder his brother to possess his brother's land. Let him not breed in great numbers, for he will make a desert of his home and yours....
– The Lawgiver, (Cornelius in Planet of the Apes).

At the close of World War II, in May of 1945 Erich Traub and the staff at Insel Riems were taken captive by the Red Army of the Soviet Union. The work was briefly halted and conditions on Riems were harsh. Traub and his staff were interrogated and then forced to continue their research again from scratch, after a steady progression from its early inception, this time under Soviet authority. As mentioned previously, the Russians hauled off the entirety of Insel Riems research up to that time, including all the ultra-secret military work for the German Reich. This brought the Soviets an undreamed-of advantage over the West. They now had the best of the best in biological weapons research.

Information on where the Riems research was brought is scarce. An American intelligence report declassified in 2006 relays that sources indicated the research was taken to Riga in Latvia, and finally to Lake Seliger, while Klaus Munk, in his *Virology in Germany*, states that it was rumored to have been brought to a facility near Ilman Lake, which is a region of Russia close to the Scandinavian countries and not far from the regions of Russia where Lake Seliger is located. He also shows the harsh conditions that followed its capture:

> In the final days of the war, the island of Riems was occupied by the Russian army. They set up an artillery observation post

in the turret on the roof of the casino and had trenches dug on the island. Waldmann was removed from his post. Numerous staff were sent to internment camps. Others put an end to their lives by suicide. Shortly afterwards, the entire facility was transported to Russia by the occupying power - it was said to be to Ilmen Lake. The institution had practically ceased to exist in its previous form. [...] [1]

Insel Riems was not an insignificant biological research facility, it was perhaps the leading biological research facility on viruses and germs in existence. In fact, when the Russians took Riems, the facility was placed under the personal protection of Joseph Stalin, according to a declassified American intelligence report.[2] Clearly, the Soviet Union had understood the significance of the facility and Intelligence reports reflect this, while the Americans downplayed its significance as much as possible.

Western Intelligence, however, had been fooled and given bad intelligence when they were told that the Riems Institute had done no research for the purpose of biological warfare, and this is evident from declassified intelligence reports, claiming that Riems never engaged in human influenza research, and that the only work with bacteria ever done at the Riems Institute was limited to brucellosis and swine erysipelas:

> The Russians have shown an interest in the production and spreading of human pest [(human influenza)]. When the Russians first came to Riems in 1945, they maintained that during the war the Institute had done research on human pest [(human influenza)]. with a view of spreading it in enemy countries. It was very hard to convince them that actually the Institute had never engaged in such research. The only bacteriological (not virus) research ever done at Riems was with swine erysipelas and brucellosis.[3]

It was an established fact that Insel Riems had done work on human influenza, as Traub had published the research in 1946 for a human influenza vaccine with dual use potential in his publication "Immunization of mice against Influenza with Adsorbate Vaccines of Virus Concentrates."[4] Passing the virus through mice would have imparted pronounced neurotropic qualities for humans, as mouse passages mutated viruses to that effect. It is revealed in the paper that the human influenza strain had been given to them by Professor Kurt Herzberg, who had been researching the use of birds like canaries to spread biological weapons such as infectious hepatitis.[5] Herzberg was named in connection with biological weapons research and testing after interrogations by Western Intelligence. This had been revealed in a German text on the history of the University of Greifswald under National Socialism, the Institute which ran Insel Riems.

> One of the interrogations was Joachim Mrugowski, head of the Hygiene Institute of the Waffen-SS, who gave information at the trial on sera in concentration camps and was executed. The veterinarian Heinrich Kliewe, a professor at the University of Giessen, was also interviewed. Kliewe had carried out experiments with viruses in the Army Weapons Office. After a first interrogation on July 28, 1945, Kliewe's interrogators suggested, even look into "Prof. Herzberg of Greifswald," whom infected canaries. In addition, everything should be learned about the "Imperial Research Institute Insel Riems," as it stands in connection with "BW" or Biological Warfare was exclusive and collegial. For example, the director of the research institute on the island of Riems worked very closely with Eugen Haagen, head of the Department of Cell and Virus Research at the Robert Koch Institute in Berlin. Haagen later formed concentrated research for human viral diseases at the Reich University of Strasbourg.[6]

Likewise, Insel Riems had indeed worked with a considerable number of bacterial diseases, and this can be seen in the publications they released in journals which had been in the public domain. Even under Russian control, Helmut Ruska had been publishing from the Insel Riems electron microscope department about *Mycoplasma mycoides*, the agent of contagious bovine pleuropneumonia,[7] not to mention, *Streptococcus, E. coli*, and typhoid bacteria.[8] There is also evidence of further bacteriological research associated with Insel Riems which will be discussed later in this chapter.

After considerable hardship under Russian capture on Riems, the Soviets had Traub continue working on Foot-and-Mouth Disease (FMD) and other agents of biological warfare significance.[9] Stalin now had some of the best of scientists from the Reich when it came to biological weapons, Erich Traub, his star technician, Anne-Lise Bürger, and the rest of the Insel Riems staff were under Soviet control. On top of this, they had Traub's other protégé from Insel Riems, Zvonimir Dinter, and Insel Riems worked in close coordination with Dinter's other mentor in bacteriology, Dr. Joseph Fortner, through its association with the University of Berlin.[10] Insel Riems was also co-ordinating with The Kaiser-Wilhelm Institute and the University of Giessen, as is noted by the previous passage regarding Dr. Heinrich Kliewe and Professor Dr. Kurt Herzberg.[11]

Several important researchers who were at the Institute during WWII, however, returned to West Germany, and were able to escape the Russian occupation. Gernot Bergold and Gerhard Schramm also left Insel Riems for West Germany before the Russians took hold of it. It appears that the institute was coordinating with these scientists and institutes from before the Russian captivity. Traub's protégé, Werner Schäfer, returned to West Germany, but correspondence between Erich Traub and Werner Schäfer had been occurring even during the Russian occupation indicating that Schäfer was under their control during the beginning. Erich Traub writes his old student:

> "We have had difficult times behind us on the Riems, which you luckily only experienced at the beginning and in a mild form. They are not over yet, even if emotionally easier to endure. We are currently trying to rebuild. Waldmann is trying to 'rehabilitate'. I hope that he succeeds and that he can lead the reconstruction. If everything goes well, we will be ready for production again in a few months, if only on a small scale."[12]

Traub took a considerable pay cut under the Russian occupation, but nonetheless, he was still paid. He earned an additional perk for his work, he was given full professorship at the University of Berlin, and Ms. Bürger, his trusted technician, also accompanied Traub's professorship at the Institute.[13]

The work at Riems continued for several years under these less-than-optimal conditions. It was during this time the Russians were seeking war criminals they could use to either prosecute or blackmail, using war crimes as leverage. Traub certainly would have become a target, likely as a result of his experimental work on the human influenza vaccine along with other agents produced for Behringwerke AG.

Intelligence reports on the capture indicated that the Russians interrogated Traub on more than one occasion about Nazi activities looking for war crimes, and this was especially so with the female lab technicians, Miss Bürger and Miss Frank, according to a 1948 American Intelligence report:

> The Russians undoubtedly showed a desire to find war criminals, especially in the interrogation of female laboratory as-

sistants and other auxiliary staff of all kinds. They were asked principally about preparations for biological warfare. Enquiries were also made concerning research in human diseases, and whether the animal crematory was also used for the disposal of human bodies. The Russians allowed work to proceed in order to learn the current problems and laboratory methods.[14]

During Traub's time under Russian control, he published several papers on FMD,[15] Newcastle Disease,[16] brucellosis,[17] and Swine Erysipelas,[18] a bacterium that caused small diamond-shaped rashes that results in sepsis and was much like brucellosis. Perhaps the most revealing aspect of this time period in Traub's career under Russian control, were two meetings with the tick encephalitis researcher involved in Siberian tick expeditions from the late 1930s, the noted virologist, M. P. Chumakov, as American Intelligence reports indicate that Chumakov traveled to Insel Riems twice in 1947 to consult with a scientist on choriomeningitis:

> The Russians have ordered no specific work at the institute and have not assumed in any way its scientific direction, although Russians come there continuously to collect information. Among the more notable Russian visitors is Professor Tschumakov [sic], Stalin Prize winner, from the Moscow Institute for Research on Brain Disease. He came twice in 1947 to obtain information on choriomeningitis.[19]

Chumakov's interest in choriomeningitis in 1947 shows Chumakov was interested in the mechanisms of immune tolerance, stealth viral infections that produced little to no outward symptoms and no antibodies in the host. It is also highly significant that Chumakov would be looking so deeply into these mechanisms before teaming up with Albert B. Sabin to construct the polio vaccine.[20] After all, Chumakov and Sabin's oral polio vaccine was contaminated by SV40, a virus that acts much like LCM virus, all very elusive and problematic when it came to vaccines made from animal tissues during the Cold War.[21] The viral hemorrhagic fevers would equally hold a clear and present danger. These activities will be covered in a later chapter.

Most notable among Traub's Russian research, was the method for the cultivation of FMD in chicken eggs with his colleagues and lab technicians, Anne-Lise Bürger and Johanna Frank, who became greatly skilled in using this method, and a range of different techniques would be involved.[22] What was so unusual about this work was that no one had been successful in growing the virus in chicken eggs up to this point. All prior attempts by other researchers failed.

Erich Traub and Behringwerke employee, Bernard Schneider, along with his technicians accomplished this by mixing 10 strains of FMD virus in one live chicken egg and, using the infectious material isolated from it, then infect a guinea-pig with it, they then let the disease play out in the guinea-pig, re-isolate the virus from the guinea pig, then back into a live chicken egg, letting the virus accumulate in the egg, re-isolating it, then back into the guinea-pig, and it went on for a considerable number of passages before it finally took to the chicken egg and to chickens. The idea was to gradually get the virus used to the egg by alternating passages between the egg and guinea pig, who had already been susceptible to FMD virus. [23]

As Dr. Traub and his team became more proficient in this technique, they would both become valuable scientists to any country's biological weapons program in the early days of the Cold War. As noted in earlier chapters, the Soviets made up for their lack of technological advancement by concentrating their forces in the areas of intelligence, infiltration, sabotage, and biological warfare.

According to an American intelligence report on the activities undertaken at Riems and associated production facilities dated April 4, 1949, much more than FMD and rinderpest, a highly contagious and destructive virus of cattle, was researched at Riems and its associated facilities. An inventory listed in the report reveals more than two dozen serums and vaccines made by the ASID serum plant in Dessau, a facility Riems was closely working with, for a wide spectrum of different disease agents and conditions, including spirochetes. [24]

Among some of the serums listed were Diphtheria, Dysentery, Enterococcus, Erysipeloid, multiple sclerosis, Gonococcus, Meningococcus, anthrax, scarlet fever, Staphylococcus, Streptococcus, tetanus, tuberculosis, typhoid & paratyphoid, as well as Weil's serum from rams and rabbits,[25] which is a serum for *Leptospira grippotyphosa*, the spirochete that causes Weil's disease (leptospirosis).[26] It is possible that the serum listed for multiple sclerosis was based on the Lyme disease spirochetes Traub weaponized.

Often in a biological warfare program, the treatment or antidote was made in parallel to the weapon even though the treatment, vaccine, or antidote is not guaranteed to work, and in many diseases, there is no way to safely vaccinate against certain disease agents, and treatments are often ineffective, especially for viruses. It was in these preparations that Dr. Traub and Anne Bürger gained more needed experience with rickettsial and spirochetal disease.[27]

The serum production would indicate the scope of research on biological agents pathogenic to humans being conducted at Riems under the cover of animal disease, serum, and vaccines. Tick and insect-borne disease and entomological warfare studies would have also occurred under the direction of Traub and their facilities at Riems since insects and insect-borne disease are of considerable importance to agriculture.[28]

Indeed, Traub's professorship at the University of Berlin focused on Newcastle Disease Virus, fowl plague (avian influenza) and various avian diseases,[29] and this likely brought with it, additional work on the *differential diagnosis* for these agents, like we had discussed in earlier chapters, which would include avian spirochetosis (*Borrelia anserina*).

Likewise, it would include the transmitters of avian diseases like fowl ticks, mites, lice, and mosquitoes. From the early experiments on pseudorabies, Eastern Equine Encephalitis, and infectious anemia, Traub talked about beetles, horseflies, and mosquitoes in the transmission of disease.[30] Earlier research on FMD looked at the possibility of ticks to transmit FMD virus,[31] as well as migratory birds.[32]

It was Traub who would have been implicated in war crimes if they had occurred on Insel Riems. After all, it was Traub and Schäfer who had been working on the construction of human and avian influenza vaccines which certainly had offensive capabilities. His female technicians could have been particularly vulnerable during interrogation. Schäfer would have been implicated as well. Why he was allowed to return to West Germany must have had a pretty important reason, which we will return to in the next chapter.

The only ones who would have had any knowledge of such war crimes were the Russians, and those watching over the facility now under the personal protection of Joseph Stalin. They knew the value of this institute, and its acquisition was a high priority. Moreover, their Soviet handlers knew that they wouldn't be offering up skilled scientists and their technicians to be tried for war crimes when they could be put to use for the Soviet offensive, but the scientists were not entirely immune to the fear of prosecution, and this was a vulnerability Soviet Intelligence could exploit. Traub was in a vulnerable position, and he had to make up his mind what was in his best interest if he wanted to continue living the high-life of the Western lifestyle.

ESCAPE FROM THE RUSSIAN ZONE

On June 26, 1948, Traub and his family, along with Anne Bürger and his Behringwerke AG colleague Bernard Schneider made their so-called "escape" from the Isle of Riems and the greater Russian Zone of occupation with the help of British Intelligence, carrying with him cultures of freeze-dried FMD and other pathogens. Upon his return to the British Zone of Germany, Blanka and Traub's children went to an English camp in Alswede at Lübbecke, West Germany.[33] Traub may or may not have stopped here but went south past Marburg and Behringwerke, for a brief stay at Castle Kransberg, according to John Loftus.[34] Kransberg was used to shield valuable Nazis from potential prosecution at Nuremberg. However, he also listed a brief stay at a hotel Alto Post near Behringwerke in Marburg.

Traub's escape was coordinated with British Intelligence under Operation Matchbox, noted in the textbook, *Intelligence and Statecraft: The Use and Limits of Intelligence in International Society*, and the escape was coordinated from Berlin where Traub had been teaching.[35] Sources interviewed by the FBI regarding Traub's loyalties have it that, according to Traub, before the Russian occupation of Insel Riems, he was in favor of moving the laboratory equipment to Germany and fleeing to West Germany so they could be employed by either Britain, Canada, or the United States, and that he was vehemently against communism, as he thought the Russians were barbarians.[36]

However, According to Frank A. Todd, a veterinary specialist from the Pentagon, it is said that in October of 1945 Traub approached British and American Intelligence and began negotiations for employment in the West, and the FBI files show that Traub actually met with William A. Hagen, and filled out a questionnaire which was mandatory of any former Nazis seeking employment in the West. It is stated that due to Traub's association with the Air Raid Warden and the Veterinary Division, Traub would not be admitted to the West due to these associations with the Nazi Party.[37]

Soon Blanka and the family would move a little further south to another English camp at Bad Hermannsborn near Bad Driburg, just an hour-and-a-half from Behringwerke in Marburg, almost 3 hours from Castle Kransberg. Traub's personnel records indicate that he became the scientific advisor to Behringwerke, the subsidiary of IG Farben,[38] who's laboratories would, many years later be at the center of the deadly outbreak of Marburg virus in 1967.[39]

Traub's stay at Castle Kransberg, otherwise known as DUSTBIN, was likely a short stay. This was an old Nazi retreat in Hesse, a luxurious palace used by Hermann Göring and other top brass of the Reich in earlier years. After the war it became the most secure, Top-Secret holding facility for scientists and businessmen from the IG Farben

131

conglomerate, operating as a safe-house from prosecution rather than a prison for the accused at Nuremberg.[40]

While Traub was waiting for his move to the United States, he wrote and published "Advances in Active Immunization Against Animal Virus Diseases," given as a lecture at Giessen, building from similar material seen in his 1939 thesis, published in a major German medical journal with an address listed under the employment of Behringwerke.[41]

Traub also began receiving royalties for a swine erysipelas vaccine,[42] contracted through Behringwerke, which Bürger helped produce with Traub, and Bürger apparently had some of the cultures with her too when they escaped.[43] They further worked out these antigen components for Behringwerke and this would have certainly been applied to the bioweapons program of Britain, Canada, and the United States, in some form or another.

According to American Intelligence files, the location Traub listed as his address in West Germany, Hotel Alto Post, Marburg, may have been used to house him for limited work or coordination with Behringwerke labs in Marburg, after he was released from Kransberg. German archives have record of Traub's contract during the war for avian influenza, contracted with Behringwerke AG.[44] Ms. Bürger would also list a contract with Behringwerke in 1948.[45]

Traub's application also notes an invitation by the Swiss government for Traub to travel to Switzerland to advise them on problems of veterinary importance, due to the outbreaks of FMD that had been sweeping the countryside of Switzerland.[46] It was at this time that Traub was made an officer of the Food and Agriculture Organization of the United Nations, giving him a layer of diplomatic immunity in America and abroad.[47] He was in talks with the Swiss to possibly go to Canada or the United States, and the FAO is located in Geneva Switzerland, which Traub had visited in 1948.[48]

Endnotes

1   Munk K.: Virologie in Deutschland. Die Entwicklung eines Fachgebietes. Basel, Karger, 1995, pp 4-49 (DOI:10.1159/000423810)

2   Central Intelligence Agency (CIA) Intelligence Reports: THE BACTERIOLOGICAL RE-SEARCH INSTITUTE ON THE ISLAND OF RIEMS. CIA-RDP83-00415R002200020014-9. Central Intelligence Agency (CIA), Reading Room, 2011. Retrieved from: https://www.cia.gov/library/readingroom/documnt/CIA-RDP83-00415R002200020014-9

3   Ibid.

4   Traub, E. & W. Schäfer. Immunisierung von Mausen gegen Influenza mit Adsorbatimpstoffen von Viruskonzentraten. [Immunization of Mice Against Influenza with Concentrated Virus Adsorbate Vaccines]. Monatshefte fur Veterinmedizine. 1. 369-373 (1946). [Translated to English by A. Finnegan (2019)]

5   Herzberg, K. Uebertragungsversuche an Kanarienvögeln mit Hepatitis-contagiosa-Material [Transmission experiments in canaries with infectious hepatitis material]. Zbl. Bakt. Abt. I. Orig. 151: 81-106. (1944)

6   Eberle, Henrik. "Ein Wertvolles Instrument": Die Universität Greifswald Im Nationalsozialismus. Bohlau Verlag, 2015. [Translated to English by A. Finnegan (2019)]

7   RUSKA, H., & K. POPPE: Elektronenmikroskopische Untersuchungen zur Morphologie der Seiffertschen Mikroorganismen und des Erregers der Lungenseuche des Rindes. [Electron Microscopy Investigations on the morphology of Seiffert's Microorganism and the causative agent of bovine respiratory disease]. Zeitschrift für Hygiene und Infektionskrankheiten, medizinische Mikrobiologie, Immunologie und Virologie 127 (1947), S. 201-215 [Translated to English by A. Finnegan (2019)]

8   Helmut Ruska (1947). Über die Bindung des Sublimats an Bakterien und Virus [On the binding of the sublimate to bacteria and virus]., 204(4-5), 576–585. doi:10.1007/bf00245723 [Translated to English by A. Finnegan (2019)]

9   National Archives. Joint-Intelligence Objectives Agency file on Erich Traub (RG 330). NARS. Joint Intelligence Objectives Agency (JIOA), JIOA Administrative Records. (1949-54).

10   Rockborn, G., B. Liess, P.-P. Pastoret, S. Edwards, and A. San Gabriel. 1992. "Zvonimir Dinter—In Memoriam." Veterinary Microbiology 33 (1-4): 3–4. https://doi.org/10.1016/0378-1135(92)90029-

11   Eberle, Henrik. "Ein Wertvolles Instrument": Die Universität Greifswald Im Nationalsozialismus. Bohlau Verlag, 2015. [Translated to English by A. Finnegan (2019)]

12   Munk K.: Virologie in Deutschland. Die Entwicklung eines Fachgebietes. Basel, Karger, 1995, pp 4-49 (DOI:10.1159/000423810)

13   National Archives. Joint-Intelligence Objectives Agency file on Erich Traub (RG 330). NARS. Joint Intelligence Objectives Agency (JIOA), JIOA Administrative Records. (1949-54).

14   Central Intelligence Agency (CIA) Intelligence Reports: *The State Research Institute at Riems; Microbiological Research*. CIA-RDP83-00415R000900020012-6. *Central Intelligence Agency (CIA)*, Reading Room, 2011. Retrieved from: https://www.cia.gov/library/readingroom/document/CIA-RDP83-00415R000900020012-6

15   Traub, E & Z. Dinter. Uber den Einfluß der Virulenz und der Antigenstruktur von Maul- und Klauenseuche-Virusstämmen auf das Immunisierungvermögen der daraus bereiteten Vaccinen [The Influence of Virulence and Antigenic Structure of Foot-and-Mouth Disease Virus on the Immunogenicity of Vaccines Prepared from Them]. Monatshefte fur Veterinmedizine. 6. 91-96. (1946). [Translated to English by A. Finnegan (2019)]

16   Traub, E., Schäfer, W. & Schramm, G., Untersuchen uber das Virus der Atypischen Geflugelpest. [Studies of the Virus of Atypical Fowl Plague]. Z. Naturforsch B. 157-167 (1949). [Translated to English by A. Finnegan (2019)]

17   Traub, E., Immunisierung von Mausen gegen Brucellose mit Konzentrierten Adsorbatvakzinen.[Immunization of Mice Against Brucellosis by Concentrated Adsorbate Vaccines]. Monatshefte fur Veterinarmedizin. 89-94. (1948). [Translated to English by A. Finnegan (2019)]

18   Traub, E., Uber die immunbiologischen Grundlagen der aktiven Immunisierung gegen Schweinerotlauf mit konzentrierten Adsorbatimpfstoffen. [Immunobiological Foundations of Active Immunization Against Swine Erysipelas with Concentrated Adsorbate Vaccines] Monatshefte fur Veterinarmedizin 121-127. (1948). [Translated to English by A. Finnegan (2019)]

19   Central Intelligence Agency (CIA) Intelligence Reports: THE BACTERIOLOGICAL RESEARCH INSTITUTE ON THE ISLAND OF RIEMS. CIA-RDP83-00415R002200020014-9. *Central Intelligence Agency (CIA)*, Reading Room, 2011. Retrieved from: https://www.cia.gov/library/readingroom/document/CIA-RDP83-00415R002200020014-9

20   Swanson, William. "Birth of a Cold War Vaccine." Scientific American, vol. 306, no. 4, 2012, pp. 66–69., doi:10.1038/scientificamerican0412-66

21   Shah, Keerti, and Neal Nathanson. "Human Exposure to Sv40: Review And Comment." American Journal of Epidemiology, vol. 103, no. 1, 1976, pp. 1–12., doi:10.1093/oxfordjournals.aje.a112197

22   Traub E, Schneider, B., Infektion des bebruteten Huhnereies mit dem Virus der Maul- und Klauenseuche. [Infection of chicken Embryos with the Foot-and-Mouth Disease Virus]. Dtsch Tierarztl Wochenschr. 15(55). 274. 235-236 (1948). [Translated to English by A. Finnegan (2019)]

23   Traub, E., Schneider, B., Zuchtung des Virus der Maul- und Klauenseuche im bebruteten Huhnerei. [Breeding of the Virus of Foot-and-Mouth Disease Virus in Chicken Embryos]. Z Naturforsch B. May-Jun; 3 (5-6):178-87. (1948) [Translated to English by A. Finnegan (2019)]

24   Central Intelligence Agency (CIA) Intelligence Reports: *Installations of the Serum-Werk VEB Dessau (Formerly ASID), East Germany 1953 (CIA Information Report)*. *Central Intelligence Agency (CIA)*, Reading Room, 2006. Retrieved from: https://www.cia.gov/library/readingroom/document/cia-rdp82-00457r016300350010-6

25   Ibid.

26   Ido, Y, et al. "THE RAT AS A CARRIER OF SPIROCHAETA ICTEROHAEMORRHAGIAE, THE CAUSATIVE AGENT OF WEILS DISEASE (SPIROCHAETOSIS ICTEROHAEMORRHAGICA)." The Journal of Experimental Medicine, The Rockefeller University Press, 1 Sept. 1917, https://www.ncbi.nlm.nih.gov/pubmed/19868153

27   National Archives, Joint Intelligence Objectives Agency, J.I.O.A. Administrative Records. (1950). Memorandum on Anne Bürger, C. F. Berrens, Naval Medical Research Institute, to Chief of Naval Operations, 27 November 1950, Navy Escape Clause (RG 330). NARS.

28   Central Intelligence Agency (CIA) Intelligence Reports: *Installations of the Serum-Werk VEB Dessau (Formerly ASID), East Germany 1953 (CIA Information Report)*. *Central Intelligence Agency (CIA)*, Reading Room, 2006. Retrieved from: https://www.cia.gov/library/readingroom/document/cia-rdp82-00457r016300350010-6.

29   National Archives. Joint-Intelligence Objectives Agency file on Erich Traub (RG 330). NARS. Joint Intelligence Objectives Agency (JIOA), JIOA Administrative Records. (1949-54).

30   Traub, E. & K. Beller. *Untersuchungen uber die ansteckende Blutarmut der Pferde. II. Ubertragungsversuche.* [Research on equine infectious anemia. II. Transmission experiments.] Archiv fur wiss. und prakt. Tier. 77:411-422. (1942)

31   Hirschfelder, H. & J. Wolf. Die Bedeutung von Insekten und Zecken für die Epide-miologie der Maul- und Klauenseuche [The Importance of Insects and Ticks for the Epidemiology of Foot-and-Mouth Disease. Zschr. Hyg. Zool. 142-147 (1938)

32   Waldmann, O. & H. Hirschfelder. Die epizootische Bedeutung der Rattern, des Wildes, der Vögel und der Insekten für die Verbreitung der Maul- und Klauenseuche [The Epizootic Importance of Rats, the Fauna, the birds and the insects for the spread of Foot-and-Mouth Disease]. Berliner tierarztl.

33   National Archives. Joint-Intelligence Objectives Agency file on Erich Traub (RG 330). NARS. Joint Intelligence Objectives Agency (JIOA), JIOA Administrative Records. (1949-54).

34   Loftus, Personal communication. (2018)

35   Maddrell, P. Operation Matchbox and the Scientific Containment of the USSR. Intelligence and Statecraft: The Use and Limits of Intelligence in International Society (ed. Jackson, P., & J. L. Siegel), Praeger, (2005). pp. 189

36   Federal Bureau of Investigation (FBI): RG 65 Erich Traub, (Declassified FBI Investigations on the Loyalties of Erich Traub). NARA., Doc. # QO1-458431291

37   Ibid.

38   National Archives. Joint-Intelligence Objectives Agency file on Erich Traub (RG 330). NARS. Joint Intelligence Objectives Agency (JIOA), JIOA Administrative Records. (1949-54).

39   Leitenberg, Milton & R. A. Zilinskas. *The Soviet Biological Weapons Program: a History*. Harvard University Press, 2012., pp. 92-93

40   Loftus, Personal communication. (2018)

41   Traub, E., Forschritte auf dem Gebiete der Aktiven Immunisierung gegen Tierischen Viruskrankheiten. [Advances in the field of active immunization against animal virus diseases] Zentrl. Bakt. I. Orig, Bd 154. (1949).

42   National Archives. RG 65 Erich Traub, (Declassified FBI Investigations on the Loyalties of Erich Traub). Federal Bureau of Investigation (FBI): NARA., Doc. # QO1-458431291

43   National Archives. Joint-Intelligence Objectives Agency file on Erich Traub (RG 330). NARS. Joint Intelligence Objectives Agency (JIOA), JIOA Administrative Records. (1949-54).

44   Behringwerke AG. (1943, June 18). Behringwerke [Letter to The Reich Ministery of the Interior]. Insel Riems Institute, Isle of Riems, Germany.

45   National Archives, Joint Intelligence Objectives Agency, J.I.O.A. Administrative Records. (1950). Memorandum on Anne Bürger, C. F. Berrens, Naval Medical Research Institute, to Chief of Naval Operations, 27 November 1950, Navy Escape Clause (RG 330). NARS..

46   Ibid.

47   Records indicate that Traub was already a member by the time he arrived in the United States, as one month after his arrival his reports were being presented to the FMD conference in Berne, Switzerland, run by the FAO. He may have been a member as far back as the Russian occupation, but it is certain that he was by the time he reached America, indicated by the conference.

48   National Archives. *RG 65 Erich Traub,* (Declassified FBI Investigations on the Loyalties of Erich Traub). Federal Bureau of Investigation (FBI): NARA., Doc. # QO1-458431291

Chapter Nine

THE SERPENT STRIKES

THE STEALTH BIOTERRORISM OF
DR. ERICH TRAUB

Nearly all men can stand adversity, but if you want to test a man's character, give him power.

– Abraham Lincoln

On April 19, 1949, Erich Traub arrived in the United States for a high-level position under the U.S. Navy working at the Naval Medical Research Institute (NMRI) in Bethesda, Maryland, coordinating with the USDA and the U.S. Army, assisting in field studies on anti-animal agents as a supervisory bacteriologist and virologist working on a diverse range of biological agents.

An official at the Institute certified his entry and contract with the Institute, describing his importance to the United States Navy, he would "*conduct investigations* [on] *virological research with such viruses as that of lymphocytic choriomeningitis and equine encephalomyelitis. He will, with his additional background as a graduate veterinarian, assume the responsibility of specific diseases* [and] *problems as they arise in the animal colonies of the NMRI.*"[1]

The following month, Traub had a report presented in Bern, Switzerland at the 1949 conference on Foot-and-Mouth Disease (FMD) for the Food and Agriculture Organization (FAO), and the FAO presented his data on egg-adapted FMD virus.[2] Traub had been advising the Swiss government following his escape from East Germany,[3] and traveled to Switzerland in 1948 the year before his return to America.

Two months after his arrival, Traub's German Insel Riems studies of Newcastle Disease Virus and Virus N[A] from WWII with Gerhard Schramm and Werner Schäfer were completed and published as a 1949 paper "Studies on the Virus of Atypical Avian Influenza." These

---

A   Virus N is designated "N" for "negative," meaning it produced little to no antibodies

studies were mostly done in 1943 and 1944 under the Reich, but the interruption of Soviet occupation delayed its completion until 1949. In this paper, they began to characterize each component of the virus, and its antigens.[4]

This work was building off Traub's earlier work with Gottfried Pyl and Hubert Möhlmann on FMD,[5, 6] with the expertise of Schramm, who had been known for his work on the tobacco mosaic virus (TM-V).[7] By 1951, according to a declassified Intelligence report from 1952 released to this author, referring to the state of microbiological research in West Germany around that time, one section mentions the work of Schäfer and Schramm, already in the early phases of more modern genetic engineering that would have been made during the days of Insel Riems in a classified setting for the German Reich. What alarms us in this instance, however, is that both Schramm and Schäfer were still in contact with their former Insel Riems colleagues in the Soviet Zone:

> Recent work has covered the splitting of the tobacco mosaic virus, a study of the pieces, and their recombination; isolation and characterization of Newcastle disease virus and molecular [sic] of tobacco mosaic virus. Both Schramm and Schäfer, before the end of World War II, worked at the [Reich Research Institute] Reichsforschungsanstalt Insel Riems and are still in contact with members of the Riems group.[8]

There is another mention in this report which brings up an interesting parallel, to one of Erich Traub's former associates, Professor Kurt Herzberg, from the University of Greifswald, which fell under Soviet occupation with Insel Riems at the end of WWII. Herzberg, the reader may recall, was involved in experiments infecting canaries with infectious hepatitis and influenza research, which was brought up in connection with biological warfare.[9] The report reveals that Professor Herzberg was allowed to casually pack up and leave the Eastern Zone under Soviet occupation with the blessings of the government, even giving a farewell lecture before heading to West Germany. It was also thought by some that he was sent in as a scientific fifth columnist for the Soviet Union.[10] Traub's escape was equally suspect.

No suspicions were apparent to Traub's Navy superiors, however, because just six months into Traub's position at the Navy he received a favorable security progress report. Their assessment was that he posed no danger to the National Security of the United States and had a great attitude and work ethic. The Navy was obviously satisfied with the results he was producing on research & development in biological weapons.[11]

Despite this favorable security review, according to Pentagon animal disease specialist, Frank A. Todd, interviewed by the FBI in April of 1950, Erich Traub not only maintained contact with a group of his former associates in West Germany, but he maintained contact with his former Insel Riems associates still in the Soviet Zone.

Several others interviewed by the FBI, such as some of his former Rockefeller associates like Carl TenBroeck, among others, deemed Traub a definite security risk. TenBroeck was not the only one among Traub's old Rockefeller colleagues voicing a dislike of Traub, though Richard E. Shope, on the other hand, spoke of Traub in the highest of terms with great respect and admiration.[12]

Once at the Naval Institute, Traub immediately went to work on more than 40 pathogens in the realm of viruses, rickettsia, and bacteria, which had been noted by the Navy when his assistant Anne-Lise Bürger was approved to come to American shores to assist Traub.[13]

It is highly probable that Traub produced several strains of simulant germs or tracers for use in American tests, such as *Serratia marcescens*, as he often used *Serratia marcescens* in earlier experimental research to demonstrate factors about viruses like their size and filterability.[14] He also refers to vaccinia virus in comparison to his Navy studies of Newcastle Disease Virus to grow in cell-free extracts of different kinds of blood.[15] Both vaccinia virus and *Serratia marcescens* were cleared for use as standard simulants.[16] We have already discussed in earlier chapters how Traub weaponized *Serratia marcescens* (formerly called *Bacillus prodigiosis*) with Bovine Papular Stomatitis Virus in 1940,[17] a poxvirus related to the virus of smallpox and vaccinia.

Additionally, Traub began a series of experiments on Newcastle Disease Virus for the Navy with Worth I. Capps as his assistant. These were very detailed, complex studies on the immune responses and growth of Newcastle Disease Virus in the presence of different immune cells, completing several papers by 1951."[18]

Due to Traub's expertise with FMD, which became one of many effective covers for biological weapons work on Insel Riems, the same would be true for Plum Island. Traub was the godfather of Plum Island, as it had been structured after his descriptions of the setup at Insel Riems, equipped with production facilities and chicken farms nearby, as back in Germany.[19]

Not far from Plum Island, in Glastonbury, Connecticut, right next to Old Lyme, a large chicken farm, Arbor Acres, produced and supplied large quantities of chickens and eggs since WWII, and may have been supplying eggs and chickens to the USDA. It was later bought by Nelson Rockefeller in 1960. However, some years before this, and after Traub's second tenure in America, Arbor Acres, among many other chicken farms, convened with the Agricultural Research Service (ARS) to take part in special conferences by the USDA on the pathogen, *Mycoplasma gallisepticum,* and it was such a problem infecting turkeys, chickens, and contaminating eggs, that eradicating it was out of the question.[20] It is more than likely that the rise in disease was the result of Traub's live Newcastle Disease Vaccines and tests around the country with Newcastle Disease Virus feather bombs which had dropped from high altitudes laced with chicken blood infected with the virus.[21]

The Americans conducted field experiments on and around the island, as Traub had done on Riems and over foreign territory. Traub had the necessary skill, experience, and expertise to supervise biological warfare tests that mirror the tests he conducted in Germany. Kurt Blöme, the Nazi doctor in charge of biological warfare for Heinrich Himmler, revealed in earlier interviews with the Counter Intelligence Corps (CIC) that the Reich conducted field experiments with anti-crop insects like potato beetles dropped from planes,[22] and translations of historical essays on Insel Riems revealed the ongoing facilitation of FMD and rinderpest weapons.[23]

Not to mention, Traub was likewise well-equipped to supervise airborne tests with airborne pathogens, as the reader might recall that early in Traub's education in veterinary medicine, his first thesis investigated the hygiene of animal stalls in animal houses with a special focus on the air of the animal stalls, this would bring with it noteworthy experience working with airborne germs and the movement of air in certain environments.[24] He was gaining experience with this kind of work, just prior to the time that the Germans were accused of conducting clandestine airborne germ warfare tests with *Serratia marcescens* bacteria in the subways of London and Paris.[25]

Serratia marcescens was at that time thought mostly non-pathogenic but was used in open-air experiments as a simulation of how pathogenic bacteria would spread out in a given environment to show how extensive a real attack could be. In later chapters, we will cover American simulant testing activities in further depth.

These factors were relevant and form part of the reason Traub was chosen as, among other duties, a "supervisory bacteriologist" for the American military, to supervise bacterial simulant tests, listed in the JIOA (Joint Intelligence Objectives Agency) file on Erich Traub.[26]

Agents pathogenic to humans that were weaponized with antigens from FMD would also fall under the cover of agricultural research, similar to how the variants adapted to mice and chicken eggs were hidden under defense against FMD, and tested effectively as airborne mists by the Reich on Insel Riems when freeze-dried,[27] as well as carried by insects.[28] It was known that mouse passages increased the neurotropic qualities for humans and adapting it to chicken eggs could have been the method for equally adapting it to humans due to the similarities between the avian and human immune systems.[29, 30]

During WWII and the years leading up to Traub's return, British, Canadian and American personnel used Plum Island, in the Long Island Sound of New York, as well as Horn Island, off the coast of Mississippi, and a number of other state Agricultural Experiment Stations around the United States to conduct tests on anti-animal agents, with Horn Island and possibly Plum Island having worked on live agents such as brucellosis and anthrax during the war.[31, 32] The State Department then passed legislation to use Plum Island, then known as Fort Terry, to conduct work on animal diseases that could also infect humans, such as FMD Virus, Vesicular Stomatitis Virus, brucellosis, Newcastle Disease Virus, mycoplasma, among others.[33]

We know that this legislation was passed with the intention that Traub would be working there if he were brought to American shores, because during the hearing, which took place in January of 1948, a reference was made to Traub without directly naming him. It was during testimony with the Subcommittee on Foot-and-Mouth Disease of the Committee on Agriculture, between congressman Ernest K. Bramblett of California and lead scientist from the University of California, Dr. Jacob Traum, who would become one of Plum Island's early lead scientists:

> Mr. Bramblett: [...] I am rather disturbed, a little bit, but I am happy that you are in it actively, [...] because I understand we lost one of the other top world experts. He came into the American occupational zone in Germany and offered to give himself up, and he did, and they immediately took him back and gave him to one of the other countries, and since then we have not heard very much about him, if anything.
>
> Dr. Traum: Yes, he is back in the Russian zone.
>
> Mr. Bramblett: You do not hear very much from him or what he is doing there, do you?
>
> Dr: Traum: No. I think they are trying to put him to work there without any equipment. That is what I understand. I have not been there so what I tell you is just hearsay.[34]

There is no doubt that this is a direct reference to Traub because he had indeed offered himself to work for the United States, filled out a questionnaire with the veterinarian William A. Hagen, and because of his Nazi Party affiliations they gave him back,[35] he returned to the Soviet Zone and at that time, work at Insel Riems had come to a complete halt due to Stalin having his army disassemble and haul off the entire laboratory to Russia.[36]

In Michael Christopher Carroll's book on Plum Island, *Lab 257: The Disturbing Story of the Government's Secret Plum Island Germ Laboratory*, for example, he cites an unnamed source who worked at Plum Island in the early 1950s, confirming that Traub was indeed at the island conducting experiments with ticks:

> A source who worked on Plum Island in the 1950s recalls that animal handlers and a scientist released ticks outdoors on the island. "They called him the Nazi scientist, when they came in, in 1951 – they were inoculating these ticks," and a picture he once saw "shows the animal handler pointing to the area on Plum where they released the ticks."[37]

Further into the book the former Plum Island director J. J. Callis, inadvertently shoots himself in the foot, admitting to Carroll that from the early days they maintained tick colonies and had reinstated the tick colonies at the time of his interview.[38] In parallel to what Carroll brought forth in his book, the research done for this book will also show for the record that according to a 1953 University of Maryland thesis paper by Andrew J. Rogers, "A Study of the Ixodid Ticks of Northern Florida, Including the biology and Life History of Ixodes scapularis Say (Ixodidae: Acarina)," in 1951, tests and experiments with the black-legged tick were common occurrences at that time and the USDA had been collecting them routinely under their annual surveys.[39] Interestingly, it was not a known transmitter of any human disease back in 1945.[40]

Additional tests with insects through agricultural and military activities with mosquitoes can also be established as a common occurrence during this time. Plum Island was indeed breeding mosquitoes, evident in a later publication from *Mosquito News*, "*Aedes atropalpus* Breeding in Artificial Containers in Suffolk County, New York,"[41] where a mosquito survey was conducted on Plum Island, and abandoned tires still dotted the landscape from earlier tests on *Aedes atropalpus* infected with the agent of Eastern Equine Encephalitis (EEE), Venezuelan Equine Encephalitis (VEE), and avian malaria (*Plasmodium gallinaceum*).

This would indicate that Traub and the military personnel were supervising additional tests with avian malaria (*Plasmodium gallinaceum*). Traub did mention avian malaria in one of his Navy papers on Newcastle Disease Virus in different types of blood, citing the growth of it outside its normal growing conditions as a promising field for future research.[42] Additionally, he cites numerous additional insects like avian mites and lice on top of salt marsh mosquitoes as insects that transmit EEE. Since Traub was an expert on EEE, it would be unfathomable for him not to have considerable experience with insects.[43]

Additional references to his work on tickborne diseases can be found in the Navy's approval to hire his former Insel Riems technical assistant, Anne-Lise Bürger. Bürger was approved for work on American shores under contract with the Naval Research Institute to assist Traub in matters of biological warfare, with an impressive resumé in biological research, including rickettsia, a tickborne disease:

> Duties of the position to be filled by Miss Burger are concerned with the supervision of maintenance of approximately 40 strains of virus and rickettsias [sic] in serial egg and animal passages in order to provide stocks of infectious materials for experimental work in [the] virology division and other divisions of the Naval Medical Research Institute.[44]

There are, as of yet, no records showing that Bürger ever actually made it to the United States, because much of Traub's published research for the Navy lists Worth I. Capps as his technical assistant.[45] Bürger is never mentioned, nor thanked in any of his American publications, as well as the fact that Bürger published a research paper with Bernard Schneider in 1951,[46] when she had been approved in November/December of 1950. She published a follow-up paper with Schneider the same year, with her name changed to Anne-Lise Schneider, indicating she married Bernhard Schneider and stayed at Behringwerke AG.[47] It is a good probability more will be discovered at a later time, but probably not until after this book has been published.

What is significant in Bürger's file, however, is that it is here we find a direct reference to the tick-borne disease class of bacteria, rickettsia, tying a direct link to Erich Traub's Navy work, because essentially, she was to be conducting these tests *for* Erich Traub, working as his technical assistant. Moreover, this same document establishes, for the record, that there were no scientists skilled enough in America to replace the work she and Traub were doing, and this will become significant when we discuss Willy Burgdorfer's role. It states:

In view of past long association in the fields of bacteriology and virology with Dr. Erich Traub, whom she will assist at the Institute, Miss Bürger's assignment here cannot be as adequately filled by any personnel available in the United States.[48]

In Traub's declassified intelligence file from the Navy, it is once more emphasized that Traub's skill and expertise in biological warfare preparations were unmatched by anyone available in the United States:

> Dr. Traub is an eminent virologist and an authority on matters pertaining to biological warfare. His assignment to the Naval Medical Research Institute will fulfill an urgent need that cannot be met by personnel available in United States. His probable knowledge of preparations for biological warfare in other countries renders mandatory every effort to secure his services.[49]

The FBI file on Erich Traub shows that in April of 1950, he went to Washington, D.C. to attend a meeting with the National Research Council (NRC) and could be contacted through B. T. Simms, a USDA official who was involved with the research at Plum Island, whose name will come up in later chapters. However, it is here we can establish that Erich Traub was working for the USDA during his employment with the Navy.[50]

At any rate, the National Research Council was set up during war activities and put together scientific foundations which were geared toward National Defense.[51] It appears Traub was there to attend meetings and convene on the veterinary disease branch, headed by USDA officials Traub coordinated with. Additional records indicate that other branches of the NRC that worked with the Army Chemical Corps, like the Chemical-Biological Coordination Center, were focused on testing insecticides and concentrated in studies of avian malaria, indicating these were part of the animal disease tests going on at the time.[52]

In February of 1951, the FAO requested Traub's assistance in Colombia, to control an outbreak of FMD and to run an FMD laboratory for the Colombians and FAO in Bogotá. He left for several months and was planning to return in mid-summer, but returned in early September, just in time to supervise simulant tests around Plum Island as a supervisory bacteriologist and virologist for the Navy, simultaneously an employee of the USDA and FAO,[53] and it appears that this may have been done with the cooperation of the Long Island Biological Association, who was under contract with the Army

Chemical Corps steadily from October 1950 to October of 1952.[54, 55] It is interesting to note, Traub would be back and forth between Bogotá and the United States in parallel with the migratory bird patterns. In other words, he would travel to Bogotá as the birds were getting ready to migrate north, and travel north to the United States just as the birds were getting ready to fly south and this is demonstrated on an infographic that shows the migratory bird patterns between North and South America.[56]

During Traub's work in Colombia with FMD, Schäfer sends Traub cultures of FMD that had originally been given to him by Traub after his escape to West Germany. In further experiments with these cultures, Traub mentions that in the process of their experiments, the cultures had become so heavily contaminated with a certain kind of bacteria, that even heavy doses of Penicillin and Streptomycin failed to eliminate them. This would not be surprising for contamination with spirochetes, though he never mentions what the contaminating bacteria actually was.[57]

Tests with FMD and anti-animal agents were initiated in the fall of 1951, on Plum Island, and he would supervise bacterial simulant tests reaching across the United States, as well as those on crops, such as tests in the mid-West.[58] Traub also had a hand in the testing of Newcastle Disease Virus (NDV) in October that year, over chicken farms owned by the University of Wisconsin.[59]

A 1958 security investigation by the FBI can place Erich Traub on Plum Island and listed as an employee of the Greenport, Long Island, NY Agricultural Experiment Station, which is Plum Island.[60] He was also at the Beltsville, Maryland Agricultural Experiment Station for the Agricultural Research Service (ARS) of the USDA, working as an employee of the ARS when it was established in 1953, formerly known as the Bureau of Animal Industry (BAI). Traub worked on Vesicular Stomatitis Virus (VSV), a virus that is one of the *differential diagnoses* to FMD.[61] As the reader might recall, avian spirochetosis likewise served as the *differential diagnosis* to Newcastle Disease.[62]

Traub entered the testing phase for his work on vesicular stomatitis in 1950,[63] working with L.O. Mott, a top USDA official who worked with the Bureau of Animal Industry in 1950, which became the Agricultural Research Service (ARS) in 1953. Mott worked extensively on the Anaplasmosis and tick fever program the USDA had been running,[64] and they were supplied ticks from the University of Florida's tick farm, and the black-legged tick was a prime candidate since it wasn't known as a transmitter of human disease.[65] After Traub's second run on American shores, the black-legged tick would be a primary vector for some of the country's most tormenting infectious diseases.

My source John Loftus was the first to expose the Lyme disease connection to biological warfare in 1982, in *The Belarus Secret,* and even noted it was being spread by ticks before it was publicly acknowledged, and the Plum Island experiments had been directed and overseen by one of our allies in British intelligence, a man named Donald Maclean, a confirmed double agent for Soviet Intelligence when he defected to Moscow in 1951:

> A few months after it appeared in my book, scientists employed by the US Government published a report that confirmed that Lyme Disease was indeed being spread by ticks. However other government officials lied and denied any American tick experiments ever took place on Plum Island. It was a half-lie to conceal a sensitive political scandal.
>
> The Plum Island experiments had been carried out by one of our allies in British intelligence, a man named Donald MacLean. He was confirmed as a double agent for Soviet Intelligence when he defected to Moscow in 1951.[...] [66]

Donald Maclean had been instrumental in the formation of joint-agreements between Britain, Canada, and the United States to share research and collaborate on nuclear, chemical, and biological development and testing, and all Top-Secret information relevant to it. Maclean was also appointed head of Chancery at the British Embassy in Cairo, Egypt,[67] a geographic location that would become significant as an intermediary area for biological warfare research taking place in Africa under the Navy's special unit, NAMRU-3.[68] John Loftus is here saying that Maclean was directing these tests, though not actually the one physically conducting the experiments, this was being done by other scientists after WWII, under his direction, and it was Erich Traub who supervised these tests when he came to America under Operation Paperclip which Loftus revealed in *The Belarus Secret* in 1982:

> Even more disturbing are the records of the Nazi germ warfare scientists who came to America. They experimented with poison ticks dropped from planes to spread rare diseases. I received some information suggesting that the US tested some of these poison ticks on the Plum Island artillery range off the coast of Connecticut during the early 1950s. I explored the old

spies' hypothesis that the poison ticks were the source of the Lyme disease spirochete, and that migrating waterfowl were the vectors that carried the ticks from Plum Island all up and down the Eastern Seaboard. Most of the germ warfare records have been shredded, but there is a top-secret US document confirming that "clandestine attacks on crops and animals" took place at this time. The Lyme disease outbreak in America was monitored secretly under the cover of a New England health study.[69]

Their extensive expeditions collecting and cataloguing ticks and various arthropods, along with disease agents passing between the insects and host, such as the fowl tick, *Argas persica,* a natural host to the agent of avian spirochetosis, *Borrelia anserina.*[70] NAMRU-3 worked closely with the University of Cairo, and both NAMRU-3 and the University of Cairo, joined in researching agents like avian spirochetosis, having also worked closely with the University of California and the USDA.[71]

Many years earlier, in 1938, ticks and insects like biting flies were researched at Insel Riems for their potential to spread FMD, published as "The Significance of Insects and Ticks for the Epidemiology of Foot-and-Mouth Disease."[72] A second paper, "The Epizootic Significance of Rats, Game, Birds and Insects for the Spread of Foot-and-Mouth Disease," was also published.[73] In these papers, they admit the tick is a long-term carrier of FMD, claiming negative results in transmitting the disease to guinea pigs, but say nothing of testing it in cattle. They equally downplayed its significance in the wild animals and birds, though admit that birds can sometimes act as carriers. The paper also doubted their significance in the biting flies and ticks, even as they are long-term carriers. These few papers may have been intentionally misleading to deflect attention and downplay their significance in order to cloak some of their military research.

I say this because their earlier results at Insel Riems were contradicted much later. Multiple hazards in the spread of FMD had been identified by the FAO by 1994, according to an FAO publication, "Foot-and-Mouth Disease: Sources of Outbreaks and Hazard Categorization of Modes of Virus Transmission," ticks had been listed as a high hazard in the spread of the virus.[74] Traub's work at Insel Riems adapting FMD Virus to mice and chicken eggs would also bring updated mutations and new qualities with new potential in both ticks and wild animals.

ERICH TRAUB'S TICK WEAPONS & WEAPONIZED LYME DISEASE

Sometime during Traub's return to American shores putting his talents to use for the American military and their cooperation with Britain and Canada, weaponized pathogens and insects were unleashed on the very countries Traub was supposed to be helping. This will become more evident in the following chapters. On its face, researchers would face extreme difficulty pasting together the history of Traub's expertise on ticks and tick-borne disease, as the evidence is very well-hidden, scattered in obscure places, and in the German language. However, the truth will become more evident as I walk the reader through the stages that blessed these weapons with the expertise and signature of Erich Traub.

We will start with Lymphocytic Choriomeningitis Virus (LCM). When Traub discovered LCM virus, it was at a time when he realized he could awaken sleeping viruses already within the host with a foreign protein or concentrated antigens suspended in broth, injected into the mouse's brain. This caused a septic shock that awakened LCM virus from dormancy already in the mice, activating it and spreading it to the other mice and the animal keepers who worked at the Institute, causing an epidemic from scratch.

As this occurred, he noticed that after the initial illness or fever period in which the mice are visibly ill, it would recede for a time but it damaged the mouse's immune system, causing a persistent, chronic infection with little to no antibodies. This also brought on additional infections with other bacteria like mycoplasma as mixed infections. The mothers with damaged immune systems would then pass the LCM virus to their newborns, and these mice were always born infected without antibodies or noticeable signs of disease but they came down with chronic neurodegenerative diseases later in life. They could spread virulent LCM virus without any sign of disease. Cancer would also rise in the infected colonies.

He later realized that the lipid portions in the surface proteins of the virus allow for it to damage the immune system and mutate itself rapidly to escape the immune system defenses.[75] This agent, an antigen or lipoprotein (literally "lipid protein") found on the surface of certain pathogens, would later be synthesized as a biochemical adjuvant called Pam-3-Cys (P3C).[76] P3C would mimic the effect of agents carrying this lipid portion to affect the immune system in the same damaging manner by stimulating certain receptors of the immune system.[B] This is also found on the outer surface proteins of the Lyme Disease agent, *Borrelia burgdorferi*.[77]

B   These receptors are known as toll-like receptors, and there are 10 known toll-like

Eventually, what he discovered was baptized *"immune tolerance,"* but he was not credited for it and the Nobel Prize was given to two other scientists much later for what Traub discovered, which we will cover in later chapters. It is called immune *tolerance* because the immune system is suppressed and forced to tolerate harmful pathogens it should be keeping out of the body, and these pathogens then integrate into the central nervous system and brain, the core of our physical being.

When Traub returned to Germany to accept a position at the University of Giessen under Professor Dr. Karl Beller in 1938, by 1939 Traub became well-versed in tickborne diseases and those that could be transmitted by hard-bodied ticks like *Rickettsia ruminantium* (heartwater), which is closely related to the tickborne disease and common Lyme co-infection, Human Monocytic Ehrliciosis (*Ehrlicia chaffeensis*),[78] as well as the co-infecting blood parasites like *Babesia* which causes human babesiosis. He was taught about a complex disease condition that had been seen in dogs sick with a mix of infections like *Babesia, Ehrlichia, Bartonella,* and *Leishmaniasis*. With the exception of *Leishmania*, these were transmitted by hard-bodied ticks that do not feed on humans, but it served as an important animal model for a human biological weapon.[C] We know Traub was versed in this expertise because he was working directly under Beller at this time when Beller was putting the chapter together for the textbook.[79]

Beller showed Traub how this mix of infections caused a similar condition as the *immune tolerance* seen in his Rockefeller mice, how complex and challenging it became for diagnosis for the average physician and veterinarian when multiple, mixed infections produced multiple overlapping diseases simultaneously with little to no antibodies. He was also shown that the genus of relapsing fever spirochetes (*Borrelia*) could occasionally be transmitted by hard-bodied ticks like the brown dog tick, which is not a nuisance to humans.

With a few modifications however, Traub could easily adapt the spirochete to take to a hard-bodied tick that feeds on humans, such as the *Ixodes* ticks or the *Amblyomma* ticks. Likewise, other German researchers from Berlin had found the avian spirochete could even be transmitted by *Culex* mosquitoes.[80]

---

receptors in the human immune system. They are often stimulated in various combinations and pairs called ligands. The TLRs known to be responsible for immune tolerance are the combinations of TLR2/TLR1, and TLR2/TLR6.

C   It is incontrovertible that *Bartonella* can be spread by ticks, as many researchers have demonstrated it, but in other instances these can also infect as secondary, opportunistic pathogens that develop in the immunosuppressed.

The same year, Traub became focused on the study of viral diseases of birds under his German mentor. Likewise, he had to be well-versed in all of the *differential diagnoses* of these avian diseases, so he could tell the viral diseases he specialized in, apart from other diseases that produced similar symptoms. Only an expert could tell them apart. He became especially fluent in the science of avian influenza, also called fowl plague virus, and later to become an expert in its close relatives, Newcastle Disease Virus and Virus N.[81]

When Professor Beller had Traub take Werner Schäfer under his wing the same year, Traub had him procure a strain of the spirochetes that caused avian spirochetosis (*Borrelia anserina*, then known as *Spirochaeta gallinarum*) from Rockefeller funded psychiatrist Franz Jahnel, a spirochete expert at the Kaiser-Wilhelm Institute. It was brought to Traub for research and teaching purposes. It is here where Traub can be found in possession of the spirochetes used to make the agent later known as Lyme Disease.

Much later, we can see that the Lyme Disease spirochete was in fact related to the avian spirochete when comparing DNA from the flagella[D] of the spirochete. It was published in a 1989 paper "Shared Flagellar Epitopes of *Borrelia burgdorferi* and *Borrelia anserina*."[82] Furthermore, striking relationships were likewise shown in a 1995 paper "A Morphological Characterization of *Borrelia anserina*."[83] *Borrelia burgdorferi*, *Borrelia garinii*, and *Borrelia afzelii*, are the three species of *Borrelia* spirochetes known to produce Lyme Disease, and these are most closely related to the parent strain *Borrelia anserina*.[E] This was reflected in several additional publications.[84, 85] Furthermore, the Lyme disease spirochete is maintained and carried by many different birds, further proving the Lyme disease spirochete came from *Borrelia anserina*.[86]

However, as it was, *Borrelia anserina* was not normally transmitted by hard-bodied ticks, nor known to infect humans. It was also not normally infectious to cattle, livestock, rodents, or mice. The spirochete would have to infect these kinds of animals if it were to maintain itself in the environment. It had to infect these animals to provide a continuous source of disease for ticks to draw from in the environment. These animals would

D   **Flagella**: Flagella are hairlike filaments or protein structures found in bacteria, archaea, and eukaryotes, but most commonly they are found in bacteria. They are used like small whips to propel itself in its microbial environment.

E   Kathleen Dickson of TruthCures was the first to make this connection between *Borrelia burgdorferi* and *Borrelia anserina*, so that credit belongs to her, see: Dickson, K. "CRIMINAL CHARGE SHEETS JUNE 2017 Lobbying for a Hearing for Referral to the USDOJ for a Prosecution of the Lyme Disease Crimes." 2017. Published at: https://docs.wixstatic.com/ugd/47b066_01d68b1309ae457b81df1e06e6beae1e.pdf, However, I am adding to her discovery by now showing it was in Traub's possession and the agent was then in his possession and he used very original means to adapt it to new hosts before the advent of modern genetic engineering.

be important *reservoirs* of disease in the targeted environment. That way, the ticks would have an endless supply of these pathogens to infect and re-infect them so they could keep infecting their human hosts.

Franz Jahnel had noted a researcher in 1912 who was successful getting the avian spirochetes to infect mice temporarily, but it would not maintain the infection.[87] Traub would need the spirochete to infect not only the mice, but rodents, deer, livestock, and as many animals as possible that could help promote its survival and spread in the wild. If the spirochete was to become an effective weapon, it would have to show broad-spectrum pathogenicity, that is, infect a broad range of animals.

That's where Foot-and-Mouth Disease Virus comes in. FMD contains surface proteins known as *fusion proteins*,[88] which allow for it to penetrate cells by cell fusion, fusing to the cell tissue and incorporating the host carbohydrates into its own makeup. These fusion proteins are also found on a wide variety of other pathogens and viruses such as LCM Virus,[89] Newcastle Disease Virus,[90] Influenza Virus,[91] among many others.

These viruses can then be used to adapt a pathogen to a new species of animal it didn't previously infect. In fact, we can show that one of Traub's Iranian protégés, G. K. Kanhai, was later taught this method by Traub in the 1970s,[92] before Kanhai published a paper of his own using Sendai virus, an influenza virus, to adapt a rickettsia of cattle to hamsters when it didn't previously infect hamsters.[93] The mechanisms involved in this process are rather complex and esoteric as science, but it has to do with fusing different kinds of animal cells together using animal viruses, and for the sake of brevity, we will not be explaining the process in this book.[F]

In effect, these animal viruses could be used to adapt the avian spirochete (*Borrelia anserina*) to different animals that would be responsible for promoting its spread in the environment. This is the reason why viruses and viral proteins would be involved, and after all, while Traub's expertise was diverse, he was mostly focused on virus research. The lipid proteins found on the Lyme Disease spirochetes that caused immune tolerance, were also present in LCM virus, FMD virus, Influenza, Equine Infectious Anemia Virus, and many others that Traub worked with.[94]

Bovine Papular Stomatitis Virus, the poxvirus that Traub and Beller had earlier used to weaponize the simulant bacteria, *Serratia marcescens*,[95] may have equally been used to that effect. The *Borrel-*

F   If the reader is interested to learn more about this, it has to do with what are called *heterokaryons*. For more, see: HARRIS, H, and J F WATKINS. "HYBRID CELLS DERIVED FROM MOUSE AND MAN: ARTIFICIAL HETEROKARYONS OF MAMMALIAN CELLS FROM DIFFERENT SPECIES." *Nature* vol. 205 (1965): 640-6. doi:10.1038/205640a0

ia burgdorferi spirochete has unique plasmids[G] in their outer surface proteins (lipoproteins) with genetic material comparable to those of poxviruses and are unique in regard to bacterial plasmids.[96] Other researchers have suggested some of these linear plasmids consist of what are termed *proviruses* and *prophages*,[97] remnants of viruses that infect a bacteria or spirochete without destroying it and can actually help promote its survival by adding additional factors in favor of the pathogen to evade the immune system and assist the pathogen in overwhelming the host.[98, 99] An unusual paper from 1947 also demonstrated that the parasitic nematode *Trichinella spiralis* could transmit the LCM Virus to humans,[100] and this may have been another agent that Traub put his efforts into, since it can contaminate livestock and wild animals like deer and other animals eaten by hunters.

Interestingly, the late Harvard Professor and one of the world's leading experts on biological weapons once cited a Russian bioweaponeer who relayed Russian bioweapons research to create a *"double pathogen,"* a bacterial pathogen like plague (*Yersinia pestis*) harboring pathogenic virus like Venezuelan Equine Encephalitis Virus (VEE), that is activated by the antibiotic tetracycline, so that when the target becomes sick with plague bacteria and takes an antibiotic like tetracycline, it destroys the bacteria but activates virulent VEE virus from within its plasmids.[101] It is an intriguing prospect to suggest that Traub may have already accomplished this.

At any rate, the *Borrelia* genus of spirochetes, to which the agent of Lyme Disease belongs, sheds a bewildering array of these immune damaging lipids in small particles called blebs, so in some ways, there would be no need for genetically altering the *Borrelia anserina* spirochete any further if it could already infect humans, hard-bodied ticks, and all the animals responsible for its spread. Since it did not, the use of animal viruses to adapt the spirochete to a broad range of new hosts and hard-bodied ticks that feed on humans would guarantee its promotion in the environment. Over many decades, there would be a snowball effect, where the agent is thriving exponentially more with each passing decade, making some think it was a factor of climate change rather than nefarious biowarfare activities.[102]

Additionally, since Traub was putting a virtual cocktail of disease in these ticks, he would not only need to adapt the spirochete to these new ticks and new animal hosts to become reservoirs of disease, but likewise the tick-borne co-infections like rickettsia, protozoal blood

---

G **Plasmid**: a small cellular inclusion consisting of a ring of DNA that is not in a chromosome but is capable of autonomous replication

parasites (*Babesia*, avian malaria), *Bartonella*, *Leptospira*, and any other co-infection, would be helpful in creating an environment in which the cocktail of pathogens are able to act in synergy and overwhelm the host together while benefitting each other. Evidence suggests these tickborne co-infections came from diverse animals such as horses, dogs, and cattle.[103, 104] Therefore, he would also have to adapt these agents to birds so they could be carried and spread by the birds, and thus, a virus like Newcastle Disease Virus or avian influenza could be used to adapt a pathogen only affecting cattle to a new host in birds. The possibilities were endless.

If Traub wanted to use ticks that feed on humans, he would need to adapt the cocktail of disease agents to the other animals and birds that it feeds on.[105] Certain animal viruses could be used with ease for this process, and it became easier when multiple disease agents were used simultaneously because they tended to act synergistically in each other's benefit once the host's immune system defenses were overwhelmed by the mix of infections.

Most of the pathogens Traub worked with had nasty lipid components that suppressed and evaded the immune system, while some like *Bartonella* had very toxic proteins called endotoxin that made the host feel horrible,[106] but yet, ironically, the damaged immune system allowed for minimal antibodies and very little visible signs of disease as it integrated into the lymph nodes, brain, and central nervous system. Even routine bloodwork would not reveal the multiple disease agents overwhelming the host. Traub later published about this lack of abnormal bloodwork and absence of antibodies in mice chronically infected with LCM virus in 1960.[107]

It can be said with confidence that Traub's weaponized ticks and tick-borne disease had several developments, resulting in several circulating strains. When Russia took Insel Riems, they took strains with them. European strains of the Lyme disease agent were already spreading in Germany and Eastern Europe before he came to American shores and produced the American strains. Furthermore, Donald Maclean and British Intelligence would have been given cultures from what Traub took with him in 1945 when applying for work in the West, as well as in 1948 when he made his escape. Donald Maclean is said to have been directing Plum Island tests just after WWII up to 1948 when he left for Cairo, Egypt, and was vacationing on Long Island, NY, just south of Plum Island, during his work in America.

Therefore, the presence of the Lyme disease agent just after 1945 or before Traub's return to American shores would still be in line with this story, that British Intelligence took strains from him early on when WWII just ended and Traub continued developing and spreading it when he returned to American shores for full-time work. Other researchers have also suggested tick-infested hides that were sent to American ports just after WWII, and since they took his strains to Russia when they captured Insel Riems, this would also still be in line with this story.[108] It served as the largescale biological terrorism against the West by Stalin and the communists, the "Day X" described by the former KGB agent turned defector, Alexander Kouzminov.[109] Attempts to disprove the biological warfare connection by academic researchers like Sam Telford and David H. Persing, will be covered in later chapters.

In regard to Willy Burgdorfer, he was not the man responsible for weaponizing Lyme spirochetes, as he did not have the skill and understanding of animal disease and their hosts like Traub and his technical assistants had. In fact, it is clear that Burgdorfer did not know what he was dealing with initially, since he accidentally infected himself in the laboratory early on in his work with the agent.[110] As we have covered previously, Anne Bürger's approval stated that there were no scientists in America with the level of skill that Traub and Bürger held.[111] Moreover, we will later see how an important poultry conference discussing avian spirochetosis and bioterrorism against the United States in 1953,[112] already took place before Burgdorfer was able to sign on to biodefense work in 1954.[113] It is possible that he could have taken part in later simulant testing that spread Traub's weaponized ticks, but he was probably an unwitting participant. Furthermore, Burgdorfer would be the last person chosen to publicly discover the agent if he had been involved in the blunder.

The weapon, in essence, was the lipid portion found in the outer surface proteins of certain pathogens and viruses that stimulated the respective immune system receptors responsible for throwing the immune system into disarray.[114]

Traub did not create them, per se, but he stumbled upon their effects in LCM Virus and manipulated what nature provided to make very effective weapons for crippling populations with incapacitating strategic bioweapons. The spirochetes would deliver the toxic surface proteins which then would awaken the many sleeping viruses within us, causing complex, chronic neurodegenerative diseases, while equally promoting psychiatric disorders, mental health problems, and cancers, just like Traub had done to his little mice back at the Rockefeller Institute in 1935.[115, 116, 117]

Endnotes

1   National Archives. Joint-Intelligence Objectives Agency file on Erich Traub (RG 330). NARS. Joint Intelligence Objectives Agency (JIOA), JIOA Administrative Records. (1949-54).

2   Traub, E. La Culture du Virus Aphtheux sur Embryons de Poulet. Proceedings of the Conference on production of foot and mouth disease vaccines at Berne 1949, convened by the Office International des Epizootics Bull. Off. internat. Epiz, 31: 470-483. 1949

3   National Archives. Joint-Intelligence Objectives Agency file on Erich Traub (RG 330). NARS. Joint Intelligence Objectives Agency (JIOA), JIOA Administrative Records. (1949-54).

4   Traub, E., Schäfer, W. & Schramm, G., Untersuchen uber das Virus der Atypischen Geflugelpest. [Studies of the Virus of Atypical Fowl Plague]. Z. Naturforsch B. 157-167 (1949).

5   Traub, E. & G. Pyl. Untersuchungen über das komplementbindende Antigen bei Maul-und Klauenseuche. [Studies on the complement-binding antigen in foot-and-mouth disease] Z. Immun. Forsch.104, 158-165. (1943).

6   Traub, E. & H. Möhlmann. Typenbestimmung bei Maul- und Klauenseuche mit Hilfe der Komplementbindungsprobe. I. Mitt.: Versuche mit Seren und Antigenen von Meerschweinchen. [Type determination in foot-and-mouth disease with the help of the complement fixation sample. I. Communication. Experiments with serums and antigens of guinea pigs.] Zbl. Bakt., Abt. I Orig. 283–298 (1943).

7   Schramm, Gerhard, and Hans Friedrich-Freksa. 1941. "Die Präcipitinreaktion Des Tabakmosaikvirus Mit Kaninchen- Und Schweineantiserum." Hoppe-Seyler´s Zeitschrift Für Physiologische Chemie 270 (5-6): 233–46. https://doi.org/10.1515/bchm2.1941.270.5-6.233.

8   Central Intelligence Agency (CIA) Intelligence Reports: Microbiology Research and Laboratories from Cities in West Germany. C06492381. Central Intelligence Agency (CIA), Declassified and released directly to A. Finnegan 2023.

9   Eberle, Henrik. "Ein Wertvolles Instrument": Die Universität Greifswald Im Nationalsozialismus. Bohlau Verlag, 2015., pp. 537

10   Central Intelligence Agency (CIA) Intelligence Reports: Microbiology Research and Laboratories from Cities in West Germany. C06492381. Central Intelligence Agency (CIA), Declassified and released directly to A. Finnegan 2023.

11   National Archives. Joint-Intelligence Objectives Agency file on Erich Traub (RG 330). NARS. Joint Intelligence Objectives Agency (JIOA), JIOA Administrative Records. (1949-54).

12   National Archives. RG 65 Erich Traub, (Declassified FBI Investigations on the Loyalties of Erich Traub). Federal Bureau of Investigation (FBI): NARA., Doc. # QO1-458431291

13   National Archives, Joint Intelligence Objectives Agency, J.I.O.A. Administrative Records. (1950). Memorandum on Anne Bürger, C. F. Berrens, Naval Medical Research Institute, to Chief of Naval Operations, 27 November 1950, Navy Escape Clause (RG 330). NARS.

14   Traub, E. A Filterable Virus Recovered from White Mice. Science, 81. (2099), 298-299. doi:10.1126/science.81.2099.298. (1935).

15   Traub, E., & W.I. Capps. Studies on the in vitro multiplication of Newcastle disease virus in chicken blood. III. A stablizing substance for Newcastle disease virus present in chicken and mammalian blood cells. NMRI Research Report. National Naval Medical Center. Bethesda, MD. (1951) NMRI Research Report. Project NM 005 048.11.03.

16   Department of National Defence (Canada), Biological Warfare. OPERATION LAC correspondence. Tripartite Reports pp. 233 (000232) http://data2.archives.ca/e/e443/e011063033.pdf

17   Traub, E., et al. Untersuchungen über die Stomatitis papulosa des Rinde. [Studies on bovine papular stomatitis] Zeit. Infek. Krank. Hyg. Haus. 56 (2): 85-103. (1940). [Translated to English by A. Finnegan, 2019]

18   Traub, E., & W.I. Capps. Studies on the in vitro multiplication of Newcastle disease virus in chicken blood. III. A stablizing substance for Newcastle disease virus present in chicken and mammalian blood cells. NMRI Research Report. National Naval Medical Center. Bethesda, MD. (1951) NMRI Research Report. Project NM 005 048.11.03.

19   Memorandum "Conversation Between Doctors H. W. Schoening, M. S. Shahan and Erich Traub," M. S. Shahan, 10 December 1952.

20   Mycoplasma Gallisepticum Infection in Chickens and Turkeys : Report of the Second Study Gruop Conference : United States. Agricultural Research Service. Internet Archive, [Washington, D.C.] : U.S. Dept. of Agriculture ; 1 Jan. 1965, Retrieved from: http://www.archive. org/details/mycoplasmagallis9155unit/page/n1

21   United States, Congress, DEPARTMENT OF THE ARMY. "U.S ARMY ACTIVITIES IN THE UNITED STATES BIOLOGICAL WARFARE PROGRAMS 1942-1977." U.S ARMY ACTIVITIES IN THE UNITED STATES BIOLOGICAL WARFARE PROGRAMS 1942-1977, vol. 1, Dept. of the Army; Fort Detrick, 1977.

22   National Archives. Joint intelligence Objectives Agency (JIOA), JIOA Administrative Records. (n.d.). Interview of ALSOS Scientists: Dr. Kurt Blöme (RG 330 INSCOM dossier XE001248). NARS.

23   Lichte, J. U. (1983). Die Forschung auf der Insel Riems von 1933 bis 1945 unter besonderer Berücksichtigung der NS-Zwangsarbeiter (Inaugural Dissertation). Nordenham, Germany: The Medical Faculty of the Ernst-Moritz-Arndt University of Greifswald.

24   Traub, E. Hygienische Untersuchungen in Tierställen unter besonderer Berücksichtigung der Stalluft. [Hygienic Investigations of Animal Stables with Special Consideration for Stable Air.] Zeitschrift für Infektionskrankheiten. Haus. Vol. 45, No. 1. 1-35. (1932). [Translated to English by A. Finnegan, 2019]

25   H.W. Steed, 'Aerial Warfare: Secret German Plans'. The Nineteenth Century and After, 116 (7) (1934), pp. 1–16

26   National Archives. Joint-Intelligence Objectives Agency file on Erich Traub (RG 330). NARS. Joint Intelligence Objectives Agency (JIOA), JIOA Administrative Records. (1949-54).

27   Eberle, Henrik. "Ein Wertvolles Instrument": Die Universität Greifswald Im Nationalsozialismus. Bohlau Verlag, 2015. [pp. 538-541]

28   "Regional Project for the Eradication of Amblyomma Variegatum/Heartwater from the Caribbean. Project Profile : IICA-Guyana : Free Download, Borrow, and Streaming." Internet Archive, IICA Biblioteca Venezuela, Retrieved from: http://www.archive.org/details/bub_gb_QzwqAAAAYAAJ/page/n1

29   Kohonen, P., et al. "Avian Model for B-Cell Immunology ? New Genomes and Phylotranscriptomics." Scandinavian Journal of Immunology, vol. 66, no. 2-3, 2007, pp. 113–121., doi:10.1111/j.1365-3083.2007.01973.x.

30   Weill, Jean-Claude et al. "A bird's eye view on human B cells." Seminars in immunology vol. 16,4 (2004): 277-81. doi:10.1016/j.smim.2004.08.007

31   Cochrane, Raymond C. "DTIC ADB228585: History of the Chemical Warfare Service in World War II. Biological Warfare Research in the United States, Volume 2: Defense Technical Information Center: Free Download, Borrow, and Streaming." Internet Archive, 1 Nov. 1947, Retrieved from: http://www.archive.org/details/DTIC_ADB228585/page/n27

32   United States, Congress, DEPARTMENT OF THE ARMY. "U.S ARMY ACTIVITIES IN THE UNITED STATES BIOLOGICAL WARFARE PROGRAMS 1942-1977." U.S ARMY ACTIVITIES IN

THE UNITED STATES BIOLOGICAL WARFARE PROGRAMS 1942-1977, vol. 1, Dept. of the Army; Fort Detrick, 1977.

33   "The National Animal Disease Laboratory : United States. Agricultural Research Service. Animal Disease and Parasite Research Division : Free Download, Borrow, and Streaming." Internet Archive. January 01, 1961. Accessed August 03, 2019. https://archive.org/details/nationalanimaldi871unit. pp. 1

34   United States, Department of Agriculture. (1970, January 1). Legislative history, public law 496 - 80th Congress, Chapter 229 - 2D session, S. 2038 : United States, Department of Agriculture, office of the general counsel. Internet Archive. https://archive.org/details/PL80496/page/n51/mode/2up

35   National Archives. RG 65 Erich Traub, (Declassified FBI Investigations on the Loyalties of Erich Traub). Federal Bureau of Investigation (FBI): NARA., Doc. # QO1-458431291

36   Central Intelligence Agency (CIA) Intelligence Reports: THE BACTERIOLOGICAL RESEARCH INSTITUTE ON THE ISLAND OF RIEMS. CIA-RDP83-00415R002200020014-9. Central Intelligence Agency (CIA), Reading Room, 2011. Retrieved from: https://www.cia.gov/readingroom/document/cia-rdp83-00415r002200020014-9

37   Carroll, M. C. (2004). Lab 257: The disturbing story of the governments secret and deadly virus research facility. New York: Morrow., pp. 15-16

38   Ibid., pp. 23-24

39   Rogers, Andrew Jackson. "A Study of the Ixodid Ticks of Northern Florida, Including the Biology and Life History of Ixodes Scapularis Say (Ixodidae: Acarina)." University of Maryland & University of Florida, University of Maryland, 1953

40   Bishopp, F. C., & Trembley, H. L. (1945). Distribution and Hosts of Certain North American Ticks. The Journal of Parasitology, 31(1), 1. doi:10.2307/3273061

41   White, D. J., and C. P. White. "Aedes Atropalpus Breeding in Artificial Containers in Suffolk County, New York." Internet Archive, Mosquito News Vol. 40 No. 1, 1 Jan. 1980, Retrieved from: http://www.archive.org/details/cbarchive_117472_aedesatropalpusbreedinginartif1980/page/n1

42   Traub, E., & W.I. Capps. Studies on the in vitro multiplication of Newcastle disease virus in chicken blood. III. A stablizing substance for Newcastle disease virus present in chicken and mammalian blood cells. NMRI Research Report. National Naval Medical Center. Bethesda, MD. (1951) NMRI Research Report. Project NM 005 048.11.03.

43   Traub, E. & F. Kesting. Ueber die Ausscheidung des E.E.E.-Virus und das gelegentliche Vorkommen von Kontaktinfektionen bestimmter Art bei Mausen. [Secretion of the EEE-virus and occasional incidence of certain contact infections in mice]. Zbl. bakt. Abt. I. Orig. 166 (6). 462-475. (1956). [Translated to English by A. Finnegan (2019)]

44   National Archives, Joint Intelligence Objectives Agency, J.I.O.A. Administrative Records. (1950). Memorandum on Anne Bürger, C. F. Berrens, Naval Medical Research Institute, to Chief of Naval Operations, 27 November 1950, Navy Escape Clause (RG 330). NARS.

45   Traub, E., & Capps, W. I. Experiments with chick embryo-adapted foot-and-mouth disease virus and a method for the rapid adaptation. National Naval Medical Center. Bethesda, MD. (1953) U.S. NAVY Project NM. NMRI Memorandum Report. Project NM 000 018.07

46   Schneider, Bernard, and Anne L. Bürger. "Uber Das Serologische Verhalten Des Maul- Und Klauenseuche-Huhnereivirus Und Seine Verwendung in Form Der Adsorbat-vakzine Zur Immunisierung Von Rindern [Serological Behavior of Foot-and-mouth Disease Hen-egg Virus and Its Use in the Form of Absorbate Vaccine to Immunize Cattle]." Mh Prakt. Tier 3, no. 35 (1951): 35-40. Accessed August 3, 2019

47   Schneider, B. & A. L. Schneider. Züchtung des Virus der Maul- und Klauenseuche vom Typ A (Vallée) im bebrüteten Hühnerei. Mhefte prakt. Tierhk. 3, 206. (1951)

48   National Archives, Joint Intelligence Objectives Agency, J.I.O.A. Administrative Records. (1950). Memorandum on Anne Bürger, C. F. Berrens, Naval Medical Research Institute, to Chief of Naval Operations, 27 November 1950, Navy Escape Clause (RG 330). NARS

49   National Archives. Joint-Intelligence Objectives Agency file on Erich Traub (RG 330). NARS. Joint Intelligence Objectives Agency (JIOA), JIOA Administrative Records. (1949-54).

50   National Archives. RG 65 Erich Traub, (Declassified FBI Investigations on the Loyalties of Erich Traub). Federal Bureau of Investigation (FBI): NARA., Doc. # QO1-458431291

51   National Academy of Sciences - http://www.nasonline.org. (n.d.). History of the National Research Council. Organization of the National Research Council. https://www.nasonline.org/about-nas/history/archives/milestones-in-NAS-history/organization-of-the-nrc.html

52   National Research Council; Chemical-Biological Coordination Center. (n.d.). First symposium on chemical-biological correlation, May 26-27, 1950. The National Academies Press. https://nap.nationalacademies.org/catalog/18474/first-symposium-on-chemical-biological-correlation-may-26-27-1950

53   National Archives. Joint-Intelligence Objectives Agency file on Erich Traub (RG 330). NARS. Joint Intelligence Objectives Agency (JIOA), JIOA Administrative Records. (1949-54)., see also: National Archives. RG 65 Erich Traub, (Declassified FBI Investigations on the Loyalties of Erich Traub). Federal Bureau of Investigation (FBI): NARA., Doc. # QO1-458431291

54   Milislav. "Annual Report of the Biological Laboratory 1951." CSHL Scientific Digital Repository, Long Island Biological Association, 1 Jan. 1970, repository.cshl.edu/36632/. Retrieved from: http://repository.cshl.edu/36632/1/CSHL_AR_1951.pdf

55   MacDowell, E. Carleton (October 1952) First quarterly progress report of research carried out by Long Island Biological Association for the Biological Department, Chemical Corps, Camp Detrick. Project Report. Carnegie Institution of Washington, Cold Spring Harbor, New York.

56   Powell, Hugh. "Mesmerizing Migration: Watch 118 Bird Species Migrate Across a Map of the Western Hemisphere." All About Birds. November 22, 2017. Accessed August 21, 2019. https://www.allaboutbirds.org/mesmerizing-migration-watch-118-bird-species-migrate-across-a-map-of-the-western-hemisphere/

57   Traub, E., & W.I. Capps. Report to the Government of Colombia on the Experiments with chick embryo-adapted foot-and-mouth disease virus. FAO Report Number: AN-EPTA 178 TA/272/S/2/, Accession Number: 050178. (1953)

58   U.S. Army. U.S Army Activity in the U.S. Biological Warfare Programs, pp. 90-91, Retrieved from: https://archive.org/details/U.SArmyActivityInTheU.S.BiologicalWarfarePrograms/page/n34 [Long Island Biological Association Contracts]

59   Ibid

60   National Archives. RG 65 Erich Traub, (Declassified FBI Investigations on the Loyalties of Erich Traub). Federal Bureau of Investigation (FBI): NARA., Doc. # QO1-458431291

61   Traub, E., Jenney, E. W., & Mott, L. O. Serological studies with the virus of vesicular stomatitis. I. Typing of vesicular stomatitis viruses by complement fixation. Am J Vet Res, 73, 993-998. (1958).

62   Traub, E. & K. Beller. Geflügelpest und ahnliche Viruskrankheiten der Vögel. [Fowl Pest and Related Viral Diseases of Birds]. Handbuch der Viruskrankheiten, herausgegeben von Gildemeister, Haagen u. Waldmann. Bd. 1, Ch. 7. 590–606. Jena: Gustav Fischer (1939).

63   Traub, E., Jenney, E. W., & Mott, L. O. Serological studies with the virus of vesicular stomatitis. I. Typing of vesicular stomatitis viruses by complement fixation. Am J Vet Res, 73, 993-998. (1958).

64   Proceedings : National Research Conference on Anaplasmosis in Cattle (3d : 1957 : Kansas State College) : Free Download, Borrow, and Streaming. Internet Archive, ARS, USDA, 1 Jan. 1970,Retrieved from: http://www.archive.org/details/CAT10678552/page/n11

65   Rogers, Andrew Jackson. "A Study of the Ixodid Ticks of Northern Florida, Including the Biology and Life History of Ixodes Scapularis Say (Ixodidae: Acarina)." University of Maryland & University of Florida, University of Maryland, 1953

66   John Loftus, Taken from the rough draft of Introduction to The Sleeper Agent [personal communication] 2022.

67   Philipps, Roland. *A Spy Named Orphan: the Enigma of Donald Maclean*. Vintage, 2019.

68   "A Brief History Of The NAMRU-3 Medical Zoology Program : U.S. Naval Medical Research Unit No. 3." Internet Archive, U. S. Navy , 1 June 1968, https://www.archive.org/details/BriefHistoryOfTheNAMRU3MedicalZoologyProgram

69   Loftus, John. Americas Nazi Secret: an Insiders History of How the United States Department of Justice Obstructed Congress by: Blocking Congressional Investigations into Famous American Families Who Funded Hitler, Stalin and Arab Terrorists ; Lying to Congress, the GAO, and the CIA about the Postwar Immigration of Eastern European Nazi War Criminals to the US ; and Concealing from the 9/11 Investigators the Role of the Arab Nazi War Criminals in Recruiting Modern Middle Eastern Terrorist Groups. TrineDay LLC, 2011.

70   Hoogstraal, Harry. "African Ixodoidea. I. Ticks of the Sudan.. : Hoogstraal, Harry, 1917- : Free Download, Borrow, and Streaming." Internet Archive, U.S. Navy , 1 Jan. 1970, https://www.archive.org/details/africanixodoidea00hoog

71   Ibid.

72   Hirschfelder, H. & J. Wolf. Die Bedeutung von Insekten und Zecken für die Epizoologie der Maul- und Klauenseuche. [The Significance of Insects and Ticks for the Epidemiology of Foot-and-Mouth Disease,] Zschr. Hyg. Zool. 1938, 142-147.

73   Waldmann, O. & H. Hirschfelder. Die epizootische Bedeutung der Ratten, des Wildes, der Vögel und der Insekten für die Verbreitung der maul- und Klauenseuche. [The Epizootic Significance of Rats, Game, Birds and Insects for the Spread of Foot-and-Mouth Disease.] Berliner tierärztl. Wschr. 1938, 229

74   Food and Agriculture Organization (FAO). (1994). Foot-and-mouth disease: Sources of outbreaks and hazard categorization of modes of virus transmission. Fort Collins, CO: USDA, APHIS, VS, Centers for Epidemiology and Animal Health.

75   Zhou, Shenghua et al. "Lymphocytic choriomeningitis virus (LCMV) infection of CNS glial cells results in TLR2-MyD88/Mal-dependent inflammatory responses." Journal of neuroimmunology vol. 194,1-2 (2008): 70-82. doi:10.1016/j.jneuroim.2007.11.018

76   Zeng, W et al. "Totally synthetic lipid-containing polyoxime peptide constructs are potent immunogens." *Vaccine* vol. 18,11-12 (2000): 1031-9. doi:10.1016/s0264-410x(99)00346-1

77   Toledo A, Pérez A, Coleman JL, Benach JL. The lipid raft proteome of Borrelia burgdorferi. Proteomics. 2015;15(21):3662-3675. doi:10.1002/pmic.201500093

78   van Vliet, A H et al. "Phylogenetic position of Cowdria ruminantium (Rickettsiales) determined by analysis of amplified 16S ribosomal DNA sequences." *International journal of systematic bacteriology* vol. 42,3 (1992): 494-8. doi:10.1099/00207713-42-3-494

79   Beller, K. Herzwasser und sonstige tierische Rickettsiosen [Heartwater and other animal rickettsioses]. Handbuch der Viruskrankheiten (Ed. E. Gildermeister, E. Haagen, O. Waldmann). Vol. 2, Section 7, chapter 3, pp. 606-623. (1939) [Translated to English by A. Finnegan, 2021]

80   Zuelzer, M. Culex, A New Vector of Spirochaeta gallinarum. The Journal of Tropical

Medicine & Hygiene. Vol. 39, 204 (1936)

81   Traub, E., Schäfer, W. & Schramm, G., Untersuchen uber das Virus der Atypischen Geflugelpest. [Studies of the Virus of Atypical Fowl Plague]. Z. Naturforsch B. 157-167 (1949). [Translated to English by A. Finnegan (2019)]

82   Walker, R., Greene, R., Nicholson, W., & Levine, J. (1989). Shared flagellar epitopes of Borrelia burgdorferi and Borrelia anserina. Veterinary Microbiology, 19(4), 361-371. doi:10.1016/0378-1135(89)90101-6

83   Hovind-Hougen, K. "A Morphological Characterization of Borrelia Anserina." Microbiology (Reading, England). U.S. National Library of Medicine, January 1995. https://www.ncbi.nlm.nih.gov/pubmed/7894723

84   Marconi, R T et al. "Identification of novel insertion elements, restriction fragment length polymorphism patterns, and discontinuous 23S rRNA in Lyme disease spirochetes: phylogenetic analyses of rRNA genes and their intergenic spacers in Borrelia japonica sp. nov. and genomic group 21038 (Borrelia andersonii sp. nov.) isolates." Journal of clinical microbiology vol. 33,9 (1995): 2427-34. doi:10.1128/jcm.33.9.2427-2434.1995

85   FUKUNAGA, M., OKADA, K., NAKAO, M., KONISHI, T., & SATO, Y. (1996). Phylogenetic Analysis of Borrelia Species Based on Flagellin Gene Sequences and Its Application for Molecular Typing of Lyme Disease Borreliae. International Journal of Systematic Bacteriology, 46(4), 898–905. doi:10.1099/00207713-46-4-898

86   Sahgun, Louis. "Many California Bird Species Host the Lyme Disease Bacterium, Study Finds." Los Angeles Times, 25 Feb. 2015, www.latimes.com/science/sciencenow/la-sci-sn-california-birds-lymedisease-20150225-story.html

87   Jahnel, Franz. "Uber Das Verhalten Der Geflügelspirochäten Zum Zentralnervensystem." Medical Microbiology and Immunology, vol. 112, no. 4, Aug. 1931, pp. 613–622., doi:10.1007/BF02177222.

88   Shire, S J et al. "Purification and immunogenicity of fusion VP1 protein of foot and mouth disease virus." Biochemistry vol. 23,26 (1984): 6474-80. doi:10.1021/bi00321a031

89   Borrow, P, and M B Oldstone. "Mechanism of lymphocytic choriomeningitis virus entry into cells." Virology vol. 198,1 (1994): 1-9. doi:10.1006/viro.1994.1001

90   Treeve, P, and G Poste. "Cell fusion by Newcastle disease virus in the absence of RNA synthesis." Nature: New biology vol. 229,5 (1971): 157-8. doi:10.1038/newbio229157a0

91   White, J et al. "Cell fusion by Semliki Forest, influenza, and vesicular stomatitis viruses." The Journal of cell biology vol. 89,3 (1981): 674-9. doi:10.1083/jcb.89.3.674

92   Traub, E et al. "Behavior of foot-and-mouth disease virus on serial passage in different kinds of cells. A contribution to experimental epidemiology at cell level." Zentralblatt fur Veterinarmedizin. Reihe B. Journal of veterinary medicine. Series B vol. 15,5 (1968): 525-39. doi:10.1111/j.1439-0450.1968.tb00327.x

93   Kanhai, GK et al. "Cell fusion, using Sendai virus, to effect inter-species transfer of a cell-associated parasite (Theileria parva)." International journal for parasitology vol. 4,5 (1974): 519-21. doi:10.1016/0020-7519(74)90070-8

94   Jung, G., Wiesmuller, K.-H., Metzger, J., Buhring, H.-J., & Bessler, W. (2015, February 15). Membrane anchor/active compound conjugate, its preparation and its uses

95   Traub, E., et al. Untersuchungen über die Stomatitis papulosa des Rinde. [Studies on bovine papular stomatitis] Zeit. Infek. Krank. Hyg. Haus. 56 (2): 85-103. (1940). [Translated to English by A. Finnegan, 2019]

96   Hinnebusch, J, and A G Barbour. "Linear plasmids of Borrelia burgdorferi have a telomeric structure and sequence similar to those of a eukaryotic virus." Journal of bacteriology vol. 173,22 (1991): 7233-9. doi:10.1128/jb.173.22.7233-7239.1991

97   Mehdi S. Ferdows and Alan G. Barbour (1989). Megabase-Sized Linear DNA in the Bacterium Borrelia burgdorferi, the Lyme Disease Agent. Proceedings of the National Academy of Sciences of the United States of America, 86(15), 5969–5973. doi:10.2307/34243

98   Babb, Kelly et al. "Borrelia burgdorferi EbfC, a novel, chromosomally encoded protein, binds specific DNA sequences adjacent to erp loci on the spirochete's resident cp32 prophages." Journal of bacteriology vol. 188,12 (2006): 4331-9. doi:10.1128/JB.00005-06

99   Hovis, Kelley M et al. "Selective binding of Borrelia burgdorferi OspE paralogs to factor H and serum proteins from diverse animals: possible expansion of the role of OspE in Lyme disease pathogenesis." Infection and immunity vol. 74,3 (2006): 1967-72. doi:10.1128/IAI.74.3.1967-1972.2006

100   Syverton, J. T. et al. "The transmission of the virus of lymphocytic choriomeningitis by Trichinella spiralis." Journal of bacteriology vol. 54,1 (1947): 59.

101   Leitenberg, Milton, et al. The Soviet Biological Weapons Program: a History. Harvard University Press, 2012., pp. 196

102   Couper, Lisa I et al. "Impact of prior and projected climate change on US Lyme disease incidence." Global change biology vol. 27,4 (2021): 738-754. doi:10.1111/gcb.15435

103   Beller, K. Herzwasser und sonstige tierische Rickettsiosen [Heartwater and other animal rickettsioses]. Handbuch der Viruskrankheiten (Ed. E. Gildermeister, E. Haagen, O. Waldmann). Vol. 2, Section 7, chapter 3, pp. 606-623. (1939) [Translated to English by A. Finnegan, 2021]

104   Beller, K. & K. Bauer. Vorkommen und Bedeutung von Rickettsien auf den Lidbindehauten von Tieren. [Occurrence and importance of rickettsiae on the eyelid conjunctivitis of animals]. Zbl. Bakt. I. Abt. Orig. 158: 174-177. (1949) [research from 1944]

105   Rogers, Andrew J. "A Study of the Ixodid Ticks of Northern Florida, Including the Biology and Life History of Ixodes Scapularis Say (Ixodidae: Acarina)." University of Maryland & University of Florida, University of Maryland, 1953. Retrieved from: https://drum.lib.umd.edu/bitstream/handle/1903/16865/931201.pdf

106   Popa, Calin et al. "Bartonella quintana lipopolysaccharide is a natural antagonist of Toll-like receptor 4." Infection and immunity vol. 75,10 (2007): 4831-7. doi:10.1128/IAI.00237-07

107   Traub, E. Observations on immunological tolerance and "Immunity" in mice infected congenitally with the virus of lymphocytic choriomeningitis (LCM). Archiv Fur Die Gesamte Virusforschung, 10(3), 303-314. doi:10.1007/bf01250677. (1960).

108   Verdon, Rachel. Lyme Disease and the SS Elbrus: Collaboration between the Nazis and Communists in Chemical and Biological Warfare. Elderberry Press, 2006

109   Kouzminov, Alexander. Biological Espionage: Special Operations of the Soviet and Russian Foreign Intelligence Services in the West. Manas Publications, 2006., pp. 34-36

110   Bonnie. "Correspondence from Bonnie Bennett to Willy Burgdorfer about His Chronic Borreliosis." Utah Valley Digital Collections. Accessed July 28, 2019. https://contentdm.uvu.edu/digital/collection/Burgdorfer/id/33

111   National Archives, Joint Intelligence Objectives Agency, J.I.O.A. Administrative Records. (1950). Memorandum on Anne Bürger, C. F. Berrens, Naval Medical Research Institute, to Chief of Naval Operations, 27 November 1950, Navy Escape Clause (RG 330). NARS.

112   "Proceedings : Collaborator's Meeting on Foreign Poultry Diseases (1953 : Washington)." Internet Archive, United States Department of Agriculture (USDA) Washington, 1 Jan. 1970, www.archive.org/details/CAT10678555/page/n15

113   Boggs, D., and Willy Burgdorfer. "Interview with Willy Burgdorfer by Deirdre Boggs." NIH Intramural Research Program, National Institutes of Health (NIH), 15 Feb. 2015, Retrieved from: http://www.history.nih.gov/archives/downloads/wburgdorfer.pdf Accessed 19 May 2019.

114   Agents with these lipid portions in their surface antigens that stimulate Toll-Like Receptors (TLRs) in the pairs TLR2/TLR1, as well as TLR2/TLR6

115   Traub, E. Ueber den Einfluß der latenten Choriomeningitis-Infektion auf die Entstehung der Lymphomatose bei weißen Mause [On the Influence of Latent Choriomeningitis Infection on the Development of Lymphomatosis in White Mice]. Zentrl. Bakt. I. Orig. 147 (16). 1-25. (1941). [Translated to English by A. Finnegan, 2019]

116   Traub, E. Observations on "Late onset disease" and Tumor Incidence in Different Strains of Laboratory Mice infected Congenitally with LCM Virus I. Experiments with Random-bred NMRI Mice. Zentralblatt Für Veterinärmedizin Reihe B, 22(9), 764-782. (1975, 2010). doi:10.1111/j.1439-0450.1975.tb00643.x

117   Traub, E., & Kesting, F. Age Distribution and Serological Reactivity of Viral Antigen in Brains of Mice Infected Congenitally with LMC Virus. Zentralblatt Für Veterinärmedizin Reihe B, 24(7), 548-559. (1975, 2010). doi:10.1111/j.1439-0450.1977.tb01024.x

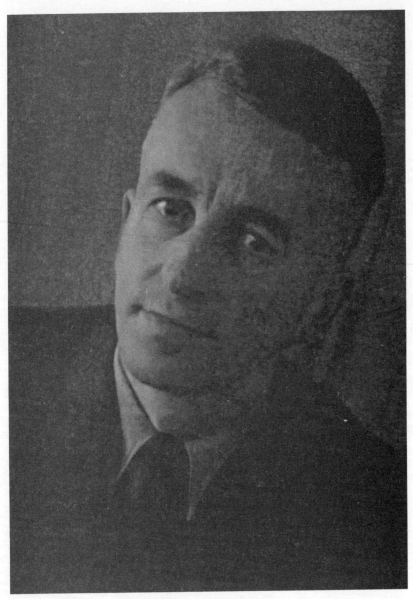

Erich Traub (1906-1958)

Chapter Ten

A Sleeper in the Ranks

The Loyalties of Erich Traub and his Mission in America

What destroys us most effectively is not a malign fate but our own capacity for self-deception and for degrading our own best self.
— George Eliot

W hen Erich Traub began his work for the U.S. Military in 1949, it was at a time when concentrated efforts at a biological warfare program were in full swing. The Cold War was well-underway, and by the following year, the tripartite cooperation between the United States, Britain, and Canada, saw an expansion and the establishment of the North American Treaty Organization (NATO), and the United Nations (UN) had been created in 1945. Cooperation between the Western countries had its benefits, but certainly came with risks. Especially when it came to espionage.

On the global battlefield, proxy wars would continue to be fought through armed conflict up to the present time, but direct wars between global superpowers would change dramatically. Newer, unconventional weapons and ways of fighting wars were rapidly developing. Nuclear weapons were becoming far too risky and destructive to use in wars. Therefore, alternatives like chemical and biological warfare were seen as a more acceptable solution.

As demonstrated in the previous chapter, Traub was instrumental in the biological weapons programs of tripartite countries, especially the American program. Despite his status as a veterinarian, he was the most skilled bioweaponeer available to the Americans and his position could not be matched by any other person in the military or academic circles within the United States. He was very high up in the American program and supervised many of the germ warfare tests on Plum Island, at Fort Detrick, and other sites.

In 1950, the Korean War began, and the United Nations and American military attempted to fend off the North Koreans from invading South Korea. However, the war was a complete disaster for the West. As the communists fighting in the Korean War were obliterating the strategy of American and U.N. forces in South Korea by the North, according to John Loftus, a decision was made to employ Traub's weaponized germs and insects as a last-ditch effort, to sway the war in their favor.[1] Big mistake. Somehow the Chinese and North Koreans were prepared for the attack and intercepted the tick and insect bombs as they were dropped from the planes, while several American planes were shot down and their pilots taken prisoner. While they were not able to stop the diseases from spreading in the decades to come, they had numerous countermeasures and spotted the planes as they were being deployed to minimalize the effect and spread of these insects and germs.[2] John Loftus, says of the Korean War:

> Traub and Maclean helped designed the insect bombs that the Americans and British military had just dropped on North Korea and China. This was a clear violation of the International Treaty prohibiting the development or use of biological weapons. This violation allowed the Russians to blackmail several key members of the Eisenhower administration into silence.[3]

According to declassified CIA intelligence reports, the Soviet Union supplied the North Koreans and Chinese with various medical prophylactics, like sera and vaccines, but with the vaccines, this was followed by nasty reactions.[4] According to a Soviet analysis of biological warfare and its response in Korea, it was noted that many agents cannot be immunized against because they fail to have any effect.[5] According to other researchers, what prevented these large epidemics was a combination of insecticides, prophylactics, and medical prevention teams deployed to intercept the bug bombs dropped on Chinese and Korean soil.[6] It would appear that someone within the ranks had indeed been tipping them off before the bug bombs were dropped.

This was no surprise, since Donald Maclean had suddenly disappeared from the ranks of British Intelligence in 1951.[7] After an intensive search and investigation, a recording was found of Maclean voicing his allegiance to the Soviet Union, declaring that, not only was he a communist, he was *"a proselytizing communist."*[8] Maclean had been a key component in the facilitation of tripartite agreements between the United States, Britain, and Canada, and was instrumental in clearing many of the Paperclip scientists for work in America, not to mention, he had been assisting Traub's escape from East Germany and testing activities on American shores.[9]

Maclean had been stationed in Cairo, Egypt since 1948 and had intelligence on the African tick and insect expeditions by the Navy's NAMRU-3 program that was initiated that year, mining disease agents and insects all over the African continent.[10] According to John Loftus, Maclean was the one responsible for getting Traub back into the United States after the War, and Maclean directed joint-British testing at Plum Island and other testing sites since World War II.[11] Plum Island was conducting biological warfare tests in 1944 with brucellosis,[12] and Maclean was stationed in Washington from 1944-1947, taking vacations on Long Island, New York, right in the vicinity of Plum Island in the Long Island Sound. Maclean would have had access to cultures of weaponized spirochetes from Traub through British Intelligence sources just after 1945 when Traub was in the British and American zone applying for work with the West, and Traub brought cultures with him in 1948 when he made his official escape. By 1952, Traub was officially offered the lead scientist position on Plum Island by Dr. Maurice Shahan, the first director of Plum Island, but Traub declined. Why was that so? Extensive background checks might be one such reason.

TRAUB'S INTERROGATION BY CIC AGENT DAN BENJAMIN

Just after WWII, the revelations of Igor Gouzenko exposed massive spy rings operating in Britain, Canada, and the United States.[13] As a result, this eventually led to the discovery of Traub's handler, the one who helped him get cleared for Operation Paperclip, Donald Maclean, of MI6, one of the key people who helped set up NATO, defecting to Russia in 1951.[14]

John Loftus says it was around this time, Traub began to get nervous, turning down top positions at the USDA's Plum Island, and this aroused the suspicion of military intelligence. Traub's release of large amounts of weaponized insects, such as ticks, mosquitoes, and mites, were carrying much more than harmless, benign tracers, and soon Traub's assistance in the States would be a cornered rat.

Author Linda Hunt was the first to bring forth the military's employment of Erich Traub and Operation Paperclip.[15] John Loftus exposed the Lyme disease connection to biological warfare in *The Belarus Secret*.[A] In 2004, author Michael Christopher Carroll likewise brought more attention to Erich Traub and the activities around

---

A   Republished as *America's Nazi Secret* (Trine Day 2010)

Plum Island in *Lab 257: The Disturbing Story of the Government's Secret Plum Island Germ Laboratory*. Now, for the first time, in this book, John Loftus further tells the story of Traub's interrogation by Counter Intelligence Corps (CIC) Agent Dan Benjamin, to bring forth these startling new revelations of Erich Traub's confession to being a Soviet double-agent of the KGB:

> Author Linda Hunt never got the credit she deserved for exposing Nazi scientists who had entered America under Operation Paperclip. Linda Hunt had been the first American journalist to visit Insel Reims, the secret island off the northern coast of Germany. This was where from 1945 onwards Nazi scientist Dr. Eric Traub and Stalin's biological warfare experts continued their joint research on immunological weapons.
>
> Linda Hunt is the giant upon whose shoulders all future biowar researchers have stood. Several authors ripped off her research into the declassified intelligence files and then published her archival discoveries without citation under their own names. But I know the truth.
>
> Ms. Hunt was first to warn the world about the dangers from the Paperclip scientists, but she was not the first one to warn me about the evil Dr. Traub. That credit belongs to Dan and Anne Benjamin, arguably the best husband-wife intelligence team before Bob Baer of CIA married a woman smarter than he was.
>
> After WWII, Dan was an agent in the US Army's elite Counter Intelligence Corps (CIC), Dan became the senior CIC agent in charge of anti-communist intelligence for the American zone of occupied Germany, a position he later held for the entire European Command (EUCOM G-2) and then finally at the Pentagon where he was a Department of Army Civilian (DAC) who liaised with CIA.
>
> The Pentagon thought that Dan's charming British wife, Anne, was "just a secretary." In fact, Anne did start as a secretary for the government in the British zone of occupied Germany. But, like her husband, her brilliance was soon recognized.
>
> What Dan's friends in the Pentagon never knew was that Anne was recruited as an officer in the British Secret Intelligence Service (SIS or MI6). It was Anne who was in charge of the British secret intelligence archives for occupied Germany.
>
> Anne received reports from Frederick "Freddy" Van Den Heuvel. Freddy was the SIS officer in charge of recruiting Nazi

scientists, many of whom the British Government protected from prosecution as war criminals. Freddy's best recruiting agent was Robert Maxwell who ran a German "publishing house" for scientific papers.

Publication was a bait no scientist could refuse. Maxwell's publishing company for scientific papers was an SIS front to lure Nazis scientists to come out of hiding before the Russians could find them and drag them off to Moscow.[B]

By 1949, as the SIS archivist in post war Germany, Anne Benjamin had probably learned all that could be learned about SIS recruitment of Nazi scientists, including the evil Nazi genius, Dr. Traub. According to the SIS reports Anne received, the Russians had held Dr. Traub in custody in communist-controlled Eastern Europe after WWII, but SIS somehow arranged Traub's miraculous "escape" to West Germany.

Anne and her American husband, Dan Benjamin, were suspicious. By 1951, it was clear to them that that the senior SIS officers who approved Dr. Traub's escape from the Soviet Army's clutches were none other than Kim Philby and Donald Maclean, the highest-ranking communist spies inside British Intelligence.

Dan and Anne suspected (correctly) that it was this same "Cambridge Ring" of communist spies inside the SIS that had arranged Dr. Traub's immigration to America under Operation Paperclip. Kim Philby's underling (and lover) Donald Maclean was the SIS's scientific liaison to the Americans advising them which Nazis were worth recruiting.

It should be no surprise that the American space program was "advised" by Maclean to recruit useless Nazi bureaucrats like Werner von Braun, while the Russians recruited the real rocket experts of the Third Reich. That is why the Russians were the first to succeed in launching their Sputnik satellite into orbit while American missiles kept exploding on the launch pad. As Khrushchev boasted to Nixon that "our Germans are better than your Germans."

As the Benjamin's had feared, several of the Nazi rocket scientists recruited under Operation Paperclip turned out to have been war criminals like Arthur Rudolf (which made him subject

---

B   John Loftus: *"Years later, Maxwell's daughter, Ghislaine was told to call me if she wanted to know how her father died. I told her SIS discovered Robert Maxwell was a double agent for the Mossad. The SIS did not push him off his boat, but they did cancel his financial credit. The SIS slowly drove Maxwell into bankruptcy which eventually forced him to jump off his boat and drown. [...]"*

to Soviet blackmail). After US intelligence officials publicly admitted to expunging the records of Nazi scientists, Arthur Rudolf agreed to surrender his American citizenship and be deported.

Another famous Nazi scientist was Ohio State University's Albertus Strughold. After he was exposed as a war criminal, the university took the professor's name off of one of their buildings. That is only the tip of Ohio State's iceberg: there are eight underground levels nearby in Columbus, Ohio built by the US military to which the students are not allowed.

No one in the Pentagon suspected at the time that Dr. Traub was perhaps the most villainous of all the Nazis to enter America. He was just a German veterinarian with some expertise in animal vaccines, a very profitable market for American pharmaceutical companies. The greed of Big Pharma to employ Nazi scientific experts like Traub led to the Benjamins' warnings being ignored. But soon the American military began to realize that Dan Benjamin may have been right to suspect that there was more to his story.

Dr. Traub had been recruited by Donald Maclean of the Cambridge Five Spy Ring inside SIS. Maclean, the communist agent, had advised the gullible Americans which German scientists should be brought to America under Operation Paperclip. When Maclean defected to Moscow in 1951, the Pentagon realized that Dan Benjamin was the only one who had been asking the right questions about the Nazi scientists whom McLean had sent to America, especially Dr. Traub.

Dan Benjamin was asked by the Department of Defense to investigate why Dr. Traub had refused three times to accept a promotion for director of the biological laboratory on Plum Island between Connecticut and New York's Long Island. Was it because the Plum Island job required an intensive investigation for a Top-Secret clearance? Was there something in Dr. Traub's past that he feared would be discovered?

Dan Benjamin personally interrogated Dr. Traub. As the CIA will attest, Dan was probably the best interrogator in American intelligence. He never used torture or truth serums. Dan simply studied everything about his subject before he ever met him. Dan was friendly to Dr. Traub but made it clear to him that the actual interview was an unnecessary formality.

Dan already knew Traub's miraculous "escape" from communist East Germany had been arranged with the help of the communist spy ring inside British SIS. Dan briefly walked Traub through a few of the many contradictions and coverups in Traub's record. Did Dr. Traub have anything he wished to say for the record before he was handed over for sentencing as a spy for the KGB?

The bluff seemed to work. Dr. Traub decided to confess. He admitted that he had been captured by the Russian army at the end of WWII. He admitted that his fake escape from East Germany was arranged by Philby and Maclean because he promised to serve the Soviet Union as a communist spy inside American intelligence.

But Traub claimed he was such an unimportant little guy that the Russians never activated him for espionage. In fact, they never even bothered him again. Traub's explanation was that Soviet intelligence must have had so many other higher-level spies among the Nazi paperclip scientists, that the KGB never needed to contact a low-level veterinarian like him.

Traub said he repeatedly refused American promotions requiring any security clearance because he wanted to keep a low profile so the Russians would not bother with a little guy like him. It was a lie, but it was one that the Eisenhower administration desperately wanted to hear. Traub's public trial could have exposed the Dulles' brothers perfidious behavior.

Instead of following Dan's recommendation to prosecute Dr. Traub as a communist spy and investigate all the other German scientists, the Eisenhower administration ordered the Pentagon to accept Traub's rather dubious explanation. Nevertheless, the Army insisted that if Traub was not going to be sent to prison, at the very least Traub should be fired from all his American contracts and deported back to Germany where he should be placed under continuous surveillance and banned from any classified research.

Instead, The Eisenhower administration allowed Traub to continue serving as a UN health inspector. This UN status plausibly afforded Traub diplomatic immunity from American arrest as a confessed communist spy. To my shame, I did not give Dan's story about this seemingly minor Nazi scientist much priority for a follow up. Even though my time and funds were limited by my health, I did not give up entirely.

In the late 1980's I asked Rachel Verdon, one of my wonderful Lyme Disease volunteers, to request declassification of government records concerning Plum Island. Rachel discovered that nearly all the records were still classified or had been destroyed, including the bioweapons master file named "clandestine attacks on crops and animals" which had been illegally shredded.

Rachel also discovered many open-source documents confirming my sources insistence that the Russians had extensively studied tick-borne disease for more than a half century. Rachel's tireless research was not wasted as it did prove beyond any doubt that the US Government had built a brick wall of secrecy around whatever the communist double agents had done at Plum Island.

I did cooperate openly with another author in a wonderful book called *Lab 257* but there was not much that I could tell him while the classification order was still in effect.

Even if Dan Benjamin had mentioned Traub's name, I had quite forgotten it for many years until I was accidentally reminded by Hollywood producers looking into Traub's background with tick experiments at Plum Island. How many German scientists under Operation Paperclip could there be who repeatedly declined promotions to be director of research at Plum Island? Traub had to be the same man who confessed to Dan that he was a spy for the KGB.

Dan and Anne had passed away before I could tell them that I had figured out why Traub never went to prison as a Nazi war criminal turned KGB spy. Traub was untouchable because he could blackmail the Eisenhower administration. It was Traub who designed the insect bombs that the US Air Force had dropped on North Korea and China. It was not his first such war crime. [16]

THE AFTERMATH: A COVERUP AND BACK TO GERMANY

By 1952, the U.S. Military and Western Intelligence had a real problem on their hands, worse, a complete embarrassment. What normally would have meant a death sentence for a confessed Soviet double agent was covered up and classified at the highest levels, most likely due to the fact that he had a lot of dirt on the biological testing activities during his time on the biological warfare program and the biological weapons used in the Korean War. To top it off, he also could have had dirt on the Rockefeller Institute. Clearly, Traub could bring others right down with him if a public trial were to follow.

This was already a nightmare situation, but they did not want the additional public scandal to follow. Bad enough that they took a Nazi bioweaponeer who was in all probability a war criminal, employed him to work on the most sensitive areas of the biological weapons program, already a dirty business to be in, but worse, Traub was also a Soviet double agent! How damaging this would be if it ever got out.[17] Furthermore, he already had diplomatic immunity due to his being an official of the Food and Agriculture Organization (FAO) of the United Nations (UN). As the story goes, they sent him back to Bogotá, Colombia until they could figure out what next to do with him.

Throughout Erich Traub's second tenure in the United States, the FBI conducted ongoing investigations into his loyalties and associations, interviewing some of his associates, such as William A. Hagen, Frank A. Todd, James D. Horton, former Rockefeller colleagues like Carl TenBroeck, Richard E. Shope, Ernest Smillie, Ralph B. Little, John B. Nelson, as well as colleagues from the Naval Institute, such as Wallace P. Rowe, Herbert Hurlbut, Worth I. Capps, and even former Reich scientist Theodore Benzinger, a high-altitude and decompression researcher, who had at one time been on the defendants list to be tried for war crimes at Nuremberg.[18]

The reactions were mixed, either having a strong dislike of Dr. Traub, indifference, or friendly to great admiration of him. Some of the more notable responses were made by former colleagues at Rockefeller Institute, such as Carl TenBroeck, Ralph B. Little, and John Nelson.

According to his former Professor, Dr. TenBroeck, Traub was a very hard worker, but described him as cocksure and arrogant.[19] He admitted that Dr. Traub never discussed politics nor expressed any opinion for or against Hitler, but he did mention that Blanka was never happy in the U.S. and always felt she had to defend herself and her homeland.[20]

Dr. Ernest Smillie, superintendent of the Princeton, NJ section of the Rockefeller Institute, on the other hand, described him as extremely pro-Nazi in a 1942 investigation, but this is contradicted in his second interview in 1950.[21]

Dr. John B. Nelson, who ran secondary studies under Traub's supervision, gave some further insight on the moral character of the German virologist and claimed his dislike of Traub on *"the fact that DR. TRAUB was a veterinarian and, he went out of his way to be cruel to animals. DR. NELSON stated that he felt that any person who is cruel to animals shows little distinction and difference in his treatment of his fellow human beings."*[22]

Another former-Rockefeller Institute colleague echoed what Nelson had to say, describing Traub as, *"a domineering German and Surly type of individual with a violent temper. He said that DR. TRAUB showed no consideration for animals while he was working with them and not much more consideration for the people he was associated with."*[23]

Traub's American counterpart, Richard E. Shope, had some commendable remarks to make about his former German colleague. Wallace P. Rowe, one of Traub's new American colleagues and virologists, recalled Traub saying that the Russians who overtook Insel Riems, *"stole his research results and claimed them as their own."*[24]

By the time of these reports, the truth about Traub's loyalties and directed bioterrorism against the Americans and Western countries probably had not been known by more than a handful of people, it does not appear that the agents used were immediately known, but they began to infect the civilians with strange mystery diseases that were complex, hard to diagnose, and even harder to treat. These weapons began to establish themselves in the environment and the momentum was sure to continue as the years carried on.

Traub was in Bogotá, Colombia periodically until the end of 1952, and returned to Maryland, and soon decisions were made for Traub to return to Germany on October 7, 1952, to lead a virus research institute in Tübingen, West Germany. Therefore, Erich Traub submitted his resignation from the position with the U.S. military, but continued research for them in Tübingen.[25, 26]

Traub set himself up at the University of Tübingen upon his return, which became the cover story for those not *"in the know"* about Traub's real purpose for leaving America. Outsiders would be told that the scientist just decided to pack up and go home.[27] Traub's repatriation was approved and on January 14, 1953, Traub and his family boarded the SS Stockholm, and sailed back to Germany, where he began his position at the University of Tübingen's Federal Research Institute for Virus Disease of Animals (*Bundesforschungsanstalt fur Viruskrankheiten*).[28]

Agreements were also made, that, upon return to Germany, Traub would have to be under surveillance for the remainder of his life.[29] This, however, did not stop Traub from continuing relations with former Insel Riems associates, persons of interest, exchanging of germs, among other activities. Nor did it keep him off American shores with further employment by the USDA, all the way up until the late 50s and possibly early 60's.[30]

Endnotes

1   Loftus, John J. "Memorandum on Biological Weapons History." 2018

2   Endicott, S. L., & Hagerman, E. (1999). *The United States and biological warfare: Secrets from the early cold war and Korea*. Bloomington, IN: Indiana University Press.

3   John Loftus, Taken from the rough draft of Introduction to The Sleeper Agent [personal communication] 2022.

4   Central Intelligence Agency (CIA) Intelligence Reports: IMMUNOLOGY - POLY-VACCINES. CIA-RDP80-00809A000600250904-0. Central Intelligence Agency (CIA), Reading Room, 2011. Retrieved from: https://www.cia.gov/library/readingroom/docs/CIA-RDP80-00809A000600250904-0

5   Central Intelligence Agency (CIA) Intelligence Reports: MEDICAL SERVICE IN MASS ATTACK USSR. "GENERAL INFORMATION ON THE BIOLOGICAL WEAPON AND PRINCIPLES OF ANTI-EPIDEMIC DEFENCE OF THE POPULATION." CIA-RDP81-01043R003800050002-9. Central Intelligence Agency (CIA), Reading Room, 2011. Retrieved from: https://www.cia.gov/library/readingroom/docs/CIA-RDP81-01043R003800050002-9

6   Endicott, S. L., & Hagerman, E. (1999). *The United States and biological warfare: Secrets from the early cold war and Korea*. Bloomington, IN: Indiana University Press.

7   "The Two Elusive Diplomats; Donald Maclean--Guy Burgess Men in the News." The New York Times, https://www.timesmachine.nytimes.com/timesmachine/1956/02/12/306141502.html

8   "LOST BRITON IS SAID TO ADMIT RED TIES; Lords Hear Missing Diplomat's Recording of the Statement Is in Hands of F. B. I." The New York Times, 29 Oct. 1952, https://www.timesmachine.nytimes.com/timesmachine/1952/10/29/93586243.html?pageNumber=11

9   Loftus, John J. (personal communication). 2018

10   Harry Hoogstraal. leader of the African insect expeditions, worked much of the time in between African tick expeditons, at the University of Cairo, coordinated with the U.S. Navy, which Maclean would have been somewhat privy to.

11   Loftus, John. (personal communication). 2018

12   Hoover, D. L., & Borschel, R. H. (2005). Medical Protection Against Brucellosis. *Biological Weapons Defense*, 155–184. doi:10.1385/1-59259-764-5:155

13   Gusenko, Igor, and Robert Bothwell. *The Gouzenko Transcripts: the Evience Pres. to the Kellock-Tascherau Royal Commission of 1946*. Deneau, 1982.

14   "LOST BRITON IS SAID TO ADMIT RED TIES; Lords Hear Missing Diplomat's Recording of the Statement Is in Hands of F. B. I." 1952. The New York Times. The New York Times. October 29, 1952.

15   Hunt, Linda. *Secret Agenda the United States Government, Nazi Scientists, 1945 to 1990*. St. Martins Pr, 1991.

16   Loftus, John. Early draft of introduction to this book. (personal communication). 2022

17   Ibid.

18   National Archives. RG 65 Erich Traub, (Declassified FBI Investigations on the Loyalties of Erich Traub). Federal Bureau of Investigation (FBI): NARA., Doc. # QO1-458431291

19   Ibid.

20   Ibid.

21   Ibid.

22   Ibid.

23   Ibid.

24   Ibid.

25   National Archives. Joint-Intelligence Objectives Agency file on Erich Traub (RG 330). NARS. Joint Intelligence Objectives Agency (JIOA), JIOA Administrative Records. (1949-54).

26   USDA and military employment and funding noted in his 1954 paper on Newcastle Disease. See: Traub, E. A booster effect of irradiated or formolized Newcastle disease virus upon the infectivity of active virus in the presence of chicken blood. National Naval Medical Center. Bethesda, MD. (1954) U.S. NAVY Project NM. NMRI Memorandum Report. Project NM 005 048.11.06

27   Loftus, John. (Personal communication)

28   National Archives. Joint-Intelligence Objectives Agency file on Erich Traub (RG 330). NARS. Joint Intelligence Objectives Agency (JIOA), JIOA Administrative Records. (1949-54).

29   National Archives. RG 65 Erich Traub, (Declassified FBI Investigations on the Loyalties of Erich Traub). Federal Bureau of Investigation (FBI): NARA., Doc. # QO1-458431291

30   Ibid.

Chapter Eleven

VECTOR WEAPONS & SIMULANT ATTACKS

THE MEANS AND METHODS OF THE AMERICAN BIOLOGICAL WARFARE PROGRAM

There is poison in the fang of the serpent, in the mouth of the fly and in the sting of a scorpion; but the wicked man is saturated with it.

– Chanakya

From 1932-1933, in the subways of London and Paris, German Intelligence had been secretly conducting open-air *simulant* tests with the so-called "harmless" bacteria, *Serratia marcescens* as a simulation of a more dangerous microbe.[A] It was published in a 1934 article by prominent British journalist Wickham Steed.[1] Although his warnings were repudiated and attempts were made to discredit the article, it was later confirmed by Soviet Intelligence.[2]

In fact, when German scientist Kurt Blöme was interviewed by the Joint Intelligence Objectives Agency (JIOA) about biological warfare and was asked about any field experiments he told his interrogators that simulant testing of this type with *Serratia marcescens* was also done by the Germans in Eastern Europe during WWII.[3] It is probably not a coincidence that after WWII, the United States and Britain would be conducting the same tests at the advice of German experts like Erich Traub playing the role of supervisory bacteriologist.[4]

In 1950, the U.S. Navy conducted open-air tests in Operation Sea Spray with *Serratia marcescens* over the city of San Francisco, California, to simulate an attack with deadly germs on American cities.[5] Before long, a man had died, and 10 others had developed unusually resistant infections with the bacterium at a nearby hospital.[6] While the Army claims it did not know the bacteria could cause human in-

---

A   Formerly called *Bacillus prodigiosis* and *Micrococcus prodigiosis*

fections, the scientific literature on the agent documents a handful of cases of illness going back to 1903.[7] Several scientific papers on the illness in man occurred at military installations published by military scientists.

In 1943, U.S. Army researchers from Fort Belvoir isolated the bacterium from a case of meningitis in an Army soldier.[8] In 1946, a station hospital at the U.S. Army's Camp Detrick noted four illnesses following exposure to the bacteria by Detrick personnel performing experiments with an air purification machine.[9]

By 1976, *The Washington Post* and other outlets caught wind of what the military was doing and reported that open-air tests in San Francisco, New York City, Key West, and Panama City, had been secretly carried out in populated areas for many years. These articles mention that tests were also conducted using *Bacillus globigii* (*Bacillus subtilis* var. *niger*) and the pathogenic fungus *Aspergillus fumigatus*.[10] *Aspergillus fumigatus* is a devious pathogen that causes aspergillosis which is often incurable,[11] while its mycotoxins can be carcinogens.[12] Yeast cells were occasionally used to simulate the spread of *Coccidioides immitis*.[13]

1977 Congressional Hearings on Simulant Testing

The allegations of secret open-air testing on populated areas led to a congressional hearing in 1977, *Biological Testing Involving Human Subjects by the Department of Defense, 1977*. Members of the U.S. Army appeared before congress and downplayed the testing and tried to maintain that there was not sufficient evidence to conclusively prove the man died from the tests, even though a handful of other cases were noted following the test when infections with *Serratia marcescens* had not been seen at the nearby hospital prior to the tests. The Army then supplied two volumes of declassified material, *U.S. Army Activity in the U.S. Biological Warfare Programs*.[14]

What is interesting to note about the 1977 congressional hearings, the U.S. Navy was never called before congress even though the San Francisco test that caused the illnesses and a man's death was a Navy test which the Army only indirectly participated. It must be asked why the Army was the only military branch at this hearing when it was being conducted by many military branches and federal agencies working together. The Navy and Air Force activity was never questioned, nor was the U.S. Department of Agriculture. The Central Intelligence Agency (CIA) was also named as participants in some of these tests, but likewise, they were never questioned by congress at this hearing either.

The Army Chemical Corps was a major participant of chemical and biological warfare activities, and it was the Army Chemical Corps who owned Plum Island before transferring the laboratory to the USDA in 1953. However, the Navy was also a major participant in the program, as Erich Traub essentially worked for the Navy and the USDA. Moreover, the USDA and other federal agencies worked with and coordinated research activities with the Army through the Chemical-Biological Coordination Center of the National Research Council, a scientific committee with scientists from academia and the military, with subdivisions like biochemistry, entomology[B], veterinary medicine, and more.[15] Through these joint committees, the biological warfare program was being developed through many channels, agencies, and outfits. It would be a grave mistake to think the material given to congress by the U.S. Army was the full scope of the biological warfare program.

To give a glimpse of the collaborative effort between different agencies and outfits, the Federal Civil Defense Agency, published an annual report in 1954 that had a special section on biological warfare, "Communicable Disease Control and Biological Warfare Defense," which states:

> Close liaison has been continued with the Department of Defense, the Department of Health, Education, and Welfare, the Department of Agriculture, the Central Intelligence Agency, and other Federal agencies, on biological warfare defense problems.[16]

The same kind of liaising was ongoing in research activities between military branches, the USDA, the CIA, academic circles, and the corporate sector, as documents supplied to congress demonstrate. Furthermore, any research that could be done by the academic circles was done by them and reflected back to the National Research Council or directly to the military.[17]

MORE OPEN-AIR SIMULANT TESTS

Sometime between 1955 and 1956, lightbulbs filled with *Bacillus globigii* (*Bacillus subtilis* var. *niger*) were thrown on the train tracks of a New York subway and carried through the subways theoretically exposing more than a million people, known as Operation Big City.[18] These mirrored the tests the Germans carried out in Paris and London subways in 1932 and 1933. Later, the health effects of exposure to *Bacillus globigii* are documented to cause detrimental health effects.[19]

B   **Entomology**: a branch of zoology that studies insects and arthropods

Tests of this nature had been ongoing since the end of WWII, and many open-air tests were conducted all over the country. In St. Louis, the fluorescent particles zinc cadmium sulfide, were sprayed all over the city in a fog, and the tests were later picked up in a *Business Insider* article in 2012, "The Army Sprayed St. Louis With Toxic Aerosol During a Just Revealed 1950s Test," with a female cancer survivor citing the sudden onset of devastating cancers, her father died of cancer in 1955, she watched four siblings die of cancer and wondered if the tests were responsible.[20]

It is certainly a possibility that toxicity to this fluorescent particle was harmful to humans, but additional tests with agents like *Aspergillus fumigatus* may have been run here as well by other outfits or agencies. The mycotoxins produced by species of *Aspergillus* are potent carcinogens,[21] including those of *Aspergillus fumigatus*,[22] and Aspergillus mycotoxins were also being considered as insecticides.[23] In 1951, a test with *Aspergillus fumigatus* listed in the 1977 hearing was conducted on African American laborers in a Navy warehouse where crates they would be handling were intentionally contaminated with the mold and it was done with race in mind.[24]

Allegations of additional tests not cited in the hearing were also said to have taken place by other outfits and agencies. For example, in 1979, *The Washington Post* published an article, "Report Suggests CIA Involvement in Fla. Illnesses" alleging the CIA was conducting tests with whooping cough bacteria in 1955, and a rise of the illness was noted in the nearby county.[25]

The incident cited in St. Louis was part of Operation LAC (Large Area Coverage), but there were additional joint-research activities between Britain, USA, and Canada, under the tripartite program not discussed in the 1977 hearing. A declassified Canadian Defense document on biological warfare in relation to Operation Large Area Coverage shows that this program must have been a much broader program than the relatively minor St. Louis tests. The extensive documentation with numerous simulant agents and live pathogens indicates that Operation Large Area Coverage was far more than these initial tests with fluorescent particles.[26]

According to the Canadian document on Large Area Coverage, some of the simulants that were researched on a routine to semi-routine basis included *Serratia marcescens, Bacillus subtilis* var. *niger* (*Bacillus globigii*), *Escherichia coli, Sarcina lutea*, vaccinia virus, *Staphylococcus citreus, Aspergillus fumigatus*, along with the addition of fluorescent particles of Zinc Cadmium Sulfide.[27]

Since it was indicated in the correspondence that many of these strains were found in the environment and thought to be non-pathogenic, it is probable they were used in a similar capacity to *Serratia marcescens* and *Bacillus subtilis*.

From 1948-1953 open-air tests using live pathogens over animals on rafts in the ocean were tested by the British with cooperation from the United States in Operation Harness, Operation Cauldron, Operation Hesperus, Operation Negation, and Operation Ozone.[28] These mirrored the tests on Norwegian reindeer conducted by the Germans over Lake Peipus in Estonia.[29]

In a tripartite report from 1955 cited in the Canadian document, vaccinia virus (smallpox vaccine) was proposed and agreed upon to be used as a simulant and had been used in field trials in all countries involved in the tripartite research, indicating this was done routinely on a large scale:

> Tenth Tripartite Report – Sept. 55
>
> UK outlined the work done on vaccinia, emphasizing that this was very much an interim report. Because vaccinia was relatively safe, easy to produce and easy to assess, it was used as a simulant in both laboratory and field trials in order to gain information on the use of smallpox virus (Variola) as a [biological warfare] agent. The vaccinia material was stable at – 60 Degrees C, stood up well under freezing and thawing and could be freeze-dried without reduction in titer. In the spray work it was found that the virus was as stable as Bg spores, although the spray factor varied with different batches.[30]

Additionally, they used tularemia, *Brucella suis*, and Venezuelan Equine Encephalitis (VEE), at least in some of the field experiments near the Bahamas:

> UK Annual Report – Sept. 55
>
> Test Sphere - Nearly 100 experiments have been conducted, sometimes lasting over 2-3 days and on other occasions, more than one per day. The first object was correlation with the last field tests using the same four agents, B. suis, Bact. tularense, Venezuelan equine encephalomyelitis virus, and vaccinia virus. The selected temperatures and humidities included those of the Bahamas "night" trials done in the absence of ultraviolet light and the same spray device was used.[31]

Decades later, tripartite activity shows that in 1993, simulants were still being tested and it was decided that *Bacillus subtilis* and vaccine strains of Newcastle Disease Virus had been decided on for standard simulants. This report was also deciding on what vaccine viruses could be used as simulants, and in stark contrast to the 1955 tripartite report agreeing on vaccinia virus as a safe simulant, this report assesses it once again, concluding:

> Despite its extensive use for immunization of the human population against smallpox, vaccinia virus is a virus of relatively high pathogenicity with a long, if sporadic history of lethal infections and postvaccinial encephalitis. Even more serious than the standard complications listed in the Submission is the prospect of vaccinial pneumonia in a population now almost devoid of the individual or herd immunity resulting from smallpox vaccination.
>
> Vaccinia virus must unquestionably, therefore, be excluded. [...] [32]

Open-air tests on populated areas with dubious simulants have been consistently carried out since the biological warfare program was an offensive program and these simulants were dispersed through airborne routes on a frequent basis, and records indicate that this is still going on today.

"On July 30, 1977, Congress passed Title 50 section 1520, "which involve the use of human subjects for the testing of chemical or biological agents." Under this law, the Department of Defense would be allowed to test chemical and biological agents on civilians conducting experiments deemed necessary to the Department of Defense. The only consent necessary in the law were if "local civilian officials in the area in which the test or experiment is to be conducted are notified in advance of such test or experiment." This meant that they would at the bare minimum notify some of the officials in government positions like the federal agencies, but none of the general population who might be subjects in the experiment had to be notified.[33]

In 1996, this law was repealed, and a new law replaced the original section 1520, which became 1520a, *Restrictions on the — Use of Human Subjects for Testing of Chemical or Biological Agents.* This new law made informed consent on its subjects necessary, with several loopholes. The new law allowed as exceptions to the new law *"(1) Any peaceful purpose that is related to a medical, therapeutic, pharmaceutical, agricultural, industrial, or research activity. (2) Any purpose that is directly related to protection against toxic chemicals or biological weapons and agents."*[34]

Nearly all biological warfare research has been conducted under the guise of peaceful *"medical, therapeutic, pharmaceutical, agricultural, industrial, or research activity,"* and therefore all that had to be done for the Department of Defense or participating agencies involved was to say that it was defensive work or related to peaceful research activity and they would be able to legally continue experiments and tests over populated areas. The other loopholes to this were the "War Powers Resolution" and "National Emergencies" section of Title 50, which meant the new 1520a law could be suspended in times of war and national emergency, and we have been under many since 1997, especially after September 11, 2001.

With the 1520a law in place, they could continue their simulant activities under so-called peaceful scientific and medical research, or biodefense activities claiming to protect the population from biological warfare. With this in mind, expansions were also made on older laws like Title 42 of 1944, which had to do with public health, social welfare, and civil rights. Under this law, much could be done through scientific research addressing public health. It was under this law that saw the creation of the Biomedical Advanced Research and Development Authority (BARDA), a section of the Department of Health and Human Services (HHS) that oversaw the research and development of what is termed medical countermeasures, measures to protect against biological warfare agents, pandemic influenza, and emerging diseases of all kinds.[35] Under this law, and under the cover of benign or defensive scientific and medical research, the activities under the original Title 50 law could not only continue, but be greatly expanded and taken to new heights never before seen under the original law.

INSECT AND ARTHROPOD VECTOR RESEARCH

The American biological warfare program was not only concerned with the study of airborne pathogens dispersed by way of the air, but also by insects and arthropods. What has been declassified by the U.S. Army has been minimal, but so far there have been several programs declassified and released to the public. There were other experiments conducted through dispersal by insects.[36, 37]

These would carry simulants in insects and through the natural chain of transmission in a given ecosystem. A modern day example is the so-called harmless rickettsia, *Wolbachia pipientis*, in *Aedes aegyptii* mosquitoes, released by the millions over the last few years, touted as an insecticide that unsurprisingly failed to have the desired effect.[38] Like the airborne tests, simulant testing with insects were also taking place since the end of WWII and does not seem to have stopped.

In 1992, hundreds of ticks infected with wasp eggs to allegedly "breed them out" were being released on Martha's Vineyard by academic researchers by the hundreds,[39] while simulant tests with the genetically engineered mosquitoes infected with *Wolbachia* seems to have actually expanded the insect simulant program to become the Operation LAC of insect simulant testing.[40] It does not appear that the *Wolbachia* are as harmless and non-transmissible as they thought, because there is some evidence that *Wolbachia* antigens are being found in people with cancer,[41] and the bacteria has also been given antigens from the herpes-simplex virus which would certainly help it acquire human pathogenicity.[42]

According to John Loftus, the classified files have shown him that the Germans were conducting studies with ticks in North Africa during WWII by tracking their spread through the bullseye rash and other symptoms associated with spirochetes and tick-borne disease. As we have shown in earlier chapters, his sources were saying that joint testing with the British at Plum Island was ground zero for the Lyme disease spirochetes in America, with ticks attached to shore-birds used as simulant tests of an entomological warfare attack with what were claimed as harmless ticks and a harmless rash, when in fact it was sabotage. The most likely candidate was the black-legged tick as it was not thought to transmit any known disease at the time. These ticks then carried the hidden cocktail of disease all over the country.[43] All evidence would certainly reflect what has been said by Loftus, despite several attempts by academicians and government researchers to disprove it.

Later in the book, I will walk the reader through some of these attempts, they are easy to refute, and at least one scientific publication used to dispel the Lyme Disease connection to biological warfare actually supports the story you are reading in this book.[44] Needless to say, many well-funded public relations campaigns, front organizations, and think-tanks of all kinds have been devoted to reinforcing the official position and keeping the truth about Soviet biological terrorism on Americans concealed.

Firstly, we can demonstrate the history of active research to develop and test insects and arthropod delivery systems in the American biological warfare program. We can also see that key officials from the USDA and military associated with Erich Traub were actively involved in tick and tick-borne disease research at the time, coordinating with the Army Chemical Corps, the U.S. Navy, and academic universities. Secondly, we can demonstrate that the military, the Smithsonian Institute, and a significant number of academic, military, and USDA researchers were tracking the migration of birds and the diseases they carried as an official program. In a later chapter, we will see that these surveillance programs were also run on the human population to monitor the problem rather than try to solve it.

In 1954, Operation Big Itch assessed the use of fleas to transmit disease to an enemy by munitions or bug bombs and this was deemed a success.[45] In 1955, Operation Big Buzz field tested mosquitoes dispersed in similar munitions and dispersed over large areas, with equally favorable results.[46] In 1956, the mosquito trials expanded to test a variety of different methods of dispersal in Operation Drop Kick to the desired end.[47] Operation May Day was run in parallel to Operation Drop Kick the same year but baited the mosquitoes with dry ice traps to further assess the effectiveness.[48] In all instances, the tests were deemed successful and followed with more, but remain classified.

As noted previously, the U. S. Navy began a large-scale tick and arthropod-borne disease collection program through the special Navy unit headed by Harry Hoogstraal called the Naval Medical Research Unit No. 3 (NAMRU-3). This project began in 1948 from the University of Cairo, Egypt, but expeditions were sent to different areas of Africa to collect ticks and insects of all kinds and catalogue both the ticks and the diseases they harbored. [49] These results were then shared with the British, as British scientist Don Arthur published the data in "Studies on Exotic Ixodes Ticks (Ixodoidea, Ixodidae) from United States Navy and Army Activities."[50]

Prior to this, the U.S. military and USDA had also done surveys in North America since at least 1945, cataloguing the ticks and their hosts by two USDA scientists F. C. Bishopp and Helene Louis Trembley, published a lengthy paper, "Distribution and Hosts of Certain American Ticks," and it is here they mention that the USDA was collecting the black-legged tick annually.[51]

These studies then produced additional work on more specific locations like Long Island and New York, as shown by researcher George Anastos from the Harvard Biological Laboratory who published "Hosts of Certain New York Ticks" in 1947.[52] Anastos was well-connected with other names from the biological warfare program like C. M. Clifford from the Rocky Mountain Laboratory,[53] as well as Harry Hoogstraal of NAMRU-3.[54] Additional researchers added to these North American studies in 1949 with "Some Host Relationships of Long Island Ticks,"[55] and "Further Notes on the Host Relationships of Ticks on Long Island."[56] All of these papers contained study of the black-legged tick, among others.

In 1951, Andrew J. Rogers of the University of Maryland wrote a dissertation on the black-legged tick (*Ixodes scapularis*) mentioning that "[a]*lthough it is not known to be a vector of any disease in nature, its abundance and wide range of hosts among the larger mammals, including man, makes this species a very important pest.*"[57] However, by 1958, *The Reporter Dispatch* reported on July 16, 1958, with an article "Ticks Repulsive, but You Must Respect 'Em!," showing the black-legged tick was named alongside the lone-star tick as a serious transmitter of disease, saying, "[t]*he Lone Star tick, a tick not found around here, is also a serious disease carrier, as is the black-legged tick. The dog tick and the black-legged tick are found in the East. All are loosely called 'wood ticks.' for they are found in woodland areas.*"[58]

In 1952, the USDA was actively engaged in tick-borne anaplasmosis research, with annual conferences and a lead USDA official H. W. Schoening was discussing strains of *Anaplasma* not being "inoffensive" and that isolation of the *Anaplasma centrale* pathogen was not going to be possible on Plum Island for a long time:

> Schoening: Does [*Anaplasma*] centrale exist in the United States? Blood brought from South Africa would also bring other diseases. Also, [*Anaplasma*] centrale blood may not be inoffensive under our conditions; there will be no room for isolation of it at Plum Island for a long time to come.[59]

This statement shows that tick-borne diseases were normally fair game on Plum Island, but construction was underway and did not have adequate facilities and was by that time supposed to be doing defensive work. Traub's colleague L. O. Mott, who worked with Traub at the Beltsville Station of the USDA, was also very involved in tick and anaplasmosis research.[60] Recall that author Michael C. Carroll in his book about Plum Island has already documented former Plum Island director J. J. Callis admitting that tick colonies were in fact kept there and used in experimental research at that time.[61]

In 1961, L.O. Mott participated in an annual committee on exotic diseases of animals, alongside Col. Frank A. Todd and Plum Island's first director, Dr. M. S. Shahan, and other members. Mott presented a report "Anaplasmosis Experimental Field Trial Activities" discussing field trial work on the tick-borne disease *Anaplasma* that had been ongoing since the early 1950s at many stations across the country, leading it from the USDA's experimental research division at Beltsville, Maryland.[62] Erich Traub was at Beltsville with Mott in 1950 when the program was active, indicated by Traub's paper on Vesicular Stomatitis Virus (VSV), co-authored with Mott, from work done in 1950.[63]

Frank Todd, another of Traub's associates we have already discussed in earlier chapters, presented an opening paper to this committee, "Defense Against Biological Warfare on Livestock," making it clear the committee was concerned with aspects of biological warfare.[64] Field trials and transmission experiments with *Anaplasma* were part of the areas covered by the committee on exotic agents relevant to biological warfare, as research from the Beltsville station of the USDA shows.[65] Not surprisingly, *Anaplasma* is now a co-infection of Lyme Disease that is found in the black-legged tick, *Ixodes scapularis*.[66]

The USDA's Animal Disease Eradication Division (ADE) begins to mention diseases of the black-legged tick in a 1962 publication, *Manual on livestock ticks for animal disease eradication division personnel*, demonstrating that the tick was *"not a known vector of any disease although experimentally it has transmitted bovine anaplasmosis. I. scapularis is an experimental vector of tularemia and has been found infected in nature."*[67]

In 1952, Plum Island director M.S. Shahan, has an early USDA publication on Foot-and-Mouth Disease (FMD) which mentions that FMD Virus could be transmitted to ticks and mentions British experiments with the sheep tick (*Ixodes Ricinus*) and the fowl tick (*Argas persicus*).[68] The only dilemma with FMD virus in these ticks was that the virus would not maintain itself in the host since it would not pass to the next generation of ticks. This of course, was one of Traub's specialties.

Traub utilized viruses like LCM for its ability to transmit through generations from mother to newborns due to it having an affinity for the ovaries.[69] He realized the potential for using certain viruses like LCM to adapt other viruses to new hosts and impart new qualities, disable the immune system, and maintain steady infection transmission from mother to newborns.[70] LCM could likewise be used to adapt FMD virus to ticks since he noted the ability for LCM virus to grow in tick cells in 1972, indicating he was already doing this in his own work.[71]

By 1986, a report from the Caribbean on Heartwater (*Rickettsia ruminantium*) lists FMD as a disease that can be transmitted by ticks,[72] and by 1994, the Food and Agriculture Organization (FAO) of the United Nations lists ticks as a high hazard in the spread of FMD.[73]

However, M. S. Shahan published a report from Plum Island in 1959, "Exotic Diseases," discussing some of the newer diseases that were becoming a problem for the USDA and public health service, mentioning the spirochete *Leptospira* as a major disease hitting the livestock and farming industry, as well as the *Babesia*-like blood parasite *Theileria parva* (East Coast Fever) and *Ehrlicia ruminantium* (heartwater),[74] the rickettsia of cattle that is related to human monocytic ehrliciosis,[75] both transmitted by ticks, and were treated in Karl Beller's 1939 chapter on heartwater while Traub was his assistant.[76]

The USDA was also working extensively with *Babesia* parasites, testing ticks infected with babesiosis (formerly piroplasmosis) with public research from 1963 at the Beltsville station, noted in USDA publication *Agricultural Research Vol. 11, No. 10.*, with tests from the Beltsville, USDA station on the equine babesiosis agents *Babesia equi* and *Babesia caballi* in *Dermacentor* ticks:

Ticks are tested as carriers

> Veterinarian T. O. Roby and entomologist D. W. Anthony [had] tested the ticks for their ability to transmit piroplasmosis. The ticks were kept in a jar having a constant humidity until they deposited their eggs, the eggs hatched, and the larvae (seed ticks) appeared ready to feed.
> Approximately 1,000 seed ticks were placed on the ear of a horse that had been born and raised at Beltsville and had not been used for studies of this kind. A linen bag was placed over its ear and attached with cement to prevent the ticks from moving over the animal. The horse was placed in an isolation building designed for tick transmission work.[77]

Mosquito simulant tests and live agent tests would have been a part of the early experiments when Traub was at Plum Island running these tests with the Navy, USDA, and the Army Chemical Corps. 30 years later, a 1980 issue of *Mosquito News* indicates that abandoned tires and animal cages were found on Plum Island, probably from earlier testing phases, and were inadvertently breeding mosquitoes shown to be species that served as important transmitters of Eastern Equine Encephalitis virus (EEE) and avian malaria, along with additional moquitoes of concern, like the *Culex* mosquitoes,[78] which were demonstrated by Germans in 1937 to transmit *Borrelia anserina* spirochetes.[79]

In 1955, field experiments at the University of Wisconsin demonstrated the ability for biting flies (*Diptera*) and mosquitoes to transmit Vesicular Stomatitis Virus (VSV),[80, 81] and the following year, Plum Island presented at their 1956 conference on vesicular diseases, new insects that could experimentally transmit VSV.[82]

Avian Vector Research

As insect research was thoroughly investigated for its applications in biological warfare and its defense, the birds that insects fed on were also investigated for their role in transporting disease to the enemy and vis versa. In 1942, Erich Traub mentioned the role of migratory birds in the spread of diseases like Newcastle Disease Virus.[83]

Insects that fed on birds were studied and reared in laboratory settings for experimental research by academic institutes that worked with the Navy, Army, and U.S. Department of Agriculture. R. E. Kissling, who worked with the USDA and University of California on *Borrelia anserina* in 1949,[84] conducted other areas of avian research on the spread of diseases with biological warfare significance.

In 1951, he and other researchers were publishing on EEE virus recovered from a purple grackle bird,[85] and again in the "Isolation of a psittacosis-like agent from the blood of snowy egrets."[86] In 1953, he was publishing on birds as winter hosts for Eastern and Western Equine Encephalitis Virus (EEE & WEE) with the support of the Army Chemical Corps.[87] In 1954, the studies concerned arthropod-borne EEE in wild birds.[88] In 1956, Venezuelan Equine Encephalitis Virus (VEE) was assessed in wild birds.[89] Studies like these, connected with scientists of military or biological warfare backgrounds from the time Traub assisted in the setup of the American program and decades beyond it can be found in multitudes in the scientific literature.

In the following decade, a large-scale surveillance program known as Project Starbright was initiated in the Pacific Ocean to study migratory birds and the diseases they harbored. According to a published journal article by Roy MacLeod, "'Strictly for the Birds': The Military and the Smithsonian's Pacific Ocean Biological Survey Program, 1963-1970," the Smithsonian Institute held military contracts for the Army Chemical Corps from 1963-1970, spending considerable time in the Pacific to study the annual patterns of bird life, and the staff was even asked to feed mosquitoes on the birds and have the blood sent in for analysis without an explanation why.[90]

The bird survey was a joint-military operation of the U.S. Army Chemical Corps, the Office of Naval Research, and the Smithsonian Institute. Word broke about the large, ongoing survey sometime in the 60s, and by the end of the 60s they received a considerable amount of public backlash, even sparking protests against the Smithsonian Institute for having military contracts.[91]

Results can be found from the Hawaiian studies that were obviously included in the overall objective for Project Starbright, with participation from R.E. Kissling, later published in "Arthropod-borne Virus Survey on the Island of Oahu, Hawaii," with several other scientists tracking the viral disease agents in the birds of the Hawaiian islands.[92] Among some of the agents they were either testing for or discovered in the birds were: Japanese B Encephalitis, St. Louis Encephalitis, Western Equine Encephalitis, Eastern Equine Encephalitis, and Dengue Fever.[93]

Another study by Richard E. Warner of the University of California, an institute that was associated with the Navy, conducting research and activity with them, along with the USDA, published in 1968, a detailed report on bird diseases in the Hawaiian Islands in "The Role of Introduced Diseases in the Extinction of the Endemic Hawaiian Avifauna," showing several diseases that could have been introduced into Hawaii, such as avian malaria and bird-pox.[94] Warner also discusses work being done by his group in the Marshall Islands, which could only have been part of the Starbright program.[95]

Endnotes

1   Steed, H. W. *Aerial Warfare: Secret German Plans. The Nineteenth Century and After*, 116 (7) (1934), pp. 1–16.

2   Central Intelligence Agency (CIA) Intelligence Reports: PROSPECTIVE USES OF BACTERIOLOGICAL WARFARE IN FUTURE WARS. CIA-RDP80-00809A000600120022-4. Central Intelligence Agency (CIA), Reading Room, 2011. Retrieved from: https://www.cia.gov/readin-groom/document/cia-rdp80-00809a000600120022-4

3   National Archives. Joint intelligence Objectives Agency (JIOA), JIOA Administrative Records. (n.d.). Interview of ALSOS Scientists: Dr. Kurt Blöme (RG 330 INSCOM dossier XE001248). NARS.

4   Joint Intelligence Objectives Agency (JIOA), JIOA Administrative Records. (1949-54). Joint-Intelligence Objectives Agency file on Erich Traub (RG 330). NARS.

5   Cole, Leonard A. (1988). *Clouds of Secrecy: The Army's Germ Warfare Tests Over Populated Areas*. Rowman & Littlefield. pp. 75–84.

6   WHEAT, R. P. (1951). INFECTION DUE TO CHROMOBACTERIA. A.M.A. Archives of Internal Medicine, 88(4), 461. doi:10.1001/archinte.1951.03810100045004

7   Bertarelli, E.: Untersuchungen und Beobachtungen über die Biologie und Pathogenität des Bacillus prodigiosus, Zentralbl. Bakt. 34:193 and 312, 1903.

8   Aronson, L C, and S I Alderman. "The Occurrence and Bacteriological Characteristics of S. marcescens from a Case of Meningitis." *Journal of bacteriology* vol. 46,3 (1943): 261-7. doi:10.1128/jb.46.3.261-267.1943

9   Paine, T F. "Illness in man following inhalation of Serratia marcescens." *The Journal of infectious diseases* vol. 79,3 (1946): 226-32. doi:10.1093/infdis/79.3.226

10   Cole, Leonard A. *Clouds of Secrecy: the Army's Germ Warfare Tests over Populated Areas*. Rowman & Littlefield, 1990

11   The Aspergillosis Trust. (n.d.). Raising Awareness of Aspergillosis. Aspergillosis Trust. https://www.aspergillosistrust.org/

12   Navale, Vishwambar et al. "Aspergillus derived mycotoxins in food and the environment: Prevalence, detection, and toxicity." *Toxicology reports* vol. 8 1008-1030. 2 May. 2021, doi:10.1016/j.toxrep.2021.04.013

13   Cochrane, Raymond C. "DTIC ADB228585: History of the Chemical Warfare Service in World War II. Biological Warfare Research in the United States, Volume 2: Defense Technical Information Center: Free Download, Borrow, and Streaming." Internet Archive, 1 Nov. 1947, pp. 395 Retrieved from: https://archive.org/details/DTIC_ADB228585/page/n395

14   Committee on Human Resources. 1977. Biological Testing Involving Human Subjects by the Department of Defense, 1977: Hearings before the Subcommittee on Health and Scientific Research of the Committee on Human Resources, United States Senate, Ninety-Fifth Congress, First Session ... March 8 and May 23, 1977. S7-857 O. Washington: U.S. Govt. Print. Off. pp. 17, Retrieved from: https://archive.org/details/biologicaltestin00unit/page17

15   Chemical-Biological Coordination Center; National Research Council. (n.d.). Chemical-Biological Coordination Center of the National Research Council. The National Academies Press.   https://nap.nationalacademies.org/catalog/21524/chemical-biological-coordination-center-of-the-national-research-council

16   Federal Civil Defense Agency (FCDA). (n.d.). Civil defense papers (Annual Report 1954). Internet Archive. https://archive.org/details/CivilDefense_201901/Fcda-1954-Annual-ReportFor1954/page/n4/mode/1up

17   War Bureau of Consultants Committee, and George W. Merck. 1945. Report to the Secretary of War by Mr. George W. Merck, Special Consultant for Biological Warfare. Report to

the Secretary of War by Mr. George W. Merck, Special Consultant for Biological Warfare. National Acadamy of Science (NAS) Online Collections. Retrieved from: http://www.nasonline.org/about-nas/history/archives/collections/organized-collections/1945merckreport.pdf

18   The Washington Post. (1979, December 4). CIA may have tested biological warfare in New York in '50s, Church says. The Washington Post. https://www.washingtonpost.com/archive/politics/1979/12/04/cia-may-have-tested-biological-warfare-in-new-york-in-50s-church-says/0872f274-58c6-4184-bde3-50d1ecef0573/

19   HEALTH EFFECTS OF PROJECT SHAD BIOLOGICAL AGENT: BACILLUS GLOBIGII, (Bacillus licheniformis), (Bacillus subtilis var. niger), (Bacillus atrophaeus) National Academies. 2004. Contract No. IOM-2794-04-001

20   Salter, J. (n.d.). The army sprayed St. Louis with toxic aerosol during a just revealed 1950s test. Business Insider. https://www.businessinsider.com/army-sprayed-st-louis-with-toxic-dust-2012-10

21   Perrone, Giancarlo, and Antonia Gallo. "Aspergillus Species and Their Associated Mycotoxins." Methods in molecular biology (Clifton, N.J.) vol. 1542 (2017): 33-49. doi:10.1007/978-1-4939-6707-0_3

22   Pepeljnjak, S et al. "The ability of fungal isolates from human lung aspergilloma to produce mycotoxins." Human & experimental toxicology vol. 23,1 (2004): 15-9. doi:10.1191/0960327104ht409oa

23   Insecticidal Mycotoxins Produced by Aspergillus Flavus Var. Columnaris : Beard, Raimon L. (Raimon Lewis). Internet Archive, New Haven : Connecticut Agricultural Experiment Station , 1 Jan. 1971, Retrieved from: http://www.archive.org/details/insecticidalmyco00bear

24   Cole, Leonard A. Clouds of Secrecy: the Army's Germ Warfare Tests over Populated Areas. Rowman & Littlefield, 1990, pp. 45-46

25   Richards, Bill. 1979. "Report Suggests CIA Involvement In Fla. Illnesses." The Washington Post. WP Company. December 17, 1979. https://web.archive.org/web/20161022051613/https://www.washingtonpost.com/archive/politics/1979/12/17/report-suggests-cia-involvement-in-fla-illnesses/5b10205e-170b-4e38-b64e-2e9bca8f50df/

26   Department of National Defence (Canada), Biological Warfare. OPERATION LAC correspondence. Tripartite Reports pp. 000232 http://data2.archives.ca/e/e443/e011063033.pdf

27   Ibid.

28   Regis, Edward. The Biology of Doom: The History of Americas Secret Germ Warfare Project. New York: H. Holt, 2000.

29   Eberle, Henrik. "Ein Wertvolles Instrument": Die Universität Greifswald Im Nationalsozialismus. Bohlau Verlag, 2015.

30   Department of National Defence (Canada), Biological Warfare. OPERATION LAC correspondence. Tripartite Reports pp. 000232 http://data2.archives.ca/e/e443/e011063033.pdf

31   Ibid.

32   Ho, J., et al. "DTIC ADA593829: A Safety and Environmental Assessment of the Biological Simulants Bacillus Subtilis and Newcastle Disease Virus. Volume 1: Discussion : Defense Technical Information Center." Internet Archive, 1 Jan. 1993, Retrieved from: http://www.archive.org/details/DTIC_ADA593829/page/n3

33   50 USC 1520

34   50 USC 1520a

35   42 U.S. Code § 247d–7e - Biomedical Advanced Research and Development Authority

36   DTIC AD0596046: Outdoor Mosquito Biting Activity Studies, Project BELLWETH-ER-I, BW 459 : Defense Technical Information Center., U.S. Army Chemical Corps. Research & Development Command, 1 Dec. 1960, Retrieved from: http://www.archive.org/details/DTIC_AD0596046

37   Committee on Human Resources. 1977. Biological Testing Involving Human Subjects by the Department of Defense, 1977: Hearings before the Subcommittee on Health and Scientific Research of the Committee on Human Resources, United States Senate, Ninety-Fifth Congress, First Session ... March 8 and May 23, 1977. S7-857 O. Washington: U.S. Govt. Print. Off. pp. 17, Retrieved from: https://archive.org/details/biologicaltestin00unit/page17

38   McCall, Rosie. "Plan to Crush Native Mosquito Population with Gene-Edited Strain Fails-May Have Made Them Stronger Instead." Newsweek, Newsweek, 19 Sept. 2019,   https://www.newsweek.com/plan-crush-native-mosquito-population-gene-edited-strain-fails-1459619

39   Donn, Jeff. "Scientists Use Wasps to Kill Disease-Carrying Tick." AP NEWS. September 12, 1992. Accessed August 22, 2019. https://www.apnews.com/cfcf511f5e214fb-154de187879e8c796

40   Fitzsimons, T. (2022, March 12). EPA Oks Plan to release 2.4 million more genetically modified mosquitoes. NBCNews.com. https://www.nbcnews.com/news/us-news/epa-oks-plan-release-24-million-genetically-modified-mosquitoes-rcna19738

41   Chen, X.-P., Dong, Y.-J., Guo, W.-P., Wang, W., Li, M.-H., Xu, J., ... Zhang, Y.-Z. (2015). Detection of Wolbachia genes in a patient with non-Hodgkin's lymphoma. Clinical Microbiology and Infection, 21(2), 182.e1–182.e4. doi:10.1016/j.cmi.2014.09.008

42   "Tetracycline (Tet) Inducible Expression." Addgene, https://www.addgene.org/tetracycline/

43   Loftus, John. Americas Nazi Secret: an Insiders History of How the United States Department of Justice Obstructed Congress by: Blocking Congressional Investigations into Famous American Families Who Funded Hitler, Stalin and Arab Terrorists ; Lying to Congress, the GAO, and the CIA about the Postwar Immigration of Eastern European Nazi War Criminals to the US ; and Concealing from the 9/11 Investigators the Role of the Arab Nazi War Criminals in Recruiting Modern Middle Eastern Terrorist Groups. TrineDay LLC, 2011.

44   Persing, D., Telford, S., Rys, P., Dodge, D., White, T., Malawista, S., & Spielman, A. (1990). Detection of Borrelia burgdorferi DNA in museum specimens of Ixodes dammini ticks. Science, 249(4975), 1420–1423. doi:10.1126/science.2402635

45   Rose, William H. "An Evaluation of Entomological Warfare as a Potential Danger to the United States and European NATO Nations," U.S. Army Test and Evaluation Command, Dugway Proving Ground, March 1981

46   Ibid.

47   "Summary of Major Events and Problems: (Reports Control Syrnbol CSHIS-6) United States Army Chemical Corps, Fiscal Year 1959." United States Army Chemical Corps. pp. 101–104.

48   Rose, William H. "An Evaluation of Entomological Warfare as a Potential Danger to the United States and European NATO Nations," U.S. Army Test and Evaluation Command, Dugway Proving Ground, March 1981

49   Hoogstraal, Harry. "African Ixodoidea. I. Ticks of the Sudan." Internet Archive, U.S. Navy , 1 Jan. 1970, Retrieved from: www.archive.org/details/africanixodoidea00hoog

50   Arthur, Don R. "Studies on Exotic Ixodes Ticks (Ixodoidea, Ixodidae) from United States Navy and Army Activities." The Journal of Parasitology 43, no. 6 (1957): 681. doi:10.2307/3286566.

51   Bishopp, F. C., & Trembley, H. L. (1945). Distribution and Hosts of Certain North

American Ticks. *The Journal of Parasitology*, 31(1), 1. doi:10.2307/3273061

52   Anastos, George. "Hosts of Certain New York Ticks." Psyche: *A Journal of Entomology*, vol. 54, no. 3, 1947, pp. 178–180., doi:10.1155/1947/81979.

53   CLIFFORD, C M, and G ANASTOS. "The use of chaetotaxy in the identification of larval ticks (Acarina: loxodidae)." The Journal of parasitology vol. 46 (1960): 567-78.

54   Hoogstraal, H et al. "Haemaphysalis (H.) sumatraensis sp. n. (Ixodoidea: Ixodidae), a tick parasitizing the tiger, boar, and sambar deer in Indonesia." *The Journal of parasitology* vol. 57,5 (1971): 1104-9.

55   Collins, D. L., Nardy, R. V., & Glasgow, R. D. (1949). "Some Host Relationships of Long Island Ticks." Journal of Economic Entomology, 42(1), 110–112. doi:10.1093/jee/42.1.110

56   Collins, D. L., Nardy, R. V., & Glasgow, R. D. (1949). "Further Notes on the Host Relationships of Ticks on Long Island." *Journal of Economic Entomology*, 42(1), 159–160. doi:10.1093/jee/42.1.159

57   Rogers, Andrew Jackson. "A Study of the Ixodid Ticks of Northern Florida, Including the Biology and Life History of Ixodes Scapularis Say (Ixodidae: Acarina)." University of Maryland & University of Florida, University of Maryland, 1953. Retrieved from: https://drum.lib.umd.edu/bitstream/handle/1903/16865/931201.pdf

58   "Ticks Repulsive, but You Must Respect 'Em!," The Reporter Dispatch (White Plains, New York) · Wed, Jul 16, 1958 · Page 28, Downloaded on May 30, 2023, retrieved from: https://www.newspapers.com/image/909653950

59   United States Department of Agriculture (USDA). (1970, January 1). Proceedings of the Second National Research Conference on Anaplasmosis in Cattle (2D : 1953 : Oklahoma A & M College) . Internet Archive. https://archive.org/details/CAT10678553/page/n23/mode/2up

60   Proceedings : National Research Conference on Anaplasmosis in Cattle (3d : 1957 : Kansas State College) : Free Download, Borrow, and Streaming. Internet Archive, ARS, USDA, 1 Jan. 1970,Retrieved from: http://www.archive.org/details/CAT10678552/page/n11

61   Carroll, M. C. (2004). Lab 257: The disturbing story of the governments secret and deadly virus research facility. New York: Morrow.

62   Mott, L. O. Anaplasmosis Experimental Field Trial Activities. Proc 64th Ann. Meet. U.S. Livestock Sanit. Ass. Charleston 1961. 95-101

63   Traub, E., Jenney, E. W., & Mott, L. O. Serological studies with the virus of vesicular stomatitis. I. Typing of vesicular stomatitis viruses by complement fixation. Am J Vet Res, 73, 993-998. (1958).

64   Todd, F. A. Defense Against Biological Warfare on Livestock. Proc 64th Ann. Meet. U.S. Livestock Sanit. Ass. Charleston 1961. 70-80

65   Dikmans G (1950) The transmission of anaplasmosis. Am J Vet Res 11:5-16.

66   Bush, Larry M, and Maria T Vazquez-Pertejo. "Tick borne illness-Lyme disease." Disease-a-month : DM vol. 64,5 (2018): 195-212. doi:10.1016/j.disamonth.2018.01.007

67   USDA, Animal Disease Eradication Division (ADE), et al. "Manual on Livestock Ticks for Animal Disease Eradication Division Personnel." Manual on Livestock Ticks for Animal Disease Eradication Division Personnel, U.S. Dept. of Agriculture, Agricultural Research Service, 1965. Retrieved from: https://archive.org/details/manualonlivestoc9149unit/page/68/mode/2up?q=scapularis

68   Shahan, M. S. (1970, January 1). Foot-and-mouth disease : A threat to the United States . Internet Archive. https://archive.org/details/CAT31411369/page/n14/mode/1up

69   Traub, E.: Panel discussion, Symposium on Latency and Masking of viruses VII. Internat. Congr. für Microbiol. Stockholm 1958

70   Traub, E. Observations on immunological tolerance and "Immunity" in mice infected congenitally with the virus of lymphocytic choriomeningitis (LCM). Archiv Fur Die Gesamte Virusforschung, 10(3), 303-314. doi:10.1007/bf01250677. (1960).

71   Traub, E. LCM Virus Research, Retrospect and Prospects. Lymphocytic Choriomeningitis Virus and Other Arenaviruses, 3-10. doi:10.1007/978-3-642-65681-1_1. (1973)

72   "Regional Project for the Eradication of Amblyomma Variegatum/Heartwater from the Caribbean. Project Profile : IICA-Guyana." Internet Archive, IICA Biblioteca Venezuela, Retrieved from: http://www.archive.org/details/bub_gb_QzwqAAAAYAAJ/page/n1

73   Food and Agriculture Organization (FAO). (1994). Foot-and-mouth disease: Sources of outbreaks and hazard categorization of modes of virus transmission. Fort Collins, CO: USDA, APHIS, VS, Centers for Epidemiology and Animal Health.

74   SHAHAN, M S. "Exotic diseases." *Journal of the American Veterinary Medical Association* vol. 135,1 (1959): 57-9.

75   van Vliet, A H et al. "Phylogenetic position of Cowdria ruminantium (Rickettsiales) determined by analysis of amplified 16S ribosomal DNA sequences." *International journal of systematic bacteriology* vol. 42,3 (1992): 494-8. doi:10.1099/00207713-42-3-494

76   Beller, K. Herzwasser und sonstige tierische Rickettsiosen [Heartwater and other animal rickettsioses]. Handbuch der Viruskrankheiten (Ed. E. Gildermeister, E. Haagen, O. Waldmann). Vol. 2, Section 7, chapter 3, pp. 606-623. (1939) [Translated to English by A. Finnegan, 2021]

77   USDA, "Agricultural Research : United States. Science and Education Administration. 'Horse Tick Fever' ." 1963. Internet Archive. [Washington, D.C. : Science and Education Administration], U.S. Dept. of Agriculture : [Supt. of Docs., U.S. G.P.O., distributor]. January 1, 1963. https://archive.org/details/CAT90891937124/page/6

78   White, D. J., and C. P. White. "Aedes Atropalpus Breeding in Artificial Containers in Suffolk County, New York." Internet Archive, Mosquito News Vol. 40 No. 1, 1 Jan. 1980, Retrieved from: http://www.archive.org/details/cbarchive_117472_aedesatropalpusbreedinginartif1980/page/n1

79   Zuelzer, Margarete. "Culex, a New Vector of Spirochaeta Gallinarum." Jour Trop *Med And Hyg* 39, no. 17 (1938): 204.

80   Ferris, D. H., Hanson, R. P., Dicke, R. J., & Roberts, R. H. (1955). Experimental Transmission of Vesicular Stomatitis Virus by Diptera. *Journal of Infectious Diseases*, 96(2), 184–192. doi:10.1093/infdis/96.2.184

81   Roberts, R. H., Dicke, R. J., Hanson, R. P., & Ferris, D. H. (1956). Potential Insect Vectors of Vesicular Stomatitis in Wisconsin. *Journal of Infectious Diseases*, 98(2), 121–126. doi:10.1093/infdis/98.2.121

82   USDA. "Proceedings of Symposium on Vesicular Diseases : Plum Island Animal Disease Laboratory September 27-28, 1956 : Symposium on Vesicular Diseases (1957 : Plum Island, N.Y.) ." 1970. Internet Archive. [Washington, D.C.] : Agricultural Research Service, U.S. Dept. of Agriculture. January 1, 1970., pp. 46-47. Retrieved from: https://archive.org/details/CAT31325716/page/46/mode/2up

83   Traub, E., Eine atypische Form der Geflügelpest in Hessen-Nassau. [The Atypical Form of Fowl Pest in Hessen-Nassau] Tierarztl Rundschau : 42-45. (1942a) [Translated to English by A. Finnegan, 2019]

84   Hinshaw, W. R., et al. "A Study of Borrelia Anserina Infection (Spirochetosis) in Turkeys." J. Bacteriology, vol. 57, 1948, pp. 191–206.

85   KISSLING, R E et al. "Recovery of virus of Eastern equine encephalomyelitis from blood of a purple grackle." Proceedings of the Society for Experimental Biology and Medicine. Society for Experimental Biology and Medicine (New York, N.Y.) vol. 77,3 (1951): 398-9.

doi:10.3181/00379727-77-18791

86   RUBIN, H et al. "Isolation of a psittacosis-like agent from the blood of snowy egrets." Proceedings of the Society for Experimental Biology and Medicine. Society for Experimental Biology and Medicine (New York, N.Y.) vol. 78,3 (1951): 696-8. doi:10.3181/00379727-78-19185

87   Kissling, R. E., et al. "Birds As Winter Hosts For Eastern And Western Equine Encephalomyelitis Viruses." *American Journal of Epidemiology*, vol. 66, no. 1, 1957, pp. 42–47., doi:10.1093/oxfordjournals.aje.a119883.

88   KISSLING, R E et al. "Studies on the North American arthropod-borne encephalitides. III. Eastern equine encephalitis in wild birds." *American journal of hygiene* vol. 60,3 (1954): 251-65. doi:10.1093/oxfordjournals.aje.a119718

89   CHAMBERLAIN, R W et al. "Venezuelan equine encephalomyelitis in wild birds." *American journal of hygiene* vol. 63,3 (1956): 261-73. doi:10.1093/oxfordjournals.aje.a119810

90   Macleod, Roy. "'Strictly for the Birds': Science, the Military and the Smithsonian's Pacific Ocean Biological Survey Program, 1963–1970." Science, History and Social Activism Boston Studies in the Philosophy of Science, 2001, pp. 307–337., doi:10.1007/978-94-017-2956-7_19

91   Ibid.

92   Wallace, Gordon D., et al. "Arthropod-Borne Virus Survey on the Island of Oahu, Hawaii ." *Hawaii Medical Journal*, vol. 23, no. 5, 1964, pp. 364–368.

93   Ibid.

94   Warner, Richard E. "The Role of Introduced Diseases in the Extinction of the Endemic Hawaiian Avifauna." *The Condor*, vol. 70, no. 2, 1968, pp. 101–120., doi:10.2307/1365954.

95   Macleod, Roy. "'Strictly for the Birds': Science, the Military and the Smithsonian's Pacific Ocean Biological Survey Program, 1963–1970." Science, History and Social Activism Boston Studies in the Philosophy of Science, 2001, pp. 307–337., doi:10.1007/978-94-017-2956-7_19

Chapter Twelve

CORPORATE INTEGRATION, COVERUP, AND THE PUBLIC HEALTH CONTINGENCY PLAN

STEALTH BIOTERRORISM & THE DECLINE OF WESTERN CIVILIZATION

He who permits himself to tell a lie once, finds it much easier to do it the second time.
–Thomas Jefferson, Founding Father of the United States, 1743-1826

In the time following the bioterrorism on American shores through the simulant program, a number of things transpired to substantiate that this covert war of biological sabotage was fully underway. With the Germans defeated, the Soviet Union began to turn their new weapons against the West, while the American officials suddenly began to realize that they were being attacked many times over in a short period of time through multiple channels of attack.[1]

This biological sabotage was occurring from within during Top-Secret germ warfare tests and research activities that were carried out on a national scale, some of which were open-air tests with so-called "harmless" bacterial simulants, the very biodefense activities that were supposed to be protecting the country from germ warfare. The military had been intensifying this kind of research heavily after the War, with help from the scientific and academic circles. [2]

The effects would steadily gain momentum over the years, overlapping the simulant tests under joint-British and Canadian research, while the academic circles like Cold Spring Harbor geneticists and affiliates began integrating studies on resistance, genetics, mutation and adaptation.[3] Spies from within like Erich Traub and Donald Maclean began to effectively hijack the activities and attacked its civilians with stealth bioterrorism.[4,5,6] This was the inevitable result of Western Intelligence failing to understand the Soviet biological weapons threat, and the failure of the State Department to allocate any resources for it.[7]

The Soviet moles in MI6 like Donald Maclean and the extensive spy network's participation in helping to facilitate joint-research, led to the setup of NATO agreements and working with United Nations organizations like the Food and Agriculture Organization (FAO) and the World Health Organization (WHO). It kept an excellent channel and cover for Soviet operatives,[8] people like Erich Traub,[9] who's FAO status acted as a protective blanket for his activities, providing its safeguarding through diplomatic immunity status which made him less likely to be hauled off and executed as a spy.

In fact, in 1951, an intelligence estimate had laid out in precise terms, a close parallel to what was occurring, so the State Department's failure to allocate any funding and resources to address the Soviet biological weapons threat is almost inconceivable:

> 57. Many types of BW agents are well-suited for clandestine attack, and could be employed by the USSR even well in advance of D-Day as part of an over-all plan to impair the military effectiveness of the US. In contrast to clandestine attack with atomic and chemical weapons, clandestine employment of certain BW agents would entail much less risk of identification as enemy action.
>
> a. Very small amounts of these agents would be required initially. Such amounts would be almost impossible to detect when being brought into this country under the cover of diplomatic immunity or through smuggling operations. In addition, it would not be difficult to have some BW agents procured and cultured locally by a trained bacteriologist who was immunized against and simply equipped to handle dangerous pathogens.
>
> b. BW agents do not produce immediate symptoms and their effects are not apparent until hours or days after dissemination.
>
> c. The results of some BW agents resemble natural outbreaks of disease, and it would be difficult to connect clandestine employment of such agents with a hostile act.[10]

Beginning in 1953, the USDA began holding conferences alluding to the attacks of bioterrorism through sabotage and other means, perpetuated from many different directions and sources. They realized the numerous attacks were camouflaged within the simulant program,[11] yet at the same time, who could really say the simulants weren't actually harmful?[12]

They had a serious dilemma under discussion for some time throughout the 1950s, before arriving at the inevitable conclusion as to what they wanted to do about these unfavorable problems. The most important of these conferences was the *Proceedings of Collaborators' Meeting on Foreign Poultry Diseases, November 16-17, 1953,* in which the problem of biological warfare directed against humans through the poultry industry was treated with lengthy discussions, introducing the harsh reality that the poultry industry and United States as a whole, are particularly susceptible to biological warfare attack, and had already occurred.[13]

Col. Frank A. Todd, a biodefense specialist and veterinarian with the USDA[14] and the Pentagon,[15] whom also appeared in interviews and reports from the FBI investigations of Erich Traub's loyalties, Todd was an important contact for Traub, who had become familiar with him while in Germany.[16] Todd was perhaps the most revealing in his assessment of what would have been the main channels for bioterrorism on the United States soil against agricultural animals and human targets. Some of the excerpts from his discussion detailed the methods that were used:

> We know that there always exists the threat of the accidental introduction of foreign diseases of animals and poultry into this country in spite of all the precautions that we can take. An absolute protection against the entrance of a foreign disease into this country is impossible. Foreign diseases have gained entrance in the past and will continue to appear from time to time in spite of our efforts.
>
> It must be remembered that in addition to this normal peacetime menace there is the current biological warfare threat dealing with the possibility of the deliberate introduction and spread of disease. The willful introduction of disease into this country can cause many problems. An enemy can select the host, disease, time and place. He can also distribute unusually large numbers of organisms and pests, utilize more effective methods of dissemination, as well as unusual portals of entry. An enemy can increase the problem by using several agents of similar diseases, simultaneously. The combining of disease agents of different types might produce more than one disease in the individual host with contradictory symptoms

and varying incubation periods. Such combinations might even act synergistically to make others more effective.

Unfortunately, there are a number of animal diseases, native and foreign, benign and highly fatal, that present similar symptoms, all of which increase the diagnostic problems. It is important that we keep this in mind. The presence or the suspected presence of one of these diseases that may be thought of as only a common endemic disease may in reality be masking a more serious foreign animal disease.

I believe that records indicate that several foreign poultry diseases have gained entrance into this country by the importation of undeclared laboratory cultures, from smuggled birds, and from importing insect vectors and birds during the carrier stage or during the incubation period. We also know that raw garbage, contaminated feeds and veterinary biologics have been factors in spreading disease in this country.[17]

This conference, perhaps more than any other, serves as a good illustration of what was on their minds at the time, when Traub was just finishing up his second American run. The concern was mostly centered around poultry disease, as the avian diseases seem to have a close affinity for human hosts due to the similarities of their immune systems.[18, 19]

The pathogens that the USDA officials were most concerned about in 1953, included fowl plague virus, Newcastle Disease Virus (NDV), avian spirochetosis (*Borrelia anserina*), avian malaria (*Plasmodium gallinaceum, Plasmodium lophurae*), Eastern Equine Encephalitis Virus (EEE), ornithosis (*chlamydia pneumoniae*, psittacosis), and botulism.[20] Spirochetosis appeared to be a major concern in poultry,[21] for perhaps the only time they admit it on record from that point forward, and a main part of the attack had a lot to do with Traub's weaponized spirochetes.

From very early on they began to realize the extent was much larger than they were anticipating or competent to stop, stating many thousands of imported birds entered quarantine and were released, coming down with disease after the fact, indicating insufficient quarantine periods.[22]

The underlying theme of the entire conference was biological warfare, setting in an esoteric tone, that several attacks had been discovered and the disease agents were spreading through the population against humans and animals alike. This conference indicates that at least a few people understood specific methods being employed to carry out attacks of sabotage:

Enemy airplanes could try to spread disease to farm animals and poultry by using bombs or spray tanks modified to create clouds of the infectious agents over limited targets or to blanket large areas. Aircraft and balloons could launch similar attacks using a wide variety of devices. More likely, however, attacks against farm animals would be carried out by secret acts of sabotage.

Sabotage would certainly be conducted at livestock and poultry concentration centers such as stockyards, railroad terminals, sales barns, hatcheries, biological plants, feed production plants or feed mixing establishments. It is conceivable that a clever saboteur might use biological products as a means of spreading destructive diseases to this country's poultry population [...]. [23]

Traub's experimental research on Newcastle Disease and FMD were carried out with *biological products* like vaccines, which Traub always used to carry out his dual-purpose research.[24] The conference continued on:

Several persons have suggested that bacterial diseases such as fowl cholera and fowl typhoid might be used for sabotage purposes in feed mixing establishments, especially when they are located near or in centers of heavy poultry concentrations. Chemical poisonings from this source should not be overlooked.

Danger of introducing and spreading disease is always present in raw garbage feeding. Tuberculosis, Newcastle disease and other diseases and parasites can be spread by this means.[25]

Other participants included William R. Hinshaw, the USDA official and biological warfare specialist from Fort Detrick, who gave considerable advice on the subjects of exotic disease in poultry, urging for more first-hand experience acquired through funding of post-graduate students in foreign countries and getting quality scientists from the academic world.[26] In 1961, Support was given by Hinshaw to USDA researchers investigating an outbreak of avian spirochetosis (*Borrelia anserina*) on poultry farms in Arizona, with the authors thanking William R. Hinshaw of the biological warfare laboratory at Camp Detrick for assistance.[27]

Frank A. Todd addressed the participants with "Problems Relating to the Deliberate Introduction of Foreign Poultry Diseases." B.T.

Simms gave an introductory speech, H.W. Schoening addressed the attendees with "The Problem of Diagnosis and Control of Foreign Poultry Diseases." Main officials from the sides of both the military and USDA equally participated in the conference.

These outfits worked together to come up with new ways to handle the ever-growing threats to the agricultural populations and established methods for rapid discovery of disease agents. George Cottral and M. S. Shahan from the Plum Island Animal Disease Laboratory also attended this conference. B. T. Simms also worked with Plum Island and was listed as the contact who Traub would be with in Washington during his 1950 conference with the National Research Council.

In 1955, there was a second meeting suggesting that there were a number of attacks on American soil published in *Report of the Meetings on Foreign Animal Diseases Attended by State and Federal Regulatory Officials During February and March 1955*, with opening discussion by C.D. Van Houweling noting the significance of arthropod transmission in the spreading of exotic foreign diseases:

> We must recognize that an absolute protection against the entrance of foreign animal diseases into this country is impossible. Diseases travel as man and his animals travel – as they travel faster, infection does likewise. Today's rapid intercontinental air transport, and its rapidly increasing volume, are greatly increasing the hazard of accidental disease transmission. The threat of deliberate spread and introduction of these diseases might also be a factor.
>
> Investigations of past outbreaks of foreign animal diseases in this country have indicated that disease can be introduced and spread, by means of raw garbage (foot-and-mouth disease and vesicular exanthema), contaminated animal feeds (anthrax), and other materials (hides and wool), undeclared importation of cultures (fowl plague), biologics (foot-and-mouth pullorum and anthrax), smuggled livestock and birds (psittacosis), insect vectors (Venz. EE), and animals imported in a carrier stage (bluetongue), or during the period of incubation (scrapie).[28]

From the looks of it, they may not have discovered the weaponized Lyme disease until some years later, but they knew full well that the introduction of disease by insects was a serious problem that could not necessarily ever be eradicated:

The control and eradication of some diseases is relatively simple, and others of course much more difficult. The eradication of diseases in which wild animals, other species of domestic animals and birds act as reservoirs and insects act as vectors may be extremely difficult.[29]

Interestingly, that conference included the presentation noted in early chapters, indicating Britain may have been an attacker in earlier years, when in the 1850s a British ship stopped in the port of New York to trade an older cow for a newer cow, and after the ship sailed away, they had a sudden outbreak of contagious bovine pleuropneumonia, a bovine mycoplasma (*Mycoplasma mycoides*).

In a third conference, the following year in 1956, *Proceedings of the 1956 Regional Meetings on Foreign Animal Diseases* with Col. Frank Todd discussed further the insect and avian transmissions, reservoirs, and means of spreading disease in the United States:

> We are becoming more aware of the fact that most disease agents may affect or may reside in several host species and that this may be accomplished by the organism selectively adapting itself to new hosts. This emphasizes the complicated problems associated with animal disease control and preventive medicine. These facts should also remind us that the approaches to disease control and preventive medicine are very seldom accomplished on a single species basis and that these problems cannot be immediately nor [definitively placed] into areas of human or veterinary medicine.[30]

Another revealing part of the presentation shows that vaccines were another concern for the spread of new diseases to animals, whether by accident or intentional sabotage: :

> Contaminated biologics have been incriminated in several instances as a factor in introducing and spreading animal diseases. An outbreak of foot-and-mouth disease in the United States followed the importation of a culture of smallpox vaccine from Japan.
>
> Gregg of England describes an experience in Scotland where scrapie appeared in several flocks of sheep following the use of Louping-ill vaccine. Investigations revealed that sheep used to prepare a particular lot of the vaccine in question were the progeny of scrapie infected ewes.

201

Outbreaks of Newcastle disease have followed the use of the biologics intended to prevent the disease. On one occasion in the Midwest, a widespread outbreak of pullorum disease followed the use of Newcastle disease vaccine and it was found in flocks that had been pullorum free for a number of years. Investigations in this case showed that the eggs used in the preparation of the Newcastle vaccine had originated in pullorum diseased flocks.[31]

Migratory birds to spread disease were also well-understood to be transmitters of diseases and used as reservoirs and vectors to attack a target, exclusively in biological warfare:

Migratory birds have been incriminated in a number of cases as a means of introducing and spreading disease. Outbreaks of foot-and-mouth disease in England have been associated with the flight or the presence of birds from the European continent. The fact that birds are considered a reservoir for the encephalidities [sic] makes them an ever present potential source of this infection so that migratory birds may be looked upon as another means for the introduction and spread of disease.[32]

That same year, another conference was held, this time at Plum Island Animal Disease Center (PIADC) for its opening day ceremony, with Dr. Erich Traub as one of the guests at this conference for Plum Island.[33] Michael Carroll previously described the events in his Plum Island exposé.[34] This was one of many instances where Traub, confessed Soviet double agent, was allowed back on American soil to attend symposiums and events at the USDA.

The Animal Disease Eradication (ADE) unit was put together as a special division within the Agricultural Research Service (ARS) of the USDA in 1958,[35] later setting up additional organizations to assist them.[36]

Food safety and security was top priority in the 1960s, especially when the silent attacks began to hit one-by-one, and the industry began reeling in the condemnation and destruction to their poultry and livestock industry.[37] The USDA decided agriculture needed a new image of disease,[38] or in other words, redefining of what disease really means in relation to food safety, and ultimately, human health, along with the economic, yet in the process, short-sighted the moral significance.

A dilemma was fast-approaching indeed, because regardless of what one thinks of the USDA or agricultural businesses, it is no understatement to say they had a lot on their plate when it came to the many dozens of problems sweeping the poultry and livestock industries and how to keep it afloat, keeping its food safe, minimalizing losses, keeping up with regulatory standards, pest control, cleanliness, and on and on.[39] Chemical applications like DDT and organophosphates seemed promising as pesticides at the time but were later found to potentially cause cancer in humans,[40] yet resistance in insects.[41] Breeding procedures and strict feeding practices only went so far, and soon the diseases just overcame the measures imposed.

In 1961, a large symposium on poultry health *Disease, Environmental, and Management Factors Related to Poultry Health*, held from March 20-22, 1961, at the Jefferson Auditorium, USDA in Washington D.C. It is interesting to note in this conference, they admit that the rise in poultry losses from disease and condemnation was equally exhibited in the human health of the American population:

> Conversely, what can we do about the apparent capacity of a parasite to accommodate itself through mutation? Insects resistant to pesticides have become too commonplace. Bacteria have developed resistance to sulfas. The facility of the common Staphylococcus, Micrococcus aureus, to thrive in the presence of many broad-spectrum antibiotics is well known. It is no comfort to learn that deaths from infection in man are increasing just as Broiler [chicken] condemnation losses seem to be. Dauer (1961) reported that mortality from all types of septicemia has been increasing steadily since 1948 particularly septicemia caused by staphylococci.[42]

Inspection and mandatory regulatory procedures, while seeming to be in place to safeguard the population from infectious disease, were in many ways ensuring continual exposures to the disease microbes of a chronic nature, for a small band-aid effect to the industry. They began to change their tone to see immune tolerance as an acceptable immunity, even though it meant chronic, persistent infection.[43]

Immune tolerance was overtaking the animals and humans through the diseases unleashed as well as the vaccines used to prevent them. The immune system was being overthrown to keep the diseases inapparent and unnoticeable, but in the end could have spread the diseases even more widely than it would have otherwise, and he cites F. Macfarlane Burnet and Peter B. Medawar who were given the Nobel Prize instead of Erich Traub:

That the [immune] tolerance of the embryo can at least in limited measure be prolonged through its lifetime has been demonstrated through many researchers, culminating in those of Medawar (1961) and Burnet, for which they were awarded the 1960 Nobel Prize in medicine and physiology. Medawar has suggested foreign antigens entering the fetus from the mother might weaken its resistance in later life to infectious disease. Can egg-transmitted pathogens thus gain the tolerance of the developing chick and prevent chicks thus infected from developing effective antibodies against such pathogens? And thus becoming disease carriers? [44]

A report published in the supplemental conference material, presented a post-mortem examination of condemned poultry by the USDA, showing an unprecedented number of cases were due to septicemia and toxemia, in 1959, the number of condemned poultry due to septicemia and toxemia was at 8,818,628 animals, and in 1960 that number was 11,475,815. In 1959, septicemia was the largest factor in poultry condemnation, while in 1961 airsacculitis became the leading cause of condemnation, with *Septicemia and Toxemia* and *inflammatory processes* following in 2nd and 3rd.[45] All of the condemnation causes were symptoms from infectious origins.

They began to come to the realization that the poultry diseases were much more pronounced due to respiratory pneumonia and pleuropneumonia-like organisms (*Mycoplasma*). While some of this was noted following immunizations, it was further enhanced by the fact that they had been conducting large-scale, open-air tests on a regular basis in Operation LAC and similar programs, using pneumonia-like organisms such as *Serratia marcescens*.[46] These problems became very destructive, and yet no one wanted to admit that it might be that the military made some really big errors in the vaccine and simulant programs.

Endnotes

1   Wildlife surveys, tracking of birds, mosquito and tick surveys, public health surveillance, agricultural conferences, and so on, began to show that many diseases were proliferating heavily through the United States in the late 1940's and early 1950's.

2   Canadian Department of National Defence. Joint-Research with U.S. Army Chemical Corps and Fort Detrick on OPERATION LAC. Retrieved from: http://data2.archives.ca/e/e443/e011063033.pdf

3   Demerec, M. ""Corporate Reports Annual Reports: 1949-1960."" Cold Spring HarborLaboratory. Accessed August 22, 2019. http://repository.cshl.edu/view/subjects/Annual=-5Freports.html

4   Loftus, John J. "Memorandum on Biological Weapons History." 2018.

5   "Proceedings : Collaborator's Meeting on Foreign Poultry Diseases (1953 : Washington)." Internet Archive, United States Department of Agriculture (USDA) Washington, 1 Jan. 1970,, 1953., Retrieved from: https://archive.org/details/CAT10678555/page/n5

6   Intelligence Advisory Committee, National Intelligence Estimate: Soviet Capabilities and Probable Courses of Action through mid- 1959, NIE 11- 4- 54 (Washington, D.C., 1954) (Top Secret); Intelligence Advisory Committee, National Intelligence Estimate: Soviet Gross Capabilities for Attacks on the US and Key Overseas Installations and Forces through 1 July 1958, NIE 11- 7- 55 (Washington, D.C., 1955)

7   Zabrocka, K. (2013, May 22). Under the Microscope: Why US Intelligence underestimated the Soviet Biological Weapons Program. Retrieved February 19, 2021, from https://stacks.stanford.edu/file/druid:wk216hz5745/Zabrocka_Katarzyna_Thesis_Final.pdf

8   NATO. "Did Spies Target NATO Secrets during the Cold War?" NATO. North American treaty Organization. Espionage Uncovered Series, n.d. https://www.nato.int/cps/en/natohq/declassified_138455.htm

9   Loftus, John J., (personal communication) Loftus' late friend and CIC official Dan Benjamin, interrogated Traub to extract a confession of Soviet espionage.

10   Intelligence Advisory Committee, National Intelligence Estimate: Soviet Capabilities and Probable Courses of Action through mid- 1959, NIE 11- 4- 54 (Washington, D.C., 1954) (Top Secret); Intelligence Advisory Committee, National Intelligence Estimate: Soviet Gross Capabilities for Attacks on the US and Key Overseas Installations and Forces through 1 July 1958, NIE 11- 7- 55 (Washington, D.C., 1955)

11   "Proceedings : Collaborator's Meeting on Foreign Poultry Diseases (1953 : Washington)." Internet Archive, United States Department of Agriculture (USDA) Washington, 1 Jan. 1970,, 1953., Retrieved from: https://archive.org/details/CAT10678555/page/n5

12   Vernon, R. G., and O. E. Hepler. "Chromogenic Bacteria with a Case Report of a Fatal Infection Caused by Serratia Marcescens." Q Bull Northwest Univ Med Sch. 28, no. 4 (1954): 366-72.

13   "Proceedings : Collaborator's Meeting on Foreign Poultry Diseases (1953 : Washington)." Internet Archive, United States Department of Agriculture (USDA) Washington, 1 Jan. 1970,, 1953., Retrieved from: https://archive.org/details/CAT10678555/page/n5

14   Ibid., https://archive.org/details/CAT10678555/page/8 pp. 8-11

15   Todd, Frank A. 1951. "The Public Health Veterinarian in National Defense." American Journal of Public Health and the Nations Health 41 (9): 1059–64. https://doi.org/10.2105/ajph.41.9.1059.

16   National Archives. RG 65 Erich Traub, (Declassified FBI Investigations on the Loyalties of Erich Traub). Federal Bureau of Investigation (FBI): NARA., Doc. # QO1-458431291

17   Todd, F.A., Problems Relating to the Deliberate Introduction of Foreign Poultry Dis-

eases. "Proceedings : Collaborator's Meeting on Foreign Poultry Diseases (1953 : Washington)." Internet Archive, United States Department of Agriculture (USDA) Washington, 1 Jan. 1970, 1953., pp. 8-9, Retrieved from: https://archive.org/details/CAT10678555/page/8

18   Kohonen, P., et al. "Avian Model for B-Cell Immunology ? New Genomes and Phylotranscriptomics." Scandinavian Journal of Immunology, vol. 66, no. 2-3, 2007, pp. 113–121., doi:10.1111/j.1365-3083.2007.01973.x.

19   Weill, Jean-Claude et al. "A bird's eye view on human B cells." Seminars in immunology vol. 16,4 (2004): 277-81. doi:10.1016/j.smim.2004.08.007

20   PROCEEDINGS of COLLABORATORS MEETING on FOREIGN POULTRY DISEASES. USDA, 1953., Retrieved from: https://archive.org/details/CAT10678555/page/n16, pp. 16

21   Loomis, E. C. "Avian Spirochetosis in California Turkeys." Am. J. Vet. Res. , Oct. 1953, pp. 612–615.

22   "Proceedings : Collaborator's Meeting on Foreign Poultry Diseases (1953 : Washington)." Internet Archive, United States Department of Agriculture (USDA) Washington, 1 Jan. 1970, 1953., Retrieved from: https://archive.org/details/CAT10678555/page/4, pp. 4

23   Ibid., pp. 10, Retrieved from: https://archive.org/details/CAT10678555/page/10

24   Traub, E., & Capps, W. I. Experiments with chick embryo-adapted foot-and-mouth disease virus and a method for the rapid adaptation. National Naval Medical Center. Bethesda, MD. (1953) U.S. NAVY Project NM. NMRI Memorandum Report. Project NM 000 018.07

25   "Proceedings : Collaborator's Meeting on Foreign Poultry Diseases (1953 : Washington)." Internet Archive, United States Department of Agriculture (USDA) Washington, 1 Jan. 1970, pp. 10, Retrieved from: https://archive.org/details/CAT10678555/page/10

26   Ibid., pp. 23, Retrieved from: https://archive.org/details/CAT10678555/page/23

27   Rokey, N. W., and V. N. Snell. 1961. "Avian Spirochetosis (Borrelia Anserina) Epizootics in Arizona Poultry." J. Amer. Vet. Med. Ass. 138 (12): 648–52.

28   Van Houweling, C. D. "Report of the Meetings on Foreign Animal Diseases Attended by State and Federal Regulatory Officials During February and March of 1955." Report of the Meetings on Foreign Animal Diseases Attended by State and Federal Regulatory Officials During February and March of 1955, USDA, 1957., pp. 03 Received from: https://archive.org/details/CAT10678550/page/3

29   Ibid., pp. 14 Received from: https://archive.org/details/CAT10678550/page/14

30   Todd, F. A., et al. "Proceedings of the 1956 Regional Meetings on Foreign Animal Diseases." U.S. Government Printing Office, Proceedings of the 1956 Regional Meetings on Foreign Animal Diseases, 1956. Retrieved from: https://archive.org/details/CAT10678014/page/11

31   Ibid., pp. 14, Retrieved from: https://archive.org/details/CAT10678014/page/14

32   Ibid.

33   "Proceedings of Symposium on Vesicular Diseases : Plum Island Animal Disease Laboratory September 27-28, 1956 : Symposium on Vesicular Diseases (1957 : Plum Island, N.Y.) ." 1970. Internet Archive. [Washington, D.C.] : Agricultural Research Service, U.S. Dept. of Agriculture. January 1, 1970. https://archive.org/details/CAT31325716/page/40

34   Carroll, M. C. (2004). Lab 257: The disturbing story of the governments secret and deadly virus research facility. New York: Morrow., pp. 6-7

35   United States, Congress, Animal Disease Eradication Division (ADE). "Activities Handbook - Animal Disease Eradication Division." Activities Handbook - Animal Disease Eradication Division, 1962., pp. 61

36   Smith, J. S. "The United States Department of Agriculture Emergency Animal Dis-

ease Preparedness Program." SpringerLink. Springer, Boston, MA, January 1, 1976. https://link.springer.com/chapter/10.1007/978-1-4757-1656-6_14

37   United States, Congress, Animal Disease Eradication Division (ADE). "Activities Handbook - Animal Disease Eradication Division." Activities Handbook - Animal Disease Eradication Division, 1962.

38   Welch, Frank J., A New Image for Agriculture. Disease, Environmental, and Management Factors Related to Poultry Health: a Symposium Held March 20- 22, 1961 at the Jefferson Auditorium, USDA, Washington, D.C. : United States. Agricultural Research Service. Internet Archive, [Washington, D.C.] : Agricultural Research Service, U.S. Dept. of Agriculture, 1 Jan. 1961, pp. 1-3, Retrieved from: https://archive.org/details/CAT31325715/page/1

39   "Disease, Environmental, and Management Factors Related to Poultry Health : a Symposium Held March 20- 22, 1961 at the Jefferson Auditorium, USDA, Washington, D.C. : United States. Agricultural Research Service." Internet Archive, [Washington, D.C.] : Agricultural Research Service, U.S. Dept. of Agriculture, 1 Jan. 1961, Retrieved from: https://www.archive.org/details/CAT31325715/page/n1

40   "Exposure to Chemical in Roundup Increases Risk for Cancer, Study Finds." ScienceDaily, ScienceDaily, 14 Feb. 2019, https://www.sciencedaily.com/releases/2019/02/190214093359.htm

41   King, J. C., The Genetics of Resistance to Insecticides. Annual Report of the Biological Laboratory. Project Report. Long Island Biological Association, Cold Spring Harbor, NY., pp. 36-38

42   Ibid., pp. 7, Retrieved from: https://www.archive.org/details/CAT31325715/page/n7

43   Ibid., pp. 8, Retrieved from: www.archive.org/details/CAT31325715/page/n8

44   Disease, Environmental, and Management Factors Related to Poultry Health : a Symposium Held March 20- 22, 1961 at the Jefferson Auditorium, USDA, Washington, D.C. : United States. Agricultural Research Service." Internet Archive, [Washington, D.C.] : Agricultural Research Service, U.S. Dept. of Agriculture, 1 Jan. 1961, pp.7. Retrieved from: https://www.archive.org/details/CAT31325715/page/n1

45   Ibid., pp. 12, Retrieved from: www.archive.org/details/CAT31325715/page/n12

46   Paine, T. F. "Illness in Man Following Inhalation of Serratia Marcescens." Journal of Infectious Diseases 79, no. 3 (1946): 226-32. doi:10.1093/infdis/79.3.226.

Chapter Thirteen

THE BIOLOGICAL AND SOCIAL PHENOMENON OF LYME SURVEILLANCE

A COMPREHENSIVE DISCOURSE IN PUBLIC RELATIONS

Nothing breaks the heart, courage, and strength more quickly than a lie; a lie is the most devilish, because it is the most cowardly vice.
– Ernst Moritz Arndt, German writer, 1769-1860

D espite the common belief that the first cases of Lyme disease surfaced in 1975, it had been spreading for nearly twenty-five years before attention was finally given to Lyme disease in 1975 from a cluster of cases with an unknown arthritis.[1] The agent had been monitored secretly since it began spreading and that the government knew it was being hit with biological agents from the 1950s is evident in the 1953 *Proceedings of the Collaborator's Meeting on Foreign Poultry Diseases* we discussed in previous chapters.[2] As John Loftus had revealed in his 1982 book *The Belarus Secret*, the Lyme Disease situation was being monitored under the guise of health studies in the endemic areas.[3]

No longer confined to the realm of agriculture, what were at first glance exotic animal diseases hitting the poultry and livestock industry, were actually devious zoonotic pathogens from animals adapted to humans.[4] The reader may recall from the earlier chapters, a USDA conference in 1961, *Disease, Environmental, and Management Factors Related to Poultry Health,* where USDA officials admitted that, among other things, "*it is no comfort to learn that deaths from infection in man are increasing just as Broiler* [chicken] *condemnation losses seem to be.*"[5] The biological terrorism waged on the United States was fully underway but the public was kept in the dark.

THE BIOLOGICAL AND SOCIAL PHENOMENON OF LYME SURVEILLANCE

As the USDA began to create new divisions like the Agricultural Disease Eradication (ADE) Division,[6] the U. S. Public Health System created its own agencies in parallel to the animal disease surveillance, such as the Epidemic Intelligence Service (EIS).[7] This division kept broad surveillance on situations developing like zoonotic infections emerging as new outbreaks, and the one who created EIS, Alexander D. Langmuir, set up the EIS to also begin a surveillance program on polio and the polio vaccine after the Cutter Incident occurred causing paralytic disease from the vaccine and the contamination of the vaccines with the carcinogenic SV40 virus in both the inactivated and oral polio vaccines that were given to 98 million Americans by 1960.[8] There were many other situations developing from the start of the Cold War and new agencies like the EIS would monitor the progression as Western civilization began its steady decline.

25 YEARS LATER, LYME DISEASE OFFICIALLY DECLARED TO EXIST

The first doctors to establish the presence of the disease were from Yale, Dr. Allen C. Steere and Stephen Malawista.[9] Dr. Robert Shope, the son of Traub's American mentor Richard E. Shope, served as an advisor for the early papers on Lyme disease.[10] Robert Shope was running the Yale research on arboviruses at the time, setting up the Yale Arbovirus Research Unit (YARU).[11] He had an understanding of how these diseases worked, and he knew Traub through his father, and even had dinner with Traub several years before the German virologist's death, quoted by Michael C. Carroll in his *Lab 257: The Disturbing Story of the Governments secret Plum Island Germ Laboratory*, revealing that in the late 1970's, Shope Jr. relayed that, "*I had dinner with Traub one day – out of old time's sake – and he was a pretty defeated man by then.*"[12]

While early Lyme disease publications treated the disease as an arthritic disease,[13] soon they began to acknowledge the neurological abnormalities, the similarities to Traub's LCM virus and *immune tolerance*.[14] The cocktail of several tick-borne diseases and spirochetes like *Borrelia burgdorferi* and *Leptospira* set off toxic reactions awakening sleeping viruses within the host due to the immunosuppression,[15,16] causing a myriad of confusing, often contradictory symptoms that mirrored Lupus,[17] Multiple Sclerosis (MS),[18] among others. The early cases of Lyme disease imitated viral infections for this reason because the lipoid surface protein that was shed into the blood disabled the immune system.[19] It was this toxic lipid that caused the immune system to go haywire and awaken the sleeping viruses in the manner of Traub's LCM virus.[20]

One of the early cases of Lyme disease, Polly Murray, went on to write a memoir about her struggles and the early days of public health's official recognition of the disease, then termed *Lyme arthritis*.[21] Her memoir, *The Widening Circle: A Lyme Disease Pioneer Tells Her Story*, was perhaps the first to give an inside look at the struggle, ridicule, and denial of the complex, mysterious disease by public health officials.[22] She reveals in the beginning of the book that she became very sick in August of 1955, and this appears to have been the start of the initial infection which hit off and on through the next decade until she was permanently disabled by it in the 1960s. This would show that indeed it had been spreading by the 1950s. Polly happened to be one of the unique cases with a mix of both allergic and immunosuppressive reactions to *Borrelia burgdorferi* but from the descriptions of her illness, it sounded like Lyme disease with multiple overlapping co-infections. The book best describes what Lyme disease sufferers go through. Bad enough to have their lives turned upside down by this miserable curse, but to add insult to injury, they likewise had to contend with physicians and specialists ridiculing them as a psychosomatic illness, imagining their disease.[23] She would eventually find herself at the heart of the coming conferences to study the nature of *Lyme arthritis*.[24]

INTERNATIONAL MEETINGS AND SYMPOSIUMS ON LYME DISEASE

Lyme Disease Conferences and Symposiums in the United States and abroad were soon being organized and attended on an annual basis. *The First International Symposium on Lyme Disease* was held from November 16-18, 1983, at Yale University in Connecticut.[25] Work was presented at the conference by some of the Dutch researchers who occasionally worked in cooperation with Plum Island, some who conducted characterization studies of *Borrelia anserina*,[26] with associated researchers who worked with the East African Veterinary Research Organization (EAVRO), an organization who employed a researcher taught by Traub from Iran's Razi Institute of Serum and Vaccines.[27]

Moderating a discussion on epidemiologic studies was Robert E. Shope, who explained that relying solely on antibodies to diagnose the disease was not reliable, saying that "[s]*erological test results were not very helpful for defining cases in Minnesota. [...] In any case, we still rely on a non-serological case definition.*"[28] Despite this, Shope then proposed that antibody tests should be used to monitor the disease, saying, "[t]*he states should, however, provide serological diagnosis especially for cases with joint, cardiac, or central nervous system disease. The case definition should be continually reviewed to include possible new syndromes which can be found to correlate with positive serological test results.*" Relying on antibody tests would have the consequence of silencing many active infections of Lyme disease and other co-infections.[29] Certainly there were other biomarkers of the disease that could be used, but these were likely never explored. With a surveillance program in place, international conferences would happen annually, with many drug firms taking part.[30]

The second symposium on Lyme Disease took place in Vienna, Austria, eventually published in one book, *Lyme Borreliosis: Proceedings of the Second International Symposium on Lyme Disease and Related Disorders, Vienna, 1985.*[31] This second Lyme disease conference was attended by many participants from the first event back at Yale, with scientists Willy Burgdorfer, Allen Steere, Alan Barbour, Heinz Flamm, Klaus Weber, and many more, with funding from many drug firms around the world.

THE FIRST DEARBORN CONFERENCE ON LYME DISEASE TESTING

To establish a diagnostic test to be used as the standard test to diagnose and track *Borrelia burgdorferi*, the first conference at Dearborn was set up, with a so-called *consensus* on what defines the disease and how it should be diagnosed.

In an attempt to arrive at a standard test, they set up the first conference for diagnostic testing criteria for Lyme disease, published in the *Proceedings of the First National Conference on Lyme Disease Testing, November 1-2, 1990, Dearborn, MI.* The conference report shows that 129 registrants participated in this conference. Several participants, including co-chairpersons of the committee, were veterinarians, while some speakers were scientists from the Connecticut Agricultural Experiment Station, while others were from the public health arena.[32]

The conference began with a brief overview describing early cases, its global spread and described the disease in three stages. Stage I, which is summed up in the following paragraph:

> Accompanying symptoms of early Lyme disease include malaise, fatigue, headache, fever, chills, myalgias and regional lymphadenopathy (1, 2). Occasionally patients will develop meningitis, mild encephalopathy, migratory arthalgias, hepatitis, generalized lymphadenopathy, splenomegaly, sore throat, nonproductive cough or testicular swelling. Except for fatigue, early symptoms are intermittent and changing, occasionally lasting for months after skin lesions clear.[33]

211

In Stage II, they described neurological, cardiac, and conjunctival manifestations, while equally showing that the disease spectrum mirrored the central nervous system diseases that were being monitored in early health studies to conclude that "[a]lzheimer's disease, amyotrophic lateral sclerosis, dementia, multiple sclerosis-like syndromes, progressive encephalopathy, pseudotumor cerebri, psychosis, and subtle cognitive dysfunction have all been reported as part of the clinical spectrum of Lyme disease."[34]

Stage III included arthritis and musculoskeletal manifestations, in addition to the complaints of Stage I and II.[35] In addition to these stages, some miscellaneous manifestations of Lyme Disease included hepatitis, fatal adult respiratory distress syndrome, among other things. Pregnancy complications and congenital transmission to the infant was noted in some cases.[36]

The conference then began to shift to different speakers covering various aspects of the disease, its diagnosis, treatment, the spread of the spirochete both in humans and domestic animals, and many additional aspects of *Borrelia burgdorferi* most relevant to diagnosis and testing.[37] With all the complications inherent to this agent, the conference was followed up four years later with a second conference and a new diagnostic standard and criteria which would exclude many of those who were most affected by the disease.

THE SECOND DEARBORN CONFERENCE, NEW TEST & CASE DEFINITION

The Second National Conference on Serologic Diagnosis of Lyme Disease, the follow-up conference to the first Dearborn, took place from October 27-29, 1994. This conference brought radical changes to include a new case definition of what Lyme disease was in very specific terms, and the end result was a very different disease than what they had included prior.[38] The public health system and special interest groups from academia were planning to study the disease long-term under Lyme disease surveillance programs as it ran its natural course, just as they did to African Americans and Hispanics in the earlier Tuskegee and Guatemala syphilis studies.[39, 40]

The 1994 conference on Dearborn essentially created a new test and a new definition of Lyme disease whereby only those with robust, healthy immune systems could make the cutoff and test positive while the majority with weaker immune responses would test negative even though they were considerably sicker and not responsive to antibiotics, which Dr. Raymond Dattwyler described in a lecture:

Dr. O'BRIEN: "I was concerned about your last slide where you said there was a poor correlation between serologic [i. e. antibody] response and clinical [i.e. observable] disease. And as I heard you to say, some people who mount better immune responses get worse disease. Did I hear you say that?"

DR. DATTWYLER: "No, no, I said the reverse. The better responses tended to have better response. And I should clarify where this is from. This is from antibiotic trials. These are treatment trials of erythema migrans, in which individuals given an antibiotic regimen which was not optimal – we did not know that it was not optimal at the time – the ones that failed to mount a vigorous response tended to do worse, clinically. So, there was an inverse correlation between the degree of serologic [i. e. antibody] response and the outcome."

"So, individuals with a poor immune response tend to have worse disease." [41]

They knew about these apparent genetic factors of different types of immune systems termed HLA types,[A] which can be explained in simple terms by saying that, just as there are variants of the same kind of virus in which the properties between variants can vary considerably, so there are also variants of the human immune system between different types of people with differences in susceptibility and disease manifestations of the same disease agent that can vary profoundly in the level of disease caused between different people.[42] It was the reason that some people had fatal reactions to infection with SARS-CoV-2 virus while others had no visible signs of disease.[43] The officials involved in Lyme disease from early on explained these factors when they wrote Polly Murray to ask if they could study her immune system response for a larger study on HLA typing:

We would appreciate your continuing support for this study in 3 ways. First, we feel fortunate to have been able to arrange for a special laboratory to do a test called HLA typing. This test gives information on predisposition to certain infections. Because the test needs to be done very soon after a blood sample is drawn, we will be contacting you to see if you would be willing to have another blood sample drawn. There is no charge to you for the test. [44]

A   **HLA** stands for **Human Leukocyte Antigen**, and in simple terms, just as there are variants of viruses and their properties vary between the different variants, there are also variants of the human immune system between different types of people.

However, it is likely that HLA has some involvement in people who were infected congenitally from mother to newborn, the conferred *immune tolerance* that was present in children born infected from infected, *immune tolerant* mothers. Traub found in his mice that immune tolerant mothers would invariably bring forth infected, immune tolerant mice when she gave birth to new mice.[45] It was the phenomenon Traub had described in a 1960 paper on LCM virus that the newly infected progeny of mice would make little to no antibodies to LCM virus, even though they had active, persistent viral infections without outward symptoms.[46] These inapparently infected newborns could infect others with a virulent LCM virus despite a lack of apparent disease. The virus cleared from the blood and attacked the central nervous system and these mice would develop neurodegenerative diseases later in life.[47] The Second Dearborn Conference was essentially declaring war on the sick and defenseless.

No longer was the health and wellness of Americans a priority, but instead the majority of those cases with a more devastating disease were being silenced, the new tests would deny their disease altogether, along with the science of *immune tolerance*, Traub's major contribution to virology and immunology.[48] It stands as the basis of most forms of chronic disease and mental illness, because neurotropic effects on the brain always followed the destruction of the immune system.[49] The immune system, no longer able to fend off harmful pathogens, would tolerate them instead as they invaded the brain and nervous system of its victims.

The new system of diagnostic testing standards implemented on these newer diseases spreading in America brought a one-size-fits-all approach to public health and brought incompetent healthcare with fraudulent testing,[50] improper treatment to no treatment at all, and worst of all, the denial of illness for the most severely affected patients.[51] This brand of medicine was oftentimes referred to under the catchphrase *evidence-based medicine* because using these outdated models and incompetent testing standards for diagnosis meant a negative test for a majority of those affected, and the public health system and the monopolies that run them could say there was no evidence of infection or disease even though these patients had persistent debilitating infections in the fashion of Traub, à la mode.

The *evidence-based medicine* paradigm was bolstered and reinforced by public relations firms working for the corporate side of healthcare, big pharma start-ups and vaccine manufacturers, and of course, those with government contracts. It runs that a complicated chronic disease like Lyme disease and the cocktail of infections it often came with was a very expensive disease to address and diagnose since each case would be unique with endless variations between individuals while the complex and often contradictory symptoms meant incompetence when it came to diagnosing and treating the disease.[52]

The establishment of the American Lyme Disease Foundation (ALDF) set up to lead the official talking points under one organization,[53] backed by high-profile, heavy-hitter Wallstreet financers.[54, 55] The founder, John J. Connolly, had connections to the Carlyle group that George H. W. Bush, James Baker III, and other National Defense officials were involved with at Texas A&M and the M.D. Anderson Cancer Center, who had some level of involvement with earlier mycoplasma testing in the Texas prison system.[56] John J. Connolly set up the ALDF and it worked to implement those changes in Lyme disease to reflect the changes made at the Dearborn conference of 1994 and the paradigm of *evidence-based medicine* was the gold standard for maintaining the public health and biodefense coverup.[57]

Most interesting, is the membership of one board member from a public relations firm, Ketchum Public Relations Worldwide, contracted by the American government, including the Department of Health and Human Services (HHS), the Department of Education (DoE), the Internal Revenue Service (IRS), and the US Army.[58] They provided crisis management for HHS and Medicare, as well as promoting the benefits of drugs for pharmaceutical firms using actors posing as journalists in commercials prepackaged as legitimate news stories for HHS, noted in an article by *The Washington Post*.[59]

Much more disturbing, is the fact that Ketchum Public Relations firm was also openly contracted to work for the Russian government from 2006-2015, and according to some news outlets, took about $60 million from the Kremlin to promote a more favorable view of Russia during the Syrian crisis starting in 2013, and this is also reflected in an *International Business Times* article from 2015. [60]

LLMDS & LYME ADVOCACY: FALSE DICHOTOMY FOR LYME SURVEILLANCE

The year before the Second Dearborn conference took place, a congressional hearing took place that presented the dilemma in the treatment and diagnosis of Lyme disease.[61] The public health system and those in charge of Lyme disease surveillance knew that in wiping an overwhelming majority of chronically ill patients from the slate would inhibit the active surveillance on the disease due to the lack of personal medical records, so they let the so-called Lyme-Literate Medical Doctors (LLMDs) continue practicing their unauthorized treatments, and were able to keep surveillance on these cases.

In return, the medical records and patient data could still assess the disease progression in those being treated by these doctors, at least, those who could afford the immense burden of paying top dollar to doctors running private practices running expensive tests upon every visit and would endure intensive treatments of all kinds, but there was no guarantee they would make out any better than those who couldn't afford it and left it untreated.[62]

While some of these LLMDs would have their licenses removed or private practices closed, by and large, the public health establishment let the LLMDs continue practicing, and besides, Pharma was still banking off it through the sale of prolonged courses of antibiotics.[63] It is not to suggest that these doctors worked for the The Centers for Disease Control and Prevention (CDC) per se, but the portals used in the patient data and diagnostics would have been integrated into a system that CDC would have access to.

Before long, however, the CDC and public health system running Lyme surveillance was funding and supporting opposing sides of the equation, such as the Lyme advocacy organizations in opposition to the side Allen Steere and the ALDF was serving. SmithKline & Beecham, who would be developing the LYMErix vaccine, was also getting behind these Lyme advocates.

In 1993, for example, a surveillance report on Lyme disease published by the Bacterial Zoonoses Branch, Division of Vector-Borne Infectious Diseases, National Center for Infectious Disease, Center for Disease Control, offers a clue into what the funding of opposing groups was all about – *surveillance* – to study the short-term and long-term progression of the disease agent filtering through the population:

> Two items are presented in this issue of the Lyme Disease Surveillance Summary, an interim progress report on CDC funded Cooperative Agreements for research and education on Lyme disease, and the reprint of a recent article published in the MMWR [Morbidity and Mortality Weekly Report] on complications of treatment of suspected Lyme disease. [64]

Further into the report, under a section of the surveillance plan, Education of the Public and Health Care Providers, the Lyme Borreliosis Foundation, which later became the Lyme Disease Foundation (LDF), was listed in the surveillance program, to educate the public, while the American Lyme Foundation, which became the ALDF, played the role of educating physicians and the general public:

> The Lyme Borreliosis Foundation has developed and is distributing instructional videos aimed at school children, the general public, and workers at risk because of occupational exposures. Videos for school children based on the Muppets have been shown at the V International Conference on Lyme Borreliosis and the annual meeting of the American Public Health Association. These also serve Spanish-speaking and hearing-impaired audiences. A number of public service announcements (PSA's) have been produced and widely shown and aired in the regional media. A wide range of written materials has also been produced and distributed.
>
> The American Lyme Foundation (New York) has established a telephone information hot-line service and has produced educational videos for elementary and high school students. PSA's have also being [sic] produced. Written material is available for the lay public, and an informational brochure for physicians and other health care workers is being produced.[65]

In 1995, another report was published with reference to additional educational material that would be provided, one for the public, and one for educators, indicating the education of medical professionals, the former provided by the Lyme Disease Foundation (LDF), while the latter provided by the American Lyme Disease Foundation (ALDF), two groups that publicly oppose each other:

ADDITIONAL AVAILABLE EDUCATIONAL MATERIALS NOT INCLUDED IN LDSS V6/N1

Lyme Disease Foundation
Community Education Poster Board
Educational Material for School-Age Children
Target Audience: All Ages

American Lyme Disease Foundation
Lyme Disease: Clinical Update for Physicans
Materials for Educators
Type: Booklet [66]

In later years, the Lyme Disease Foundation (LDF) received promotional funding from drug firm SmithKline & Beecham (SKB) as the LYMErix vaccine was about to hit the market,[67] and when FDA hearings and newspaper articles show that the vaccine began causing severe reactions and illness in those receiving them,[68, 69] the LDF publicly denounced it:

> One lay advocacy organization that SKB initially supported was the Lyme Disease Foundation. At the 1998 VRBPAC meeting that ultimately gave approval to the vaccine, Karen Vanderhoof-Forschner, the foundation's president, offered passionate support for LYMErix. Similar in many ways to the SKB-sponsored clinician who addressed the meeting, Vanderhoof-Forschner argued that [Lyme disease (LD)] was a geographically widespread, underdiagnosed, chronic, devastating, and costly disease— and thus worthy of prevention by vaccination. But in 2001 she told the same advisory board that the vaccine "represents an imminent and substantial hazard to the public health and needs to be immediately recalled."[70]

THE 1997 LYME DISEASE FOUNDATION SYMPOSIUM

As the ALDF and establishment public health officials had conferences such as Dearborn to serve their aims, the Lyme Advocates and non-profits were separately organizing conferences of their own, with support of the CDC, culminating in a 1997 conference, *Basic and Clinical Approaches to Lyme Disease: a Lyme Disease Foundation Symposium, Boston, Massachusetts, 19-20 April 1997.*[71]

The conference has some of the ALDF side involved in this conference like Gary Wormser,[72] and a presentation by David H. Persing from the Mayo Foundation,[73] who we will hear more about in the following chapter. The conference also had a presentation by LLMD Sam Donta,[74] and also notable is a paper by researchers from SmithKline regarding specific issues developing and implementing a Lyme disease vaccine.[75] In one presentation, the conference saw researchers from Austria do a presentation on what made Lyme disease a chronic infection.[76]

COLLABORATION WITH RUSSIA ON LYME DISEASE TESTING

With the passing of the Dearborn standard tests for Lyme disease in the mainstream medical practice, Allen Steere carried out cooperative studies with Russia, through NIH grants on Lyme borreliosis in Russia to equally put the new guidelines in effect in there, though it is unclear that he ever travelled to Russia for these studies.[77, 78, 79] At any rate, this would essentially be covering one another's tracks through the tripartite blackmail, as the British, Germans, Canadians, United States, and now Russians, kept from addressing the dirty work of their biological war that had been ongoing since the start of World War I.[80]

LYMErix: The Great Imitator Shot

As Steere's studies of Lyme borreliosis in Russia finished up, clinical trials moved on, with two vaccines constructed for U.S. approval like a race to the finish line. One vaccine was being worked on through Connaught Laboratories, and another through SmithKline & Beecham,[81] both taking place in the United States. However, SmithKline & Beecham began a separate trial in the Czech Republic on children in collaboration with the University of Connecticut.[82] Both vaccine trials in the United States accumulated lawsuits by 1996.[83]

SmithKline, however, produced a finished product despite a lack of safety, speeding through the final phases of their American trials declaring the vaccine safe and effective. However, Connaught even pulled their vaccine after claiming "successful phase III clinical trials."[84] Something wasn't right from the start, but no one wanted to speak up about exactly what that was, and when the injuries began to surface in significant numbers, they downplayed it.[85]

More suspiciously, SmithKline and the University of Connecticut took all their subjects in the Czech trials from the same age group, ethnic background and geographic location.[86] This group may have appeared to have the best HLA type to produce the most favorable responses to push through the vaccine trial obstacles. Strangely, research by Russian and American scientists at New York Medical College (NYMC) had significant studies going on at the time on the different HLA types between ethnic populations,[87] including one specifically on the Northern European HLA makeup similar to the Czechoslovakians published the same year the trial began.[88]

The vaccine was backed and finally approved by the FDA despite the failures to properly assess the safety.[89] It was released by SmithKline & Beecham, who later became GlaxoSmithKline (GSK), a merger of SmithKline & Beecham and Glaxo Wellcome,[90] formerly Burrough's Wellcome & Co.[91]

By 1998, the vaccine manufacturers and its scientists were able to somehow pass the vaccine off as safe and effective to the FDA,[92] while

219

writing off the associated side effects as unrelated or minimal, but the public would have a different experience.[93]

Soon people started to experience severe reactions due to onset of the immunosuppression from these forms of antigen on the immune system.[94] By 2001, LYMErix vaccine reactions were making headlines, such as "Concerns Grow Over Reactions to Lyme Shots."[95] At the time of its release, SmithKline's LYMErix was promoted for use by physicians, especially in Lyme endemic areas.[96] But they were not told that the vaccine could produce the same outcome as those cases of chronic Lyme disease even without spirochetes involved, because the chronic aspect of Lyme disease is the result of what that antigen does to the immune system.[97] It is interesting to note that in a 1996 patent by David H. Persing, "Method for detecting B. burgdorferi infection" (US6045804A), he explains the ability of the outer surface protein A (OspA) antigen in LYMErix to cause exactly what would later be reported and brought out in FDA hearings, mirroring chronic Lyme disease:

> Additional uncertainty may arise if the vaccines are not completely protective; Vaccinated patients with multisystem complaints characteristic of later presentations of Lyme disease may be difficult to distinguish from patients with vaccine failure. Vaccine failures have been occasionally noted in animal models [...] and infection with antigenically variant strains of B. burgdorferi, which are being increasingly documented in the U.S., might still occur.[98]

The reactions were frequent enough to have initiated a hearing by the FDA, and this generated a testimony by a former Pfizer employee, Kathleen Dickson, a chemical analyst who worked on validation of methods for the company, testified to the nature of the outer surface protein A (OspA) antigen causing immunosuppression or immune tolerance that followed the injuries, with unreadable Western blot diagnostic tests, and attested to the fraudulent diagnostics on how the new case definition wiped out a majority of cases right off the bat, but most of all, she attested to the action of the antigen being used in the LYMErix vaccine, known for its ability to cause immune tolerance, a chronic and persistent immunosuppression.[99]

Testimonies from victims of adverse vaccine reactions to LYMErix were presented and submitted to the FDA, where typically most people could not handle more than two shots before being incapacitated, many of whom would not recover.[100] SmithKline & Beecham set up an HMO-based surveillance system to monitor the recipients regarding any damage caused by specific fractions of the lipoprotein, even long after they received the vaccine.[101]

Several years before, Alan Barbour and Wolfram Zuckert published an article in 1997 titled "New Tricks of Tickborne Pathogen," likening *Borrelia*'s immune evasion tactics to the Star Wars defense system where it keeps changing the outer surface of its makeup to avoid immune system attack. Also, this paper admits the unsettling fact that the OspA vaccines being tested were entirely experimental because in their own words, they could not arrive at a solid conclusion about what OspA is or does:

> One of the lipoproteins, OspA, has already been crystallized and structurally characterized, and it is undergoing human field trials as a vaccine against Lyme disease, although no one yet knows what it does.[102]

This was because the Americans never had the exceptional understanding or talent like the Germans did.[103] Barbour, Burgdorfer, and the rest of American biodefense, they may have had long and busy careers, and yes, they understood many aspects of the agents involved, but they were no Erich Traub. It was known from the end of the war that the immunosuppressive qualities of these toxic lipoids worked to disturb the immunization process, not confer it.[104] In comparative terms, it was the antigenic backbone of a slow-virus disease.[105]

The vaccine developers must have known the OspA antigen was going to be suppressive to the immune system but decided to push onward anyway, after all, burning out the immune system with similar vaccines to induce immune tolerance as a defense strategy worked so well in the cattle and poultry industries, but things did not go so smoothly in the human domain.[106] People can speak up about painful symptoms and discomfort from a vaccine, unlike those voiceless chickens and cows in the poultry and livestock industry in the forty years prior.[107]

During the FDA hearings, after SmithKline & Beecham told the FDA and the public that there were almost no adverse events, Dr. Ben Luft, of the Connaught vaccine project, testified to what he thought of this unusual affair:

> DR. LUFT: I just wanted to comment about the lippidation. [sic] That the actual lipoprotein, the fact that it is lippidated

[sic] does almost act as a mitogen,[B] and it gives a whole host of other -- so, I mean, that is -- In a way I feel like I'm almost in a twilight zone when we are talking about surveillance and these adverse events, and I forgot the name of the -- one of the vice presidents from SmithKline.

What disturbs me is that in the SmithKline presentation there were 950 adverse events. There was a nice presentation of that. And this afternoon we heard testimony from 20 individuals of 20, of approximately 20 people who had very significant adverse events.

And the disconnect for me is I'm hearing that, and I'm seeing that data, and I don't see any reflection of one to the other as if we were in two different universes. I'm not ascribing what the validity is to these complaints. Certainly I was moved by it. But the fact of the matter that it didn't even enter into the discussion, or into the charts, or the tables, is disturbing. And there is some problem in the actual, the adequacy of the surveillance that is currently going on, in that we are not seeing that data in the company's presentation.

And it goes back to my original point about the ICD codes, [...] you have to be able to get assurances, you have to be able to feel secure, you have to make sure that actually there is a very active surveillance system that is going to go out, that is going out and actually pulling in these types of cases.

And I think that that is something that we have to consider. I don't think the idea of a passive type of system, or a system that is going to take three to five years to kind of figure out whether we had an adequate power, or whether we had an adequate input of the right information, or whether we were -- whether we cast a wide enough net will really be adequate. And I invite the sponsors to give me some insight as to why there seems to be this discrepancy. But, in a way, I think I'm just restating the obvious. This is -- I mean, I can't...[108]

SmithKline finally withdrew the vaccine, citing low sales, but that was just the cover story.[109] GSK knew the extent of it, and it was outlined in numerous victim's testimony to the FDA, along with lawsuits. Additional testimony was given by Ms. Dickson, the former Pfizer employee brave enough to go up against the treasonous drug firms and public health system.[110]

B   Mitogen is an agent that causes mitosis, or cell division and growth factors, mutations, etc., and this can become very relevant in chronic diseases and cancers.

Endnotes

1   Steere, A C, J A Hardin, and S E Malawista. "Lyme Arthritis: a New Clinical Entity." Hospital practice. U.S. National Library of Medicine, April 1978. https://www.ncbi.nlm.nih. gov/pubmed/658948

2   USDA. "Proceedings of the Collaborator's Meeting on Foreign Poultry Diseases (1953 : Washington)." Internet Archive, United States Department of Agriculture (USDA) Washington, 1 Jan. 1970, Retrieved from: www.archive.org/details/CAT10678555/page/n15

3   Loftus, J., & N. Miller. (1982). *The Belarus secret: The Nazi Connection in America.* Paragon House.

4   Todd, Frank A. "The public health veterinarian in national defense." *American journal of public health and the nation's health* vol. 41,9 (1951): 1059-64. doi:10.2105/ajph.41.9.1059

5   "Disease, Environmental, and Management Factors Related to Poultry Health : a Symposium Held March 20- 22, 1961 at the Jefferson Auditorium, USDA, Washington, D.C. : United States. Agricultural Research Service." Internet Archive, [Washington, D.C.] : Agricultural Research Service, U.S. Dept. of Agriculture, 1 Jan. 1961, Retrieved from: https://www. archive.org/details/CAT31325715/page/n1

6   USDA, Animal Disease Eradication Division (ADE). "Activities Handbook - Animal Disease Eradication Division." Activities Handbook - Animal Disease Eradication Division, 1962. Retrieved from: https://archive.org/details/activitieshandanidiseradrich/mode/2up

7   Goodman, R A et al. "Epidemiologic field investigations by the Centers for Disease control and Epidemic Intelligence Service, 1946-87." Public health reports (Washington, D.C. : 1974) vol. 105,6 (1990): 604-10.

8   "United States Navy Medical News Letter Vol. 26, No. 11, 9 December 1955 : U.S. Navy. Bureau of Medicine and Surgery." 1955. Internet Archive. December 9, 1955. https:// archive.org/details/NavyMedicalNewsletter19551209/page/n27

9   Steere, Allen C., Stephen E. Malawista, David R. Snydman, Robert E. Shope, Warren A. Andiman, Martin R. Ross, and Francis M. Steele. "An Epidemic of Oligoarticular Arthritis in Children and Adults in Three Connecticut Communities." Arthritis & Rheumatism 20, no. 1 (1977): 7-17. doi:10.1002/art.1780200102.

10   Reik, L, A C Steere, N H Bartenhagen, R E Shope, and S E Malawista. "Neurologic Abnormalities of Lyme Disease." Medicine. U.S. National Library of Medicine, July 1979. https:// www.ncbi.nlm.nih.gov/pubmed/449663

11   Tesh, Robert B. "In Memoriam: Robert E. Shope, M.D." Vector borne and zoonotic diseases (Larchmont, N.Y.). U.S. National Library of Medicine, 2004. https://www.ncbi.nlm.nih. gov/pubmed/15228809

12   Carroll, M. C. (2004). *Lab 257: The disturbing story of the governments secret and deadly virus research facility.* New York: Morrow., pp. 11

13   Steere, A C, J A Hardin, and S E Malawista. "Lyme Arthritis: a New Clinical Entity." Hospital practice. U.S. National Library of Medicine, April 1978. https://www.ncbi.nlm.nih. gov/pubmed/658948

14   Reik, L, A C Steere, N H Bartenhagen, R E Shope, and S E Malawista. "Neurologic Abnormalities of Lyme Disease." Medicine. U.S. National Library of Medicine, July 1979. https:// www.ncbi.nlm.nih.gov/pubmed/449663

15   Elsner, Rebecca A., Christine J. Hastey, Kimberly J. Olsen, and Nicole Baumgarth. "Suppression of Long-Lived Humoral Immunity Following Borrelia Burgdorferi Infection." PLOS Pathogens 11, no. 7 (2015). doi:10.1371/journal.ppat.1004976.

16   Sausen, Daniel G et al. "Stress-Induced Epstein-Barr Virus Reactivation." *Biomolecules* vol. 11,9 1380. 18 Sep. 2021, doi:10.3390/biom11091380

17   Harley JB, James JA. Epstein-Barr virus infection induces lupus autoimmunity. Bull NYU Hosp Jt Dis. 2006;64(1-2):45-50. PMID: 17121489.

18   Hassani A, Khan G. Epstein-Barr Virus and miRNAs: Partners in Crime in the Pathogenesis of Multiple Sclerosis? Front Immunol. 2019 Apr 3;10:695. doi: 10.3389/fimmu.2019.00695. PMID: 31001286; PMCID: PMC6456696.

19   Whang, H. Y., & Neter, E. (1967). Immunosuppression by Endotoxin and its Lipoid A Component. Experimental Biology and Medicine, 124(3), 919–924. doi:10.3181/00379727-124-31886

20   Traub, E. Persistence of Lymphocytic Choriomeningitis Virus in Immune Animals and Its Relation To Immunity. Journal of Experimental Medicine, 63(6), 847-861. doi:10.1084/jem.63.6.847. (1936).

21   Steere, A C, J A Hardin, and S E Malawista. "Lyme Arthritis: a New Clinical Entity." Hospital practice. U.S. National Library of Medicine, April 1978. https://www.ncbi.nlm.nih.gov/pubmed/658948.

22   Murray, P. (1996). The widening circle: A Lyme disease pioneer tells her story. New York, NY: St. Martin's Press.

23   Tavel, Morton E. "Somatic Symptom Disorders without Known Physical Causes: One Disease with Many Names?" The American journal of medicine. U.S. National Library of Medicine, October 2015. https://www.ncbi.nlm.nih.gov/pubmed/26031885

24   Steere, A C et al. "Historical perspective of Lyme disease." Zentralblatt fur Bakteriologie, Mikrobiologie, und Hygiene. Series A, Medical microbiology, infectious diseases, virology, parasitology vol. 263,1-2 (1986): 3-6. doi:10.1016/s0176-6724(86)80093-1

25   Steere, Allen C. "First International Symposium on Lyme Disease: Yale University School of Medicine, November 16-18, 1983." The Yale Journal of Biology and Medicine, First International Symposium on Lyme Disease: Yale University School of Medicine, November 16-18, 1983, 1984.

26   Hovind-Hougen, K. "A Morphological Characterization of Borrelia Anserina." Microbiology (Reading, England). U.S. National Library of Medicine, January 1995. https://www.ncbi.nlm.nih.gov/pubmed/7894723

27   Traub, E., Kanhai, G. K., & Kesting, F. Behavior of Foot-and-Mouth Disease Virus on Serial Passage in Different Kinds of Cells. A Contribution to Experimental Epidemiology at Cell Level*. Zentralblatt Für Veterinärmedizin Reihe B, 15(5), 525-539. (1967, 2010). doi:10.1111/j.1439-0450.1968.tb00327.x

28   Shope, Robert E., Discussion: Epidemiologic Studies. The First International Symposium on Lyme Disease. The Yale Journal of Biology and Medicine. 57, 707-709. (1984)

29   Ibid.

30   Stanek, Gerold, Flamm, Heinz, Burgdorfer, Willy, Barbour, Alan. "Lyme Borreliosis: Proceedings of the Second International Symposium on Lyme Disease and Related Disorders, Vienna 1985." Fischer, Lyme Borreliosis: Proceedings of the Second International Symposium on Lyme Disease and Related Disorders, Vienna 1985, 1987

31   Stanek, Gerold. Lyme Borreliosis II: Proceedings of the Second International Symposium on Lyme Disease and Related Disorders, Vienna 1985. G. Fischer Verlag, 1990.

32   "Proceedings of the First National Conference on Lyme Disease Testing, Nov. 1-2, 1990, Dearborn, Mich." Association of State and Territorial Public Health Laboratory Directors, Proceedings of the First National Conference on Lyme Disease Testing, Nov. 1-2, 1990, Dearborn, Mich, 1991.

33   Dlesk, A. Lyme Borreliosis: Clinical Orientation, Diagnosis, and Treatment. Proceedings of the First National Conference on Lyme Disease Testing, Nov. 1-2, 1990, Dearborn, Mich." Association of State and Territorial Public Health Laboratory Directors, Proceedings of

the First National Conference on Lyme Disease Testing, Nov. 1-2, 1990, Dearborn, Mich, 1991., pp. 09

34   Ibid., pp. 10

35   Ibid., pp.10-11

36   Ibid., pp. 11-12

37   Ibid., pp. 23-108

38   Dickson, Kathleen. "Charge 2: The Patents." TRUTHCURES.ORG CRIMINAL CHARGE SHEETS JUNE 2017, 2017. https://docs.wixstatic.com/ugd/47b066_01d68b1309ae457b81d-f1e06e6beae1e.pdf

39   Reverby, Susan M. 2013. *Examining Tuskegee: the Infamous Syphilis Study and Its Legacy*. Chapel Hill: Univ. of North Carolina Press.

40   Mcneil, Donald G. "U.S. Apologizes for Syphilis Tests in Guatemala." *The New York Times*. October 01, 2010. Accessed July 27, 2019. https://www.nytimes.com/2010/10/02/health/research/02infect.html

41   Dickson, K. "CRIMINAL CHARGE SHEETS JUNE 2017 Lobbying for a Hearing for Referral to the USDOJ for a Prosecution of the Lyme Disease Crimes." 2017., pp. 23. Published at: https://docs.wixstatic.com/ugd/47b066_01d68b1309ae457b81df1e06e6beae1e.pdf

42   O'Neill, N. (2020, March 25). Genetics could play role in coronavirus deaths, health experts say. Retrieved February 15, 2021, from https://nypost.com/2020/03/25/genetics-could-play-role-in-coronavirus-deaths-health-experts-say/

43   O'Neill, N. (2020, March 25). Genetics could play role in coronavirus deaths, health experts say. Retrieved February 15, 2021, from https://nypost.com/2020/03/25/genetics-could-play-role-in-coronavirus-deaths-health-experts-say/

44   Murray, P. (1996). *The widening circle: A Lyme disease pioneer tells her story*. New York, NY: St. Martin's Press., pp. 120

45   Traub, E. LCM Virus Research, Retrospect and Prospects. Lymphocytic Choriomeningitis Virus and Other Arenaviruses, 3-10. doi:10.1007/978-3-642-65681-1_1. (1973)

46   Traub, E. Observations on immunological tolerance and "Immunity" in mice infected congenitally with the virus of lymphocytic choriomeningitis (LCM). Archiv Fur Die Gesamte Virusforschung, 10(3), 303-314. doi:10.1007/bf01250677. (1960).

47   Traub, E. Ueber den Einfluß der latenten Choriomeningitis-Infektion auf die Entstehung der Lymphomatose bei weißen Mause [On the Influence of Latent Choriomeningitis Infection on the Development of Lymphomatosis in White Mice]. Zentrl. Bakt. I. Orig. 147 (16). 1-25. (1941). [Translated to English by A. Finnegan, 2019]

48   Dinter, Z. Persönaliches, Begegnungen mit Erich Traub.[Personal Encounters with Erich Traub] Berl. Munch. Tier. Woch. 96. 70-72. (1984)

49   Traub, E., & Kesting, F. Age Distribution and Serological Reactivity of Viral Antigen in Brains of Mice Infected Congenitally with LMC Virus. Zentralblatt Für Veterinärmedizin Reihe B, 24(7), 548-559. (1975, 2010). doi:10.1111/j.1439-0450.1977.tb01024.x

50   see: TruthCures. "LYME CRYME." YouTube. YouTube, September 2, 2016. https://www.youtube.com/watch?v=f8DU1Z6R-ms&t=526s

51   Dickson, Kathleen. "Charge 2: The Patents." TRUTHCURES.ORG CRIMINAL CHARGE SHEETS JUNE 2017, 2017. https://docs.wixstatic.com/ugd/47b066_01d68b1309ae457b81d-f1e06e6beae1e.pdf

52   Dickson, K. n.d. "OspA - the Greatest Imitator." ActionLyme. TruthCures.org. Accessed July 27, 2019. http://www.actionlyme.org/Pam3Cys_Version15.htm

53   "Misinformation on Lyme Disease." American Lyme Disease Foundation (ALDF),

n.d. https://www.aldf.com/lyme-disease/#misinformation

54   "American Lyme Disease Foundation, Inc., Board of Directors, (1 of 2)." OPERATION OPENSCRIPT, n.d. https://static.secure.website/wscfus/10426050/7130095/aldf-b3-w918-o. jpg

55   "American Lyme Disease Foundation, Inc., Board of Directors, (2 of 2)." OPERATION OPENSCRIPT, n.d., https://static.secure.website/wscfus/10426050/7130096/aldf-b4-w1700-o. jpg

56   Nicolson, Garth L., and Nancy L. Nicolson. *Project Day Lily: an American Biological Warfare Tragedy*. Xlibris, 2005.

57   ALDF, "2nd Banbury Conference." American Lyme Disease Foundation (ALDF), n.d. https://www.aldf.com/2nd-banbury-conference

58   Goode, John, et al. "Ketchum PR - Everything Public Relations News." Everything, 1 Dec. 2017, https://everything-pr.com/tag/ketchum/

59   Lee, Christopher. "Medicare Drug Benefit Outlined in Campaign." Wayback Machine. The Washington Post, October 10, 2005. https://web.archive.org/web/20151011110456/ http://www.washingtonpost.com/wp-dyn/content/article/2005/10/09/AR2005100900959. html

60   Lynch, Dennis. "Russia, Ketchum End Controversial Nine-Year Public Relations Partnership." *International Business Times*, International Business Times, 11 Mar. 2015, https:// www.ibtimes.com/russia-ketchum-end-controversial-nine-year-public-relations-partner- ship-1844092

61   "Lyme Disease : a Diagnostic and Treatment Dilemma : Hearing before the Com- mittee on Labor and Human Resources, United States Senate, One Hundred Third Congress, First Session, on Examining the Adequacy of Current Diagnostic Measures and Research Activities in the Prevention and Treatment of Lyme Disease, August 5, 1993 : United States. Congress. Senate. Committee on Labor and Human Resources : Free Download, Borrow, and Streaming." Internet Archive. Washington : U.S. G.P.O. : For sale by the U.S. G.P.O., Supt. of Docs., Congressional Sales Office, January 1, 1993. https://archive.org/details/lymediseasediag- n00unit

62   This would explain the opposing arguments funded by the same source- the CDC and special interest groups

63   "Lyme Disease : a Diagnostic and Treatment Dilemma : Hearing before the Com- mittee on Labor and Human Resources, United States Senate, One Hundred Third Congress, First Session, on Examining the Adequacy of Current Diagnostic Measures and Research Activities in the Prevention and Treatment of Lyme Disease, August 5, 1993 : United States. Congress. Senate. Committee on Labor and Human Resources : Free Download, Borrow, and Streaming." Internet Archive. Washington : U.S. G.P.O. : For sale by the U.S. G.P.O., Supt. of Docs., Congressional Sales Office, January 1, 1993. https://archive.org/details/lymediseasediag- n00unit.

64   Bacterial Zoonoses Branch, Division of Vector-Borne Infectious Diseases, National Center for Infectious Disease, Center for Disease Control (CDC). "Lyme Disease Surveillance Summary." MMWR 4, no. 2 (March 1993): 1–9, see pp. 01, Retrieved from: https://stacks.cdc. gov/view/cdc/58085

65   Ibid., pp. 05, Retrieved from: https://stacks.cdc.gov/view/cdc/58085

66   Bacterial Zoonoses Branch, Division of Vector-Borne Infectious Diseases, National Center for Infectious Disease, Center for Disease Control (CDC). "Lyme Disease Surveillance Summary." MMWR 6, no. 2 (November 1995): 1–11, see pp. 06, Retrieved from: https://stacks. cdc.gov/view/cdc/58109

67   Vanderhoof-Forschner, Forschner. "Vaccination Safety, Part 1." C-SPAN. C-SPAN, n.d. https://www.c-span.org/video/?173720-1/vaccination-safety-part-1

68   FDA Vaccine Advisory Committee on LYMErix Vaccine. "LYMErix Vaccine Victim's Stories and Related Articles." 11AD, pp. 1–20. [Misc. written testimony] Retrieve from: https://web.archive.org/web/20030830064730/https://www.fda.gov/ohrms/dockets/ac/01/briefing/3680b2_17.pdf

69   Noble, Holcomb. "Concerns Grow Over Reactions to Lyme Shots." *The New York Times, The New York Times*, 21 Nov. 2000, www.nytimes.com/2000/11/21/science/concerns-grow-over-reactions-to-lyme-shots.html

70   Aronowitz, Robert A. "The Rise and Fall of the Lyme Disease Vaccines: a Cautionary Tale for Risk Interventions in American Medicine and Public Health." The Milbank quarterly. Blackwell Publishing Inc, June 2012. https://www.ncbi.nlm.nih.gov/pmc/articles/PMC3460208/.

71   Basic and Clinical Approaches to Lyme Disease: a Lyme Disease Foundation Symposium, Boston, Massachusetts, 19-20 April 1997. Chicago: University of Chicago Press, 1997.

72   Charles S. Pavia, et al. "Activity of Sera from Patients with Lyme Disease against Borrelia Burgdorferi." *Clinical Infectious Diseases*, vol. 25, 1997, pp. S25–30. JSTOR, http://www.jstor.org/stable/4460122. Accessed 4 June 2023.

73   Persing, David H. "The Cold Zone: A Curious Convergence of Tick-Transmitted Diseases." *Clinical Infectious Diseases*, vol. 25, 1997, pp. S35–42. JSTOR, http://www.jstor.org/stable/4460124. Accessed 4 June 2023.

74   Donta, Sam T. "Tetracycline Therapy for Chronic Lyme Disease." *Clinical Infectious Diseases,* vol. 25, 1997, pp. S52–56. JSTOR, http://www.jstor.org/stable/4460127. Accessed 4 June 2023.

75   François Meurice, et al. "Specific Issues in the Design and Implementation of an Efficacy Trial for a Lyme Disease Vaccine." *Clinical Infectious Diseases*, vol. 25, 1997, pp. S71–75. JSTOR, http://www.jstor.org/stable/4460130. Accessed 4 June 2023.

76   Elisabeth Aberer, et al. "Why Is Chronic Lyme Borreliosis Chronic?" *Clinical Infectious Diseases*, vol. 25, 1997, pp. S64–70. JSTOR, http://www.jstor.org/stable/4460129. Accessed 4 June 2023.

77   Steere, A. C. "Lyme Borreliosis in Russia." Grantome, NIH, 30 Sept. 1995, www.grantome.com/grant/NIH/R03-TW000514-01

78   Steere, A. C. "Lyme Borreliosis in Russia." Grantome, NIH, 30 Sept. 1996, www.grantome.com/grant/NIH/R03-TW000514-02

79   Steere, A. C. "Lyme Borreliosis in Russia." Grantome, NIH, 30 Sept. 1997, www.grantome.com/grant/NIH/R03-TW000514-03

80   starting with the details surrounding biological research at the time and the details surrounding the Spanish influenza, a hot yet occulted war of biology was kicked off to steadily gain momentum throughout the century.

81   Revkin, Andrew C. "2 Firms Seeking Approval Of Lyme Disease Vaccines." The New York Times. The New York Times, February 4, 1997. https://timesmachine.nytimes.com/timesmachine/1997/02/04/483605.html?pageNumber=28

82   Feder, Henry M., Jeri Beran, Christian Van Hoecke, Betsy Abraham, Norbert De Clercq, Charles Buscarino, and Denis L. Parenti. "Immunogenicity of a Recombinant Borrelia Burgdorferi Outer Surface Protein A Vaccine against Lyme Disease in Children." *The Journal of Pediatrics* 135, no. 5 (1999): 575–79. https://doi.org/10.1016/s0022-3476(99)70055-7.

83   Rierden, Andi. "Testing for a Lyme Disease Vaccine." The New York Times. The New York Times, December 1, 1996. https://www.nytimes.com/1996/12/01/nyregion/testing-for-a-lyme-disease-vaccine.html

84   Aronowitz, Robert A. "The Rise and Fall of the Lyme Disease Vaccines: a Cautionary Tale for Risk Interventions in American Medicine and Public Health." The Milbank

quarterly. Blackwell Publishing Inc, June 2012. https://www.ncbi.nlm.nih.gov/pmc/articles/PMC3460208/

85   The Associated Press (AP). (2002, February 28). Sole Lyme vaccine is pulled off market (published 2002). *The New York Times*. https://www.nytimes.com/2002/02/28/business/sole-lyme-vaccine-is-pulled-off-market.html

86   Feder, H M Jr et al. "Immunogenicity of a recombinant Borrelia burgdorferi outer surface protein A vaccine against Lyme disease in children." *The Journal of pediatrics* vol. 135,5 (1999): 575-9. doi:10.1016/s0022-3476(99)70055-7

87   Dickson, K. "Mysterious Russian (Defectors?) Scientists at New York Medical College Study the Cyst or Spheroplast Form of Spirochetes as Well as Human Racial Diseases Susceptibilities." ACTIONLyme, ACTIONLyme, http://www.actionlyme.org/BOGUS_RUSSIAN_NYMC_ARTICLES.htm

88   Moonsamy, P. ., Klitz, W., Tilanus, M. G. ., & Begovich, A. . (1997). Genetic Variability and Linkage Disequilibrium Within the DP Region in the CEPH Families. Human Immunology, 58(2), 112–121. doi:10.1016/s0198-8859(97)00208-5

89   Altman, Lawrence K. "F.D.A. Experts Back a Vaccine Against Lyme." The New York Times. The New York Times, May 27, 1998. https://www.nytimes.com/1998/05/27/us/fda-experts-back-a-vaccine-against-lyme.html

90   "The new alchemy – The drug industry's flurry of mergers is based on a big gamble." The Economist. 20 January 2000.

91   New "Glaxo" Company. *The Times*, Tuesday, 15 October 1935; pg. 22; Issue 47195

92   Altman, Lawrence K. "F.D.A. Experts Back a Vaccine Against Lyme." The New York Times. The New York Times, May 27, 1998. https://www.nytimes.com/1998/05/27/us/fda-experts-back-a-vaccine-against-lyme.html

93   FDA Vaccine Advisory Committee on LYMErix Vaccine. "LYMErix Vaccine Victim's Stories and Related Articles." 11AD, pp. 1–20. [Misc. written testimony] Retrieve from: https://web.archive.org/web/20030830064730/https://www.fda.gov/ohrms/dockets/ac/01/briefing/3680b2_17.pdf

94   Noble, Holcomb B. "Concerns Grow Over Reactions To Lyme Shots." *The New York Times. The New York Times*, 21 Nov. 2000, www.nytimes.com/2000/11/21/science/concerns-grow-over-reactions-to-lyme-shots.html

95   Noble, Holcomb B. "Concerns Grow Over Reactions To Lyme Shots." *The New York Times. The New York Times*, 21 Nov. 2000, www.nytimes.com/2000/11/21/science/concerns-grow-over-reactions-to-lyme-shots.html

96   Altman, Lawrence K. "Lyme Vaccine Is Approved, With Caveat." *The New York Times. The New York Times*, December 22, 1998. https://timesmachine.nytimes.com/timesmachine/1998/12/22/539830.html?pageNumber=20

97   FDA Vaccine Advisory Committee on LYMErix Vaccine. "LYMErix Vaccine Victim's Stories and Related Articles." 11AD, pp. 1–20. [Misc. written testimony] Retrieve from: https://web.archive.org/web/20030830064730/https://www.fda.gov/ohrms/dockets/ac/01/briefing/3680b2_17.pdf

98   Persing, David H., METHOD FOR DETECTING B. BURGDORFERI INFECTION (US6045804A). 2000

99   Dickson, Kathleen. TRUTHCURES.ORG CRIMINAL CHARGE SHEETS JUNE 2017, 2017. https://docs.wixstatic.com/ugd/47b066_01d68b1309ae457b81df1e06e6beae1e.pdf

100   FDA Vaccine Advisory Committee on LYMErix Vaccine. "LYMErix Vaccine Victim's Stories and Related Articles." 11AD, pp. 1–20. [Misc. written testimony] Retrieve from: https://web.archive.org/web/20030830064730/https://www.fda.gov/ohrms/dockets/ac/01/briefing/3680b2_17.pdf

101   Aronowitz, Robert A. "The Rise and Fall of the Lyme Disease Vaccines: a Cautionary Tale for Risk Interventions in American Medicine and Public Health." The Milbank quarterly. Blackwell Publishing Inc, June 2012. https://www.ncbi.nlm.nih.gov/pmc/articles/PMC3460208/

102   Barbour, Alan G., and Wolfram R. Zückert. "New Tricks of Tick-Borne Pathogen." Nature, vol. 390, no. 6660, 1997, pp. 553–554., doi:10.1038/37475.

103   Eberle, Henrik. "Ein Wertvolles Instrument": Die Universität Greifswald Im Nationalsozialismus. Bohlau Verlag, 2015. [pp. 538-541]

104   Traub, E. & W. Schäfer. Immunisierung von Mausen gegen Influenza mit Adsorbatimpstoffen von Viruskonzentraten. [Immunization of Mice Against Influenza with Concentrated Virus Adsorbate Vaccines]. Monatshefte fur Veterinmedizine. 1. 369-373 (1946). [Translated to English by A. Finnegan (2019)]

105   Whang, H. Y., & Neter, E. (1967). Immunosuppression by Endotoxin and its Lipoid A Component. Experimental Biology and Medicine, 124(3), 919–924. doi:10.3181/00379727-124-31886.

106   FDA Vaccine Advisory Committee on LYMErix Vaccine. "LYMErix Vaccine Victim's Stories and Related Articles." 11AD, pp. 1–20. [Misc. written testimony] Retrieve from: https://web.archive.org/web/20030830064730/https://www.fda.gov/ohrms/dockets/ac/01/briefing/3680b2_17.pdf

107   "Disease, Environmental, and Management Factors Related to Poultry Health : a Symposium Held March 20-22, 1961 at the Jefferson Auditorium, USDA, Washington, D.C. : United States. Agricultural Research Service." Internet Archive, [Washington, D.C.] : Agricultural Research Service, U.S. Dept. of Agriculture, 1 Jan. 1961, www.archive.org/details/CAT31325715/page/n1

108   VRBPAC (Vaccines and Related Biological Products Advisory Committee) of the Food and Drug Administration. 2001. Minutes, January 31. Retrieved from: http://www.actionlyme.org/2001_FDA_LYMErix_Transcripts.pdf, pp. 219-220

109   Hitt, Emma. "Poor Sales Trigger Vaccine Withdrawal." Nature News. Nature Publishing Group, n.d. https://www.nature.com/articles/nm0402-311b?cacheBust=1510200110898

110   Dickson, Kathleen. Testimony. VRBPAC (Vaccines and Related Biological Products Advisory Committee) of the Food and Drug Administration. 2001. Minutes, January 31. Retrieved from: http://www.actionlyme.org/2001_FDA_LYMErix_Transcripts.pdf pp. 148-154

Chapter Fourteen

THE LATE-STAGE PUBLIC RELATIONS MANIFESTATION OF LYME DISEASE

A VECTOR-BORNE VENTURE CAPITAL & PUBLIC RELATIONS CONTINUUM

In the ethical sense, propaganda bears the same relation to education as to business or politics. It may be abused. It may be used to over-advertise an institution and to create in the public mind artificial values.
— Edward Bernays, *Propaganda*

From the time the U.S. Public Health System began to acknowledge Lyme disease, the Lyme Disease Surveillance System and its associates were setting up vector-borne disease monopolies through biotech firms to serve in the public health surveillance, diagnostics, and immunotherapeutic industries, while maintaining the public image of downplaying the disease as much as possible.

Several corporate partnerships formed in the wake of the Second National Conference on Serologic Diagnosis of Lyme Disease, partnerships like Yale's L2 Diagnostics, the Massachusetts-based Imugen, Inc., a Mayo Clinic-associated firm, who was to run the diagnostic standards to be used for detection of Lyme disease by the public health system in the United States after the 1994 Dearborn set the standards in the years preceding the LYMErix vaccine.[1, 2]

A third company was set up, Corixa of Washington,[3] through scientist David H. Persing, from the Mayo Clinic non-profit, who developed recombinant vaccines and screened blood for definable biomarkers[A] as reliable criteria to help diagnose the disease in people

---

A   A **biomarker** is a biochemical substance or reaction the body produced from other stimuli that can be used to serve as criteria to indicate something that cannot be directly confirmed, *i.e.* certain viral infections or states of the immune system, so, for example, the presence

whose blood samples were complicated by other contradictory factors like having vaccine-induced antibodies already present.

In 2004, David Persing contributed to a chapter in a book from a workshop, *Infection, Cancer, and the Immune Response,* from the symposium book *The Infectious Etiology of Chronic Diseases: Defining the Relationship, Enhancing the Research, and Mitigating the Effects; Workshop Summary* describing many of the effects seen in immunosuppressive diseases and cancers passing down generations.[4] He talked about the many cancers associated with infectious diseases like SV40 virus, Epstein-Barr Virus, malaria, and other infections. Corixa also produced synthetic endotoxin under biodefense contracts that same year.[5] Corixa was active in screening blood banks in endemic areas of Connecticut for stealth pathogens like *Babesia microti,* published in a 2005 paper *"Demonstrable parasitemia among Connecticut blood donors with antibodies to Babesia microti."*[6] University of California at Davis later got into the blood bank business with Alan Barbour's assistance on the project, and the associated blood banks set-up in the areas of Washington, Oregon, and California.[7]

In the last chapter, Persing was quoted in showing that the LYMErix vaccine could cause the same complications as chronic Lyme disease, remarking that it was indistinguishable from LYMErix vaccine failure.[8] It is also rather significant that the one leading Corixa would be revealing the real mechanisms of the antigen and its effect on the immune system that was responsible for what has been termed "chronic Lyme disease,"[9] and just a year later Corixa was partnering with Stanford Rook Holdings PLC, a British biotech firm who worked in immunotherapeutics with modified-strains of *Mycobacterium* (tuberculosis) to treat immunosuppression from pulmonary tuberculosis, here working with Corixa to produce therapeutics for autoimmune disease,[10] since Steere and his other partners decided to class aspects of Lyme arthritis as an autoimmune disorder,[11, 12] when it was actually an outcome of *immune tolerance* or chronic immunosuppression instead of autoimmunity,[13] but nonetheless, a clever marketing angle indeed.

Corixa also acquired Anergen, Inc., to expand its investments in autoimmune disease therapeutics, pouring considerable resources into research on blood cancers, looking to produce cancer vaccines and biopharmaceuticals.[14] When stealth infections like Lyme disease and multiple tick-borne pathogens blunt the immune system, they cause immunosuppression and *immune tolerance,* and when the im-

---

of antibodies to some pathogen is a biomarker to indicate a pathogen is present even if the pathogen cannot be directly isolated and seen directly.

mune system is disabled it reawakens sleeping viruses, such as human herpesvirus 6 (HHV-6)[15] or Epstein-Barr Virus (EBV),[16] and this can eventually lead to cancer as these viruses are oncogenic when awakened from latency.[17]

KEEPING THE LID ON THE COVERUP

In 2019, Persing took part in a propaganda campaign with Sam Telford to deter a biological warfare connection to Lyme Disease spirochetes citing several of their older papers about genetic material found in ticks from 1945-1951,[18] and another publication about mouse skin tissue samples from 1870-1910 that show two samples of mice from 1896 having partial positive reactivity to tiny fractions of sequences from the outer surface protein A (OspA) of *Borrelia burgdorferi*.[19]

He cites those two studies to reinforce the official talking points in *The Washington Post* article, "No, Lyme Disease Is Not an Escaped Military Bioweapon, despite What Conspiracy Theorists Say," citing his two studies with Persing as though it was concrete evidence of *Borrelia burgdorferi* infection. The first study regarding tick specimen samples from 1945-1951 actually reinforces the story you are reading in this book.[20] The second paper testing mouse tissue samples,[21] however, is far less reliable and this will become evident as I walk the reader through it and show that while the first paper isn't reliable enough to conclude much, it only strengthens my argument, while the second paper on mouse tissue samples is entirely inconclusive to speak to a *Borrelia burgdorferi* infection.

However, most importantly, both papers had been refuted by Rocky Mountain Laboratory researcher Richard Marconi *et al.* saying that the primers used in the testing were not a reliable set of primers and therefore could not offer validation as to what the paper was trying to demonstrate.[22]

The paper testing ear tissue samples from the white-footed mouse collected from between 1870 and 1910 was only positive for partial sequences of outer surface protein A (OspA), tiny fractions of the overall protein DNA present in these samples, which is extracellular DNA and changes regularly and rapidly because it is constantly assimilating genetic material from foreign sources,[23, 24] including material from bacteriophages.[25] This means it contaminates the integrity of the DNA being from the actual spirochete. Also, OspA cross-reacts with surface proteins of other microorganisms and especially viruses.[26] That's not even taking into the account the possibility of false positives due to limitations inherent in the PCR testing, as the authors state in the paper itself, "*We are acutely aware of the potential for false-positive results in PCR assays.*" [27]

Not to mention, it was said that these outer surface proteins have chromosomes resembling those of vaccinia virus or other poxviruses.[28] In a paper by Persing one year after the publication on the two positive mouse sample tissues, he admitted that there is homology between plasmid DNA from *Borrelia burgdorferi* and vaccinia virus, speaking on the *"possibility of autonomous replication of plasmid DNA (which contains telomeres that are homologous to those of vaccinia virus) in human tissues independent of B. burgdorferi infection."*[29]

Therefore, it cannot be used to indicate in any reliable way to demonstrate an infection with *Borrelia burgdorferi*, let alone any other species of *Borrelia* spirochetes. They specifically address this fact in the paper on tick samples from the range of 1945-51, where they correctly test for sequences of the *Borrelia* spirochete itself but this will only indicate *Borrelia* spirochetes in general and still not conclusive to an infection with *Borrelia burgdorferi*.[30]

Telford misrepresents some of their own published research to incorrectly state they have definitively debunked the Lyme disease connection to biological warfare. The article states:

> Working with microbiologist David Persing, we found that ticks from the South Fork of Long Island collected in 1945 were infected. Subsequent studies found that mice from Cape Cod, collected in 1896, were infected.
>
> So decades before Lyme was identified — and before military scientists could have altered or weaponized it — the bacterium that causes it was living in the wild.
>
> That alone is proof that the conspiracy theory is wrong. But there are plenty of other lines of evidence that show why Lyme disease did not require the human hand changing something Mother Nature had nurtured.[31]

He goes on to say he deems *Borrelia burgdorferi* an unlikely bioweapon because of its weeklong incubation period:

> Lyme disease does make some people very sick but many have just a flulike illness that their immune system fends off. Untreated cases may subsequently develop arthritis or neurological issues. The disease is rarely lethal. Lyme has a week-long incubation period — too slow for an effective bioweapon.[32]

This entire article is laden with misleading, inaccurate statements, and stretches the truth to the point of falsehood. First, this article presupposes that in order for Lyme disease to have been a bioweapon, it had to have been done after the advent of genetic engineering technology (post-1970s), which entirely ignores the method of directing mutation by using selective animal passages.[33] Let's remember, the USA also had biological weapons in their stockpile with live agent tests in the early 1950s,[34] long before modern genetic engineering was available, so the argument that a biological weapon could only have been possible after the introduction of modern genetic engineering is not a valid argument.

Secondly, it presupposes that the only kind of effective bioweapons are only those that quickly kill or have very short incubation periods of less than a week. However, many of the biological warfare agents acknowledged in the American biological weapons stockpile have a comparable incubation period to Lyme disease, while Q fever, for example, has an incubation period of 2-3 weeks, nearly three times longer than the week-long incubation period he cites for Lyme disease.[35] Tularemia has an incubation period of 3-15 days,[36] and psittacosis has an incubation period of 5-14 days.[37] Telford also ignores the value of agents that produce slow, chronic infections that are neurotropic, that is, they deteriorate the brain and central nervous system.[38, 39]

Anyone with a halfway decent understanding of biological weapons should understand the very effective long-term strategic approach of *tire, exhaust, and overwhelm* the enemy, cripple slowly and with stealth, eventually totally overwhelming the healthcare system, sending unemployment and mental illness through the roof, destabilizing the welfare and national security of the nation. On top of that, detonate the sleeping viruses already harbored in the population with the agent and this results in profound neurotropic damage to the central nervous system of the population,[40] and watch it unravel like the mice in Traub's early Rockefeller experiments.[41]

Aside from stretching the truth regarding the samples of white-footed mice from 1870-1910, their other paper on the tick specimens from after World War II would reinforce the storyline of events within this book if it were even reliable evidence. It is possible that all samples that were positive were from 1949-1951, only two samples specifically from 1946 were positive and we have covered the probability that Donald Maclean had Traub's weaponized ticks and spirochetes brought to America by 1945 when John Loftus indicates that British Intelligence was testing these ticks at Plum Island and surrounding areas. Traub then would have updated it once again when he returned to American shores in 1949, which may be the reason for several circulating strains. That would mean the 1990 paper by Telford and Persing is merely reinforcing what is laid out here in this book.[42]

Public Relations & Socio-Political Offensives

The activities of the vector-borne monopolies and drug firms making money off tick-borne disease would greatly accelerate in the New Millennium. They would train all the doctors to accept the bogus guidelines,[43] help the perpetrators taking part of these activities brush the problem under the rug and set up a dragnet to mine new pathogens from the blood of average people through vector-borne surveillance programs and blood banks.[44] There were additional public relations people hired to slander and conduct sabotage operations against the sick who caused any unwanted noise.

One of the individuals who became somewhat well-known in the Lyme disease arena for trying to silence activists, was Edward McSweegan.[45] McSweegan worked at NMRI and NIH, and while he was at NMRI, he pulled off his first stunt, by writing Senator Goldwater to argue that the military's funding would be better spent elsewhere, under federal, academic, and corporate control.[46] This was also the year he earned himself a security clearance, likely walking onboard with some epidemiological PR firm under contract to the state department, managing science and technology (S&T) trade deals with the Soviet Union in the years leading up to its demise.[47] He visited the Vector lab in Siberia on at least one occasion.[48]

According to an interview I did of Kathleen Dickson in 2018, he went after her following her testimony to the FDA and had her arrested on trumped up charges, of which she was later cleared.[49] He spent most of his time antagonizing Lyme victims on the internet, and setting up propaganda campaigns with people such as Susan O'Connell, a British counterpart, and ruthlessly went after people like Ms. Dickson for her testimony to the FDA.[50] In a later correspondence obtained through FOIA, McSweegan can be seen discussing the extent of these campaigns much later in 2007, with numerous mainstream outlets and internet channels to keep the coverup in place:

> Dr. O'Connell:
>
> Thank you for your note.
>
> I sent a copy of it to Dr. Steve Barrett who built and manages the Quackwatch website. I have urged him to consider updating the section on Lyme disease, but I believe he has been somewhat distracted by other matters in recent years. Still, it may be possible

to update the Lyme material by copying it to another site with HTML links back to the Quackwatch index page. I'm looking into this possibility. I have already drafted some updated material just in case. If you and your colleagues would like to suggest needed changes, new data, and references please send them to me.

If outer space is the military's ultimate high ground... then cyberspace is the high ground in an information war. And what we have here is a war. Actually, a disinformation war. An insurgency against evidence-based medicine. It's time to start shooting back.

I'm vaguely familiar with your informal group to counteract misinformation. Durland Fish mentioned it to me. Sounds like a good start. Certainly, we have to do a better job of quickly responding to the accusations and antics of activists. We also have to do a better job of educating members of Congress and, in your case, Parliament. And we have to do a better job of keeping in touch with science and medical writers in the press and providing them with the necessary facts, references, quotes and sound bites.

Personally, I had been thinking that it might be useful to have a limited access website containing material to facilitate quick responses to reporters' questions and to facilitate the drafting of letters to legislators and editors. Such an online repository might contain copies of published articles on treatment trials and appropriate diagnostic methods, published commentaries on chronic Lyme disease, previously published letters to the editor, and examples of letters to send to local and national legislators. I suspect many physicians and scientists would like nothing more than to dash off a response to a newspaper or congressman, but lack the time to look up the references, dig out the quotes, and hone their message down to 300 or 400 words. This kind of repository would help.

I already have my own little repository, which I rely on for drafting letters to the editor (of *Nature, Epi & Inf, The Hartford Courant, The Washington Post,* and others), letters to congressmen (Phil Baker and I both responded to a Dec. 2006 ILADS-inspired congressional letter to the CDC), book reviews, and columns I write for a local Maryland paper. It's a lot easier to load and shoot if the ammunition is handy.

Anyway, it's one idea. Another might be to start a visible organization of researchers and ID docs with clearly stated goals and concerns similar to SEA: Scientists and Engineers for America (http://www.seform.org/). It could provide a convenient focal point for communication and strategy.

Whatever course we choose; it's going to be a long struggle. The Lymees and their parasitic LLMDs have been at this for a long time... [51]

McSweegan has just provided evidence for the reader that mainstream news outlets and online debunking sites like Quackwatch are helping to push the corporate science and public health agency talking points, by American and British public health officials through through the Ad Hoc International Lyme Disease Study Group, a working group with participation by other foreign governments, such as Susan O'Connell of Porton Down Laboratories in Britain.

Just prior to that exchange, declassified records show McSweegan can be seen again in an e-mail correspondence of a similar nature, this time with the ALDF president Phil Baker, academic professors such as Durland Fish, Allen Steere, and Henry Feder, with Barbara Johnson and Gary Wormser also on the e-mail. The e-mail was prompted by a posting of a $20,000 reward to any doctor who can prove that a patient did not still have Lyme disease following treatment with antibiotics, and this was posted by a Lyme activist Randy Sykes in Connecticut where a conference being attended to by corporate and academic professionals was to take place.[52] The exchange, begins with Durland Fish citing a lack of scientific means to counter the growing discontent and fraudulent guidelines:

> The battle cannot be won on a scientific front. We need to mount a socio-political offensive, but we are outnumbered and outgunned. We need reinforcements from outside our field. [53]

Edward McSweegan replied:

> For sick people they certainly have a lot of energy. Not to mention a lot of signs and placards.[54]

Allen Steere then returned with some recommendations:

> Ed,
>
> I have been meaning to write you about the UCS letter, and have not had a chance to do so. There is one point that I would like to emphasize. In untreated patients, there is a chronic form of Lyme disease that commonly results in Lyme arthritis, or in rare cases, Lyme encephalopathy or polyneuropathy. Our point is that subjective pain, neurocognitive or fatigue symptoms following IDSA-recommended courses of antibiotic therapy for Lyme disease are not caused by active infection.

237

Moreover, there is no peer-reviewed medical evidence that shows that months or years of antibiotic therapy is beneficial for the treatment of such symptoms. However, I think we need to be careful not to say there is no chronic form of Lyme disease. Such language has been largely removed from current draft of the letter. However, I have made a few suggestions (with track changes) for care in these statements.

I would be willing to sign the letter as long as a number of other members of the Ad Hoc International Lyme Disease Study Group do so.

Thanks for taking on this important task.

Allen [55]

The study group referred to in the aforementioned e-mail correspondence was an official International Working Group on Lyme Disease, publishing a series of papers since the very beginning to establish Lyme disease as a limited infection producing an autoimmune arthritis, curable with a few weeks of antibiotics, except for what they considered a very small minority that experienced ongoing symptoms after treatment. Their message would imply that there was nothing further that could be done aside from autoimmune management, which these biotech and drug firms would market and profit from.

Those involved in such groups would publish several papers every few years to paint for the public a misleading picture, saying that chronic Lyme disease was not a persistent *Borrelia burgdorferi* infection or an immunosuppressive disease,[56] and that post-treatment symptoms were a very rare autoimmune problem due to the initial *Borrelia burgdorferi* infection,[57] that unless patients had antibodies to meet bogus criteria for infection or autoimmune, they were psychiatric cases, as an early go at these *socio-political offensives* claimed:

> Neurologic symptoms, especially those involving changes in cognitive functions, are especially difficult to interpret [69-71]. Moreover, factors such as the premorbid personality and a tendency to somatization may determine the length of convalescence and the response to postinfection fatigue and joint aches [71,72].[58]

EVIDENCE-DEBASED MEDICINE
The science of immune tolerance as a disabling disease producing little to no antibodies nor detectable inflammation, was proven by the pioneer of German virology Erich Traub beginning

in 1936.[59] However, around the time of the emergence of Lyme disease and about 15 years before it was officially considered a disease, the infectious origins of immune tolerance were being wiped from public knowledge, with the Nobel Prize given in 1960 to Burnet and Medawar for immune tolerance, but only in organ transplant recipients, and they would ignore all the cases infected with stealth pathogens.[60] This was being done, not just with Lyme disease, but all the stealth infections that caused immunosuppression and produced chronic persistent infections.

Since these complex diseases are costly and hard to address, the medico-scientific establishment would rather not have the headache of addressing them, nor having to explain how it could be possible that an infection can occur and be spread without antibodies or outward symptoms, because the science of vaccination is supposed to assume that lack of symptoms means lack of infection, and that lack of symptoms correlates to lack of ability to spread, and immune tolerance flips that entire paradigm on its head, as Traub's published research demonstrates.[61]

Therefore, to make it more convenient for the prestige of health professionals and the profiteering of big pharma, they set-up the current public health paradigm so that the only evidence admissible in diagnosis is a standard whereby all definable and reportable diseases are only those which produce robust antibody responses and detectable inflammation. Traub's weapons do the reverse.

These immunosuppressive biological weapons demonstrate that half of the disease spectrum is marked by chronic infection and defective immune response, and the only standard used in the current paradigm of the Western public health system to detect a disease is to measure antibodies and visible inflammation. This is entirely insufficient, and this is the reason why millions are being swept under the rug and denied care for their disease, because the disease itself is being denied as illegitimate. Evidence-based medicine tells us that if cases of chronic disease and immune tolerance wish to be considered sick, they would have to demonstrate evidence of a robust immune system, lots of antibodies and inflammation, or it lacks an *evidence-based* approach. *Evidence-based medicine* is a term denoting the patient having to use the wrong tests to prove a disease it was meant to evade. It would be comparable to giving somebody exposed to asbestos a test for measuring toxic lead exposures and telling them to prove they had asbestos exposure using that test.

Endnotes

1 "New Tests Set Standard for Diagnosing Lyme Disease." *Mayo Clinic Rochester News*, Mayo Clinic Rochester, 4 Aug. 1998, https://web.archive.org/web/20000816190802/http://www.mayo.edu/comm/mcr/news/news_361.html

2 Dickson, Kathleen. "Charge 2: The Patents." TRUTHCURES.ORG CRIMINAL CHARGE SHEETS JUNE 2017, 2017. https://docs.wixstatic.com/ugd/47b066_01d68b1309ae457b81d-f1e06e6beae1e.pdf, see pp. 4-13

3 "Corixa Corporation Establishes Diagnostics Collaboration with Imugen." Corixa Corporation - News: Corixa Corporation Establishes Diagnostics Collaboration with Imugen, 7 Apr. 1998, https://www.coulterpharm.com/default.asp?pid=release_detail&id=96&year=1998

4 Persing, David H. INFECTION, CANCER, AND THE IMMUNE RESPONSE. The Infectious Etiology of Chronic Diseases Defining the Relationship, Enhancing the Research, and Mitigating the Effects; Workshop Summary. National Acad. Press, 2004., pp. 154-173

5 "Corixa Awarded $11.6 Million from NIH Biodefense Partnership to Develop Proprietary Molecules That Activate the Immune System Corixa's TLR4 Product Candidates May Provide Protective Immunity to a Wide Variety of Infectious Agents." Corixa Corporation - News: Corixa Awarded $11.6 Million from NIH Biodefense Partnership to Develop Proprietary Molecules That Activate the Immune System Corixas TLR4 Product Candidates May Provide Protective Immunity to a Wide Variety of Infectious Agents, 5 Jan. 2004, https://web.archive.org/web/20050313201650/http://www.corixa.com/default.asp?pid=release_detail&id=223&year=2004

6 David H. Persing et al. Demonstrable parasitemia among Connecticut blood donors with antibodies to Babesia microti. Transfusion, 45(11), 1804–1810. 2005 doi:10.1111/j.1537-2995.2005.00609.x

7 Brummitt, Sharon. "Ticks Carry More than Lyme Disease in California – Are Californians at Risk?" *Experiment*, 2016, https://experiment.com/projects/ticks-carry-more-than-lyme-disease-in-california-are-californians-at-risk

8 Persing, David H., METHOD FOR DETECTING B. BURGDORFERI INFECTION (US6045804A). 2000. Retrieved from: https://patents.google.com/patent/US6045804A/en

9 Ibid.

10 Corixa, Inc. "Stanford Rook Holdings PLC and Corixa Corporation Sign Agreement in Autoimmune Diseases." *Corixa Corporation News*, Coulterpharm.com, 1998, https://www.coulterpharm.com/default.asp?pid=release_detail&id=83&year=1998

11 Steere, A C et al. "Association of chronic Lyme arthritis with HLA-DR4 and HLA-DR2 alleles." *The New England Journal of Medicine* vol. 323,4 (1990): 219-23. doi:10.1056/NEJM199007263230402

12 Steere AC, Gross D, Meyer AL, Huber BT. Autoimmune mechanisms in antibiotic treatment-resistant lyme arthritis. *J Autoimmun.* 2001 May;16(3):263-8. doi: 10.1006/jaut.2000.0495. PMID: 11334491..

13 Kalish, R.S., Wood, IA., Golde, W., Bernard, R., Davis, L.E., Grimson, R.C, Coyle, P.K., Luft, B.J. Human T Lymphocyte Response to Borrelia burgdorferi Infection: No Correlation Between Human Leukocyte Function Antigen Type 1 Peptide Response and Clinical Status. (2003) Journal of Infectious Diseases, 187 (1), pp. 102-108.

14 Corixa, Inc. "Corixa Corporation to Acquire Anergen, Inc. Company Extends Product Portfolio to Include Additional Therapies for Prevention and Treatment of Autoimmune Diseases." Corixa Corporation - News: Corixa Corporation to Acquire Anergen, Inc. Company Extends Product Portfolio to Include Additional Therapies for Prevention and Treatment of Autoimmune Diseases, 1998, https://www.coulterpharm.com/default.asp?pid=release_de-

tail&id=108&year=1998

15   Broccolo, Francesco, et al. "Possible Role of Human Herpesvirus 6 as a Trigger of Autoimmune Disease." *TheScientificWorldJournal*, Hindawi Publishing Corporation, 24 Oct. 2013, https://www.ncbi.nlm.nih.gov/pubmed/24282390

16   Draborg, Anette Holck, et al. "Epstein-Barr Virus in Systemic Autoimmune Diseases." *Clinical & Developmental Immunology*, Hindawi Publishing Corporation, 2013, https://www.ncbi.nlm.nih.gov/pubmed/24062777

17   Payne, Laurence Noel, et al. "Oncogenesis and Herpesviruses: Proceedings of a Symposium Held at Christs College, Cambridge, England, 20 to 25 June 1971 ..." I.A.R.C. & World Health Organization (WHO), Oncogenesis and Herpesviruses: Proceedings of a Symposium Held at Christs College, Cambridge, England, 20 to 25 June 1971 ... 1972.

18   Persing, D., Telford, S., Rys, P., Dodge, D., White, T., Malawista, S., & Spielman, A. (1990). Detection of Borrelia burgdorferi DNA in museum specimens of Ixodes dammini ticks. Science, 249(4975), 1420–1423. doi:10.1126/science.2402635

19   Marshall, W F 3rd et al. "Detection of Borrelia burgdorferi DNA in museum specimens of Peromyscus leucopus." The Journal of infectious diseases vol. 170,4 (1994): 1027-32. doi:10.1093/infdis/170.4.1027

20   Persing, D., Telford, S., Rys, P., Dodge, D., White, T., Malawista, S., & Spielman, A. (1990). Detection of Borrelia burgdorferi DNA in museum specimens of Ixodes dammini ticks. Science, 249(4975), 1420–1423. doi:10.1126/science.2402635

21   Marshall, W F 3rd et al. "Detection of Borrelia burgdorferi DNA in museum specimens of Peromyscus leucopus." The Journal of infectious diseases vol. 170,4 (1994): 1027-32. doi:10.1093/infdis/170.4.1027

22   Marconi, R T et al. "Variability of osp genes and gene products among species of Lyme disease spirochetes." Infection and immunity vol. 61,6 (1993): 2611-7. doi:10.1128/iai.61.6.2611-2617.1993

23   Zumstein G, Fuchs R, Hofmann A, Preac-Mursic V, Soutschek E, Wilske B. Genetic polymorphism of the gene encoding the outer surface protein A (OspA) of Borrelia burgdorferi. Med Microbiol Immunol. 1992;181(2):57-70. doi:10.1007/BF00189424

24   Jing-Ren Zhang; John M Hardham; Alan G Barbour; Steven J Norris (1997). Antigenic Variation in Lyme Disease Borreliae by Promiscuous Recombination of VMP-like Sequence Cassettes. , 89(2), 0–285. doi:10.1016/s0092-8674(00)80206-8

25   Hayes SF, Burgdorfer W, Barbour AG. Bacteriophage in the Ixodes dammini spirochete, etiological agent of Lyme disease. J Bacteriol. 1983;154(3):1436-1439. doi:10.1128/jb.154.3.1436-1439.1983

26   Wojciechowska-Koszko, Iwona et al. "Cross-Reactive Results in Serological Tests for Borreliosis in Patients with Active Viral Infections." Pathogens (Basel, Switzerland) vol. 11,2 203. 3 Feb. 2022, doi:10.3390/pathogens11020203

27   Marshall, W. F., Telford, S. R., Rys, P. N., Rutledge, B. J., Mathiesen, D., Malawista, S. E., ... Persing, D. H. (1994). Detection Of Borrelia Burgdorferi Dna In Museum Specimens Of Peromyscus. Journal of Infectious Diseases, 170(4), 1027–1032. doi:10.1093/infdis/170.4.1027

28   Hinnebusch, J, and A G Barbour. "Linear plasmids of Borrelia burgdorferi have a telomeric structure and sequence similar to those of a eukaryotic virus." Journal of bacteriology vol. 173,22 (1991): 7233-9. doi:10.1128/jb.173.22.7233-7239.1991

29   Persing, D. H., Rutledge, B. J., Rys, P. N., Podzorski, D. S., Mitchell, P. D., , K. D. R., ... Malawista, S. E. (1994). Target Imbalance: Disparity of Borrelia burgdorferi Genetic Material in Synovial Fluid from Lyme Arthritis Patients. Journal of Infectious Diseases, 169(3), 668–672. doi:10.1093/infdis/169.3.668

30   Persing, D., Telford, S., Rys, P., Dodge, D., White, T., Malawista, S., & Spielman, A.

241

(1990). Detection of Borrelia burgdorferi DNA in museum specimens of Ixodes dammini ticks. Science, 249(4975), 1420–1423. doi:10.1126/science.2402635

31   Telford, Sam. "No, Lyme Disease Is Not an Escaped Military Bioweapon, despite What Conspiracy Theorists Say." The Washington Post, WP Company, 11 Aug. 2019, https://www.washingtonpost.com/health/no-lyme-diease-is-not-an-escaped-military-bioweapon-despite-what-conspiracy-theorists-say/2019/08/09/5bbd85fa-afe4-11e9-8e77-03b30b-c29f64_story.html

32   Ibid.

33   Traub, E., & Capps, W. I. Experiments with chick embryo-adapted foot-and-mouth disease virus and a method for the rapid adaptation. National Naval Medical Center. Bethesda, MD. (1953) U.S. NAVY Project NM. NMRI Memorandum Report. Project NM 000 018.07

34   Committee on Human Resources. 1977. Biological Testing Involving Human Subjects by the Department of Defense, 1977: Hearings before the Subcommittee on Health and Scientific Research of the Committee on Human Resources, United States Senate, Ninety-Fifth Congress, First Session ... March 8 and May 23, 1977. Biological Testing Involving Human Subjects by the Department of Defense, 1977: Hearings before the Subcommittee on Health and Scientific Research of the Committee on Human Resources, United States Senate, Ninety-Fifth Congress, First Session ... March 8 and May 23, 1977. S7-857 O. Washington: U.S. Govt. Print. Off. pp. 264-265, Retrieved from: https://archive.org/details/biologicaltestin00unit/page/264

35   Centers for Disease Control and Prevention (CDC). (2020). Q fever - Chapter 4 - Travel-Related Infectious Diseases. Centers for Disease Control and Prevention. Retrieved November 17, 2022, from https://wwwnc.cdc.gov/travel/yellowbook/2020/travel-related-infectious-diseases/q-fever

36   New Jersey Department of Agriculture. (n.d.). Tularemia. New Jersey Department of Agriculture . Retrieved November 17, 2022, from https://www.nj.gov/agriculture/divisions/ah/diseases/tularemia.html

37   Centers for Disease Control and Prevention (CDC). (2022, March 17). Psittacosis: Clinical features and complications. Centers for Disease Control and Prevention. Retrieved November 17, 2022, from https://www.cdc.gov/pneumonia/atypical/psittacosis/hcp/clinical-features-complications.html

38   Berth SH, Leopold PL, Morfini GN. Virus-induced neuronal dysfunction and degeneration. Front Biosci (Landmark Ed). 2009;14(14):5239-5259. Published 2009 Jun 1. doi:10.2741/3595

39   Lawson CL, Yung BH, Barbour AG, Zückert WR. Crystal structure of neurotropism-associated variable surface protein 1 (Vsp1) of Borrelia turicatae. J Bacteriol. 2006 Jun;188(12):4522-30. doi: 10.1128/JB.00028-06. PMID: 16740958; PMCID: PMC1482977.

40   Steiner I, Kennedy PG, Pachner AR. The neurotropic herpes viruses: herpes simplex and varicella-zoster. Lancet Neurol. 2007;6(11):1015-1028. doi:10.1016/S1474-4422(07)70267-3

41   Traub, E. Epidemiology of Lymphocytic Choriomeningitis In A Mouse Stock Observed for Four Years. Journal of Experimental Medicine, 69(6), 801-817. doi:10.1084/jem.69.6.801. (1939).

42   Persing, D., Telford, S., Rys, P., Dodge, D., White, T., Malawista, S., & Spielman, A. (1990). Detection of Borrelia burgdorferi DNA in museum specimens of Ixodes dammini ticks. Science, 249(4975), 1420–1423. doi:10.1126/science.2402635

43   Dickson, Kathleen. TRUTHCURES.ORG CRIMINAL CHARGE SHEETS JUNE 2017, 2017, https://docs.wixstatic.com/ugd/47b066_01d68b1309ae457b81df1e06e6beae1e.pdf

44   Brummitt, Sharon. "Ticks Carry More than Lyme Disease in California – Are Californians at Risk?" Experiment, 2016, https://experiment.com/projects/ticks-carry-more-than-lyme-disease-in-california-are-californians-at-risk

45   McSweegan, Edward. "Edward McSweegan, PhD." LinkedIn.com, LinkedIn, https://www.linkedin.com/in/edwardmcsweegan

46   McSweegan, Edward. Letter to Barry Goldwater. Received by Senator Barry Goldwater, Naval Medical Research Institute (NMRI), 13 Aug. 1986, Bethesda, MD., R https://static.secure.website/wscfus/10426050/7129340/1986-mcsweegan-goldwater.pdf

47   McSweegan, Edward. "Edward McSweegan, PhD." LinkedIn.com, LinkedIn, https://www.linkedin.com/in/edwardmcsweegan

48   McSweegan, Edward. "Sent to Siberia." The Wayback Machine, Travelmag: The Independent Spirit, 25 Sept. 2013, www.web.archive.org/web/20130925050437/http://travelmag.co.uk/?p=339 [Article originally published May 16, 2003]

49   Operation Openscript Channel. Interview with Kathleen Dickson. July 7, 2018. Available at: https://www.youtube.com/watch?v=ByuqJofLMg0&t=11s

50   Dickson, K. (personal communication). 2017

51   McSweegan, Edward. E-mail to Susan O'Connell. "Lyme vaccine article- thanks for a very useful letter." Received by Susan O'Connell, 22 Feb. 2007. Retrieved from: https://static.secure.website/wscfus/10426050/7247050/mcsweegan.pdf

52   Sykes, Randy. "Lyme Disease Exposed." YouTube, Simsbury Community Television/YouTube, 6 May 2015, https://www.youtube.com/watch?v=ow53uy1qEll

53   Fish, Durland. E-mail to Edward McSweegan, Allen Steere, Barbara Johnson, Henry Feder, Gary Wormser, et al., "Lyme rally in front of the University of CT health center." Received by Edward McSweegan, Allen Steere, Barbara Johnson, Henry Feder, Gary Wormser, et al., 07 Oct. 2007 Retrieved from: https://static.secure.website/wscfus/10426050/7266040/foia-cdc.pdf

54   McSweegan, Edward. E-mail to Durland Fish, Allen Steere, Barbara Johnson, Henry Feder, Gary Wormser, et al., "Lyme rally in front of the University of CT health center." Received by Edward McSweegan, Allen Steere, Barbara Johnson, Henry Feder, Gary Wormser, et al., 2007, Retrieved from: https://static.secure.website/wscfus/10426050/7266040/foia-cdc.pdf

55   Steere, A. C., Letter to Edward McSweegan, June 08, 2007. Retrieved from: https://static.secure.website/wscfus/10426050/7266040/foia-cdc.pdf

56   Auwaerter, Paul G, et al. "Antiscience and Ethical Concerns Associated with Advocacy of Lyme Disease." The Lancet Infectious Diseases, vol. 11, no. 9, 2011, pp. 713–719., doi:10.1016/s1473-3099(11)70034-2.

57   Feder, H. M., Johnson, B. J. B., O'Connell, S., Shapiro, E. D., Steere, A. C., & Wormser, G. P. (2007). A Critical Appraisal of "Chronic Lyme Disease." New England Journal of Medicine, 357(14), 1422–1430. doi:10.1056/nejmra072023

58   Barbour, A., and D Fish. "The Biological and Social Phenomenon of Lyme Disease." Science, vol. 260, no. 5114, 1993, pp. 1610–1616., doi:10.1126/science.8503006.

59   Traub, E. Persistence of Lymphocytic Choriomeningitis Virus in Immune Animals and Its Relation to Immunity. Journal of Experimental Medicine, 63(6), 847-861. doi:10.1084/jem.63.6.847. (1936).

60   Silverstein, Arthur M. "The curious case of the 1960 Nobel Prize to Burnet and Medawar." Immunology vol. 147,3 (2016): 269-74. doi:10.1111/imm.12558

61   Traub, E. Observations on immunological tolerance and "Immunity" in mice infected congenitally with the virus of lymphocytic choriomeningitis (LCM). Archiv Fur Die Gesamte Virusforschung, 10(3), 303-314. doi:10.1007/bf01250677. (1960).

Chapter Fifteen

The Legacy of a Sleeper Agent

Erich Traub, Pioneer of Immune Tolerance & the Slow Virus Disease

The answer is that there are two varieties of rare events: a) the narrated Black Swans, those that are present in the current discourse and that you are likely to hear about on television, and b) those nobody talks about, since they escape models.

– Nassim Nicholas Taleb, *The Black Swan*

When Erich Traub returned to Germany in 1953 to lead the Federal Research Institute for Virus Diseases of Animals in Tübingen, West Germany, records from his earlier FBI investigation and his published scientific research demonstrate that upon his return to Germany he continued collaborating and associating with the Americans for years to come. In fact, even when Traub was forced to step down as President of the Tübingen Institute for embezzlement and other charges, he was still held in the highest regard by the Americans and kept a prominent position with the Food and Agriculture Organization (FAO) of the United Nations.[1]

Despite confessing to being an agent of the KGB, which under normal circumstances would have been a death sentence, Traub was allowed to continue limited collaborative research for the U.S. Navy and USDA, and on numerous occasions the Americans sent Traub dangerous pathogens – viruses – like Eastern Equine Encephalomyelitis Virus (EEE),[2] Venezuelan Equine Encephalomyelitis Virus (VEE),[3] Lymphocytic Chroriomeningitis Virus (LCM),[4] Newcastle Disease Virus (NDV),[5] and Vesicular Stomatitis Virus (VSV).[6] Traub was then approved for several trips to re-enter the United States to take part in symposiums and conferences in the field of virology and agriculture and be a guest of honor at Plum Island's opening day ceremony in 1956.[7,8]

According to the travel logbook used by the Tübingen Institute, in spring of 1953, Traub and several colleagues from the Institute took a trip to Basel, Switzerland to visit a Swiss veterinary institute.[9] In June of that year, Werner Schäfer and his colleague Otto Armbruster, who were working with Traub from the Max Planck Institute at the time, took a trip for Traub to Berlin, East Germany to visit the Siemens and Halske, Co., the company in charge of the electron microscope department at Insel Riems and the University of Berlin.[10] The following month, Traub traveled to Rome and to Austria for the FAO, to attend a conference on Foot-and-Mouth Disease.[11]

CONTINUING RESEARCH IN TÜBINGEN

Some of Traub's American research for the U.S. Navy continued at the Tübingen Institute, demonstrating that UV radiation acts as an accelerant to Newcastle Disease Virus when the virus is not fully inactivated by the heavy doses of radiation.[12] As UV-radiation is often used to inactivate viruses in vaccine research, Traub showed that if the virus was not fully inactivated it would have a rebound effect and greatly strengthen the virus, multiplying rapidly to quickly regain itself as a more powerful virus.[13] This paper was published in 1954, concluding his Navy research once and for all. Already in 1954, Traub produced a research paper in the French language for the FAO and its associated journal, *The Bulletin of the International Office of Epizootics*, on FMD being able to survive and spread on vegetable products used in farming.[14]

In 1955, one of the first papers published by Traub as president of the Tübingen Institute, he took to studying the immune tolerance phenomenon transmitted from the mother chicken to her chicks through the chicken eggs.[15] It is noted in this paper that Wallace P. Rowe, a former colleague of Traub at the Naval Medical Research Institute (NMRI) and the National Institutes of Health (NIH) in Bethseda, Rowe sent Traub strains of LCM virus for these experiments. The same year, the USDA sent Traub a virulent strain of Eastern Equine Encephalitis virus for studies on the thermoresistence of EEE, and he was also sent a strain of Venezuelan Equine Encephalitis Virus for additional experiments in Tübingen.[16, 17]

Traub published another interesting work that year, "Effects of Salvarsan on Influenza Infection of Chick Embryos," with researcher Eva Reczko. Interestingly, Salvarsan was a treatment of choice for syphilis and spirochetal infections like relapsing fever, prior to Doxycycline.[18] Traub knew the main component of his strategic bioweapons like Lyme spirochetes were the persistent viral infections reawakened from dormancy after the onset of infection with Lyme disease and the devious cocktail of tick-borne disease it often came with.[19] These infections awakened sleeping viruses already harbored in the host and act like the foreign protein that awakened LCM virus in Traub's Rockefeller mice. In this paper, Traub was not interested in the effect of Salvarsan on spirochetes, but instead he wanted to know the effect of Salvarsan on viral infections and proceeded to study it with Influenza as a model. What Traub found was that administration of an intensive course of treatment with Salvarsan would actually greatly accelerate the viral infection:

> The following is about the effect. Salvarsan sodium […] which accelerates the infection in large but still tolerated doses and inhibits it in small doses under certain circumstances.[20]

In early 1956, Traub published a research paper on the possibility of transmission of EEE by contact between infected and uninfected mice. In this paper, he describes migratory birds and insects playing a primary role for the disease.[21] In the experiments, he notes the use of mites and lice on the mice, and also describes injecting infected mouse excrement and urine into the brains of the test mice.[22] He next mentions cannibalism in the mouse colony, whereby the uninfected would become infected after consuming the brains of other mice,[23] which resembled diseases like the transmissible spongiform encephalopathies (TSE) like Creutzfeldt-Jakob Disease (CJD), also called Kuru, seen in humans and animals after cannibalism.[24] Clearly, the nature of these experiments speak to a sadistic mindset and cruelty to animals like that described in his FBI investigations by former Rockefeller staff.[25]

In September of 1956, Traub once again set foot on American shores to attend Plum Island's opening day ceremony where the USDA hosted a conference on vesicular diseases.[26] Several years later in 1958, Traub filled out a security application to the FBI to receive special permission to enter the United States once again,[27] presumably to attend the symposium which he took part of that year, *Perspectives of Virology*,[28] in February of 1958, and in the application to the FBI, he listed employment with the Agricultural Research Service (ARS) of the USDA employed at the Greenport, Long Island station which is the Plum Island laboratory.[29] He cites Public Law 490, 80th congress as the authority for appointment, which is the 1948 legislation and congressional hearing to establish a Foot-and-Mouth Disease Virus (FMD) laboratory on an isolated island which eventually settled on Plum Island.[30]

Back at the Tübingen Institute, Traub hired a former war criminal, Eugen Haagen,[31] a prominent German virologist and bacteriologist who worked at the Robert Koch Institute and the University of Strasbourg. Like Traub, Haagen attended the Rockefeller Institute before WWII,[32] became a member of the Air Raid Protection for the German Reich. Haagen researched viruses like Influenza and epidemic jaundice,[33] typhus,[34] and took part in Nazi experiments on concentration camp inmates. During the war, Haagen coordinated with close contacts that Traub would also work with, such as Kurt Herzberg, Professor at the University of Greifswald,[35] who also worked with Insel Riems during the war, and like Traub, Haagen was also recruited to work for the Soviet Union but was arrested by British military police and was extradited to France for war crimes.[36] For Haagen's part in war crimes, he was initially sentenced to 20 years hard labor in France but for reasons unclear his sentence was communed to several years, given amnesty in 1955 and he was free by the time Traub became President of the Tübingen Institute.[37] Traub then hired Haagen, who worked at Traub's Institute from 1956-1965.[38]

HOW THE MIGHTY HAVE FALLEN: MAJOR SCANDAL AND RESIGNATION

By 1958, mounting tensions and instability at the Tübingen Institute initiated federal investigations after the dismissal of several institute employees, who wrote formal complaints to the administrative authorities of the Federal Minister for Food, Agriculture, and Forestry with pleas for investigation of misconduct, misdirection of federal money, fictitious travel expenses, and criminal actions on behalf of Traub's leadership of the Tübingen Institute.[39] The majority of complaints were directed towards Vice President Hans Melz, including sexual misconduct, but voiced Traub's complicity in the misdirection of federal money, among other things.[40]

According to the investigation, Melz had sexually assaulted some of the female staff at the Institute, including Miss Thea Hahn, an employee at the Institute. Vice President Melz was alleged to have inappropriately groped and approached numerous female employees at company outings in the years prior while inebriated, as was often the case. Melz had been cited throughout the long investigations as being an alcoholic and a womanizer.[41]

The incident involving Miss Thea Hahn, was reported to the local police in Tübingen and Stuttgart, supported by co-workers. Fearing they were soon to be fired, employees Otto Weiss and Emil Geiss followed with allegations to the authorities above the institute alleging serious mismanagement, fraud, and embezzlement were taking place. Simultaneously, reports of fictitious travel outings and fraudulent receipts to cover a complex web of financial inconsistencies were being brought up and looked at. Smaller allegations opened the door to much larger ones. Traub was being looked at in further detail because of the recklessness of Melz, while Traub could be described as a smooth criminal. However, the careless and often inebriated Vice President Melz ensured that the many years of mismanagement at the institute would soon be crashing down on both of them.

Back in America the same year, Dr. Jacob Traum retired as lead scientist for the USDA's Plum Island Animal Disease Center and the USDA once again offered Erich Traub the top position to lead Plum Island.[42] This came several months after the Federal Government of West Germany began its embezzlement investigations against Traub and Melz. Apparently, the USDA did not get that memo, and perhaps someone didn't fill them in on his espionage confession to Agent Dan Benjamin in 1952 either.

At any rate, Traub once again declined the USDA's offer. Ironically, however, the following year Traub decried his return to Germany in a letter to the Federal Minister for Food, Agriculture and Forestry in May of 1959:

> In 1952 I was working in America under very favorable conditions. The Federal Minister for Food, Agriculture, and Forestry in Bonn invited me to come back to Germany in 1952 to set up and manage a large virus institute there, especially for foot and mouth disease. Although the Federal Republic of Germany could only offer me a fraction of the income that I received in America, out of pure idealism as a German I accepted and took over the construction of the institute. For this purpose I returned to Germany in 1953.[43]

In December of 1959, during one of the proceedings against Traub and Melz, Traub was again quoted complaining about having left his position in America:

> Traub described the structure of the [federal research institute]. He pointed out that the separation in the institution between the epidemic section and the administration had been a great disadvantage for the control of the same. "If I had known that the construction would take 7 years, I would not have come back from the United States."[44]

Charges were eventually brought against both Melz and Traub, with Melz taking the bulk of responsibility and Traub coming out of it with heavy fines, a criminal record, and a semi-tarnished reputation in Germany. Most interestingly, some of the activities of Vice-President Melz speak to a high life of nightclubs, heavy drinking, strippers, prostitutes, and excessive alcohol consumption:

> Melz then reported an incident that is said to have taken place in 1957. After a night of drinking with Lilo in Cologne, he had awoken the next morning in a small town between Bonn and Cologne, without knowing in detail how that had happened. He then called the then government chief inspector Wagner from the [The Federal Minister for Food, Agriculture and Forestry] and asked him to pick him up in his private car and bring it to Bonn. Wagner did that. Wagner did not know the exact details. (RA Wagner confirmed Melz's information; when he called, he picked Melz up in his car in Uedorf in February 1957 and brought him to Bonn. Melz was very drunk and otherwise quite "disheveled." For example, he was missing a wristwatch that had apparently been taken away from him by force, and Melz only told him at the time that he had gone to Cologne with Prof. Traub and spent the last night there, and Wagner claims that Melz understood it that way as if he had somehow been abandoned by Prof. Traub.)
>
> Melz pointed out that his abnormal sexual perversions were the real motive for his behavior, which he was accused of in the process. After all, it had gone so far that he had to [please himself] at the sight of a beautiful woman on the street.
>
> The prosecutor asked Melz whether he had had intimate relationships with female [The Federal Minister for Food, Agriculture and Forestry] employees. Melz initially denied this. At the request of the public prosecutor, Melz finally admitted that he had had sexual intercourse with employee Betzel on the occasion of a private trip to Hamburg that he undertook. In response to questions from the public prosecutor, Melz said that although he had used Ms. Betzel normally, he was not satisfied. The prosecutor indicated that he did not believe this was a case of abnormal perversion for Melz. When the public prosecutor reiterated, Melz admitted that he had maintained a constant love affair with Ms. Betzel.
>
> Prosecutor: "Didn't you also bother the employee, Thea Hahn?" Melz: "I don't remember that." According to Hahn's

testimony from the public prosecutor's preliminary proceedings: "If she says so, it probably had been so."

Melz also admits at the request of the public prosecutor that he had molested Weiss' wife in her and his own apartment. Melz only disputes Ms. Weiss's testimony in the preliminary proceedings that he was very drunk. Melz: "I was often so drunk that I was unfit for service." "I also have a strong need to impress others by spending money."

Traub answered questions from the public prosecutor: "I never noticed that Melz is perverted or particularly sexually aggressive." Melz then reminds Traub of an evening spent together in a nightclub in Stuttgart, where Traub is said to have asked him not to behave so strongly towards a blonde lady, as they were already causing a commotion. Melz also reminds Traub that they were brought home together in a heavily drunk state in the motor vehicle. Traub does not deny either incident.

Melz answered the question from the defender of Traub whether Lilo even existed. "He also corresponded with her." "The money that he had misappropriated was no longer available." "I am aware that Prof. Traub is also liable for the damage caused."

Traub to Melz: "I didn't deserve that from you." [45]

In the end, Traub and Melz were both charged and convicted of several offenses, with Melz bearing the most serious offenses, while Traub's were of lesser consequence. The charges were listed as follows:

The accused Dr. Traub

1.) jointly with another
   a) intentionally abused the power granted to him by law and official mandate to dispose of third-party assets and to oblige another and violated his duty to safeguard third-party financial interests by virtue of a loyalty relationship, thereby inflicting a disadvantage on the person whose financial interests he has to look after.
   b) intending to give someone else an illegal asset advantage, damage someone else's property by making a mistake by pretending wrong facts,
2.) continued with the same action
   a) together with another with the intention of gaining an illegal asset advantage, damages the property of another by making a mistake by pretending wrong facts,

b) intentionally violated his duty to safeguard the interests of others by virtue of a loyalty relationship, thereby inflicting a certain amount on those whose interests he had to look after,

c) jointly with another the deception in legal transactions, a fake document was produced and fake documents were used.[46]

When the investigations and proceedings were concluded, Traub made out with hefty fines, and a suspended sentence of nearly 2 ½ months:

[T]he head of this research institute, President Prof. Dr. Traub, For fraud and embezzlement, instead of a prison sentence of a total of 2 months and 12 days, which was forfeited, as a replacement, given a fine of [Deutschemarks (DM)] 3,950.00 Sentenced.[47]

The embezzlement investigations contained travel logbooks from the Institute for trips taken, which indicate that Traub took several trips that deserve closer scrutiny, especially trips taken by his colleagues sent to East Germany directly for Traub. Werner Schäfer, along with Dr. Otto Armbruster, as we have mentioned, traveled to Berlin, East Germany in May of 1953, to visit the Siemens & Halske plant.[48] It is interesting to consider how they were able to travel freely between two rival superpowers who were competing for German scientists, given the sensitive positions of such scientists between the relations and Cold War developments in East and West Germany. Dr. Armbruster is repeatedly brought up in the investigations as having a *clique* against Dr. Traub, and Traub alleges they were working against him.[49]

Erich Traub also took a trip to London in 1957 for the opening of an institute, run by Dr. Ian A. Galloway, mentioned by Traub in the testimony from employees Otto Weiss and Emil Geiss, testifying to the Federal Audit Office, that Traub had been giving away free material to Galloway.[50] Traub explained that virus strains were being given to him by Dr. Galloway, apparently, Traub brought him expensive pens as a gift in return for several virus strains.[51] Dr. Galloway had been involved in the setup of the Colombian FMD lab in Bogotá for the FAO, maintaining it until Traub took it over from March 1951 to December 1952.[52]

There was also mentioned in the investigation, a trip Traub took to Venezuela, though it was not shown in the logbook.[53]

It is also interesting to note that in the early days of Traub's return, using temporary rooms for laboratory work at the Max Planck Institute, there were outbreaks with Newcastle Disease Virus in the nearby chickens as Traub resumed work, described in the investigations:

> If Ms. Hahn is accused by the Institute management of having attempted to violate the epidemiological regulations, then one must ask oneself whether Prof. Traub is not also bound by the same law, because he was in the early days of the [Federal Research Institute] responsible for the fact that the chicken plague, with which he was working, broke out in the poultry stock owned by Master baker Märkle.
>
> The laboratory, a converted bakery shop, was not shielded from the eyes at all, partly because the prescribed shut-off measures in the event of a risk of an epidemic were not taken! The outbreak of the chicken plague in the poultry population of the laboratory landlord Märkle was evidently the fault of Prof. Traub as the responsible laboratory manager and has been hushed up until today.[54]

It is also worth mentioning that several employees of Traub, a Miss Sauter and Miss Wehmaier became ill working with some of these highly infectious agents Traub had been altering, while another passed out from exposure to gases:

> Ms. Sauter, and Miss. Wehmaier were in the temporary laboratory of the [federal institute] [...] employed there she contracted a serious illness that made a long stay in a Tübingen clinic necessary. Accordingly, Dr. Wehmaier had become infected doing unfamiliar laboratory work. However, Prof. Traub understandably rejected this reason! He resigned her employment while she was ill.
>
> In these first laboratories it also happened that the first technical assistant, Miss Hilmer, had to pass out several times from escaping gas before remedial measures were taken![55]

From roughly 1955 to 1961 Traub would devote many years of further study to the mosquito-borne arbovirus Eastern Equine Encephalomyelitis (EEE). He published an entire series on the virus totaling eight publications under the title, "On the immunity of the white mouse to the EEE-virus,"[56] with additional papers like those mentioned regarding mites and cannibalism,[57] thermoresistant strains,[58] among others.[59] In between this, he also devoted time to Foot-and-Mouth Disease Virus with emphasis on increasing its neurotropic qualities,[60] and its immunosuppressive qualities.[61]

TRAUB'S STEALTH WEAPONS ON AMERICAN SHORES

As Traub had been able to pack up from American service and re-establish himself back in Germany at the Tübingen Institute, his germ weapons would not leave as easily. Like the outbreaks of Newcastle Disease Virus that followed in Traub's footsteps elsewhere, outbreaks began to plague the American continent. Notable outbreaks come to mind after his second run on American shores, such as Vesicular Stomatitis Virus (VSV), which would begin to cause outbreaks in laboratory and USDA staff, who were not sufficiently skilled to handle Traub's new pathogens.[62]

Weaponized Ticks, Lyme disease & Co-Infections. We have already covered in earlier chapters how Traub weaponized Lyme disease and weaponized ticks with additional blood parasites and rickettsia to produce the highly immunosuppressive effects and immune tolerance. There is also evidence that the *Leptospira* spirochete was included in these ticks and were isolated from the bullseye rash in early Lyme patients.[63] Insel Riems had been working with *Leptospira* spirochetes and Traub had learned of these combined infections such as *Bartonella, Babesia*, and spirochetes, in 1939 with Karl Beller, when Beller published a chapter on the nature of these diseases.[64]

Neurotropic Vesicular Stomatitis Virus (VSV). From the time of Traub's arrival in 1949 and subsequent work with the virus of Vesicular Stomatitis, outbreaks of VSV in humans began to occur at areas where he worked, supervised and instructed others for experiments with his pathogens like the University of Wisconsin,[65] the Beltsville Station of the USDA,[66] and finally, at Plum Island in 1954.[67] Michael C. Carroll had noted the outbreak in his book on Plum Island, where an infected cow coughed in a lab workers face and soon the lab worker became sick with an infection of VSV.[68]

However, this was not the first exposure to Traub's new strain of stomatitis. Several of Traub's colleagues at the USDA and military had studied the outbreak, first starting at the University of Wisconsin after five workers there contracted it in 1949 and 1950, while cases from the Beltsville station, from 1949-1958, had 100 human cases of Vesicular Stomatitis at the USDA. [69] Traub had been involved with some of the work on Newcastle Disease tested at farms owned by the University of Wisconsin,[70] and Traub's work on VSV at Beltsville had established he was there teaching the USDA researchers here how to grow purified antigen in chicken eggs.[71] Traub's signature neurotropic qualities were mentioned resulting in cases of undiagnosed encephalitis.[72] In the large majority of researchers and animal handlers, 70-96% had antibodies to VSV, 57% of those who had antibodies had symptoms of illness, while 54 human cases of vesicular stomatitis disease were diagnosed, showing that stealth outbreaks and infection with VSV was already spreading freely among the USDA.[73]

Lymphocytic Choriomeningitis (LCM) in Humans & Hamsters. In the mid-to-late 1960s, and occurring again in the mid-1970s, several outbreaks of lymphocytic choriomeningitis (LCM) virus occurred in animal colonies and laboratory personnel around New York and Maryland. In 1966, several scientists published "Epidemic Nonmeningitic Lymphocytic Choriomeningitis Virus Infection. An Outbreak in a Population of Medical Personnel."[74] This outbreak occurred in Bethesda, MD. Traub had been gone for some time at this point, but he was taking trips back to the USA and this virus could maintain itself through many generations.

Some of these scientists, such as Wallace P. Rowe, who worked with Traub early at NMRI and conducted tests with him were sending strains of LCM to Germany after his return. A second publication, "Laboratory Studies of a Lymphocytic Choriomeningitis Virus Outbreak in Man and Laboratory Animals,"[75] appeared in 1975, just as Lyme disease was being acknowledged by public health officials in the small town of Old Lyme, Connecticut. More alarming, these LCM outbreaks were not confined to these areas. On April 14, 1974, *The New York Times* published "Hamsters Killed to Prevent the Spread of Mild Meningitis," where CDC officials were frantically destroying infected hamsters around the country in a rather sudden display of concern,[76] clearly because hamsters were being used as source materials in vaccine manufacturing at the time,[77] it was generally used in vaccine research,[78] and in tissue cultures used in general academic and scientific research.[79]

Duck Virus Enteritis. Virtually the same time as the outbreak of LCM virus was occurring at New York and Maryland, ducks around Long Island and nearby Plum Island soon began to die in large numbers from the duck plague, or duck virus enteritis,[80] a herpesvirus that affects ducks and waterfowl, first seen in the 1930s and 1940s.[81] This could have been a secondary infection following an infection with spirochetes or other agents, causing an immunosuppressive reaction and reawakening the sleeping viruses like duck herpesvirus. How many animals were infected at this time is unknown, but the epidemic was a significant loss to Long Island restaurants that served the duck as a dish.[82]

Newcastle Disease Virus. While the duck plague (duck herpesvirus-1) was destroying the duck population in the Long Island sound, there had been simultaneous outbreaks across the United States of Exotic Newcastle Disease, occurring in California, and even before the duck plague hit Long Island ducks, there were reports of ducks dying from a virulent Exotic Newcastle Disease just years apart.[83] This was certainly a terrain Traub was familiar with, and much of his career during the war centered on avian influenza/fowl plague/Newcastle Disease *(Geflügelpest)*.[84] As noted earlier in this chapter, tests conducted in the mid-West gave rise to several outbreaks of Newcastle Disease through vaccination campaigns conducted around the time of Traub's employment.[85]

Foot-and-Mouth Disease Virus. In 1978, Plum Island Animal Disease Center experienced a major outbreak of Foot-and-Mouth Disease Virus on the island in which the entire stock of animals at the island had to be euthanized and incinerated. It was known that the FMD vaccines used live and inactivated virus vaccines back then, and both could revert to active virulence, and Traub had brought his freeze-dried cultures from Germany and used them in Navy work and for the USDA. Traub was already approved by the Food and Agriculture Organization to set-up other governments to produce FMD vaccine.[86]

It was also known back in Germany by Traub and his Insel Riems staff, that freeze-dried virus in vaccines could potentiate a delayed reversion back to virulent form after a considerable lapse of time.[87] Traub briefly mentioned these difficulties in a 1954 paper in French.[88] Insel Riems had already been looking into this vulnerability during WWII,[89] and Traub's freeze dried FMD cultures that were brought to America would have been used to setup Plum Island with Traub's method for producing FMD vaccines, as he was doing for the Navy.[90] What is particularly telling is that after the FMD outbreak occurred at Plum Island, they decided to hire a biotech company Genentech to create a new FMD vaccine, and one of their project scientists gave an interview about it, lending more insight into the state of FDM vaccines at the time:

What they told us was that the vaccines out there were not particularly effective in that they wouldn't give complete protection, and they would sometimes give rise to new outbreaks because the virus was not totally killed. It is an RNA virus which is constantly evolving, much like the AIDS virus. It is hard to get a good vaccine for an antigen that is constantly evolving.[91]

Echoing that sentiment, Dr. J. J. Callis, heading Plum Island at the time, told the NIH officials involved in the rolling out of recombinant DNA technologies, that producing FMD vaccines and their use could result in new outbreaks:

He suggested that recombinant technology could produce vaccine at considerably less expense as a stable product, without risk of the virus escaping from factories. Many outbreaks today result from incompletely inactivated vaccine or escape of the virus from factories.[92]

IMMUNE TOLERANCE & THE 1960 NOBEL PRIZE

In 1960, as Federal Investigations of Traub's administration and presidency of the Institute in Tübingen were reaching their peak, the Nobel Prize for *immune tolerance* was awarded to two scientists, British researcher Peter Medawar and Australian researcher Frank Macfarlene Burnet.[93] It is interesting to note several things about immune tolerance in regard to this award.

First, that these two scientists were never nominated together by anyone, nor did they work together.[94] Secondly, the Nobel Prize for immune tolerance did not include that which occurs due to infectious disease, but instead it was cited in regard to the same condition seen in organ transplants.

Moreover, there was no emphasis on infectious disease or of Erich Traub's work on LCM virus, as it was Erich Traub who had described the *immune tolerance* phenomenon in LCM virus nearly 25 years earlier.[95] Traub had already begun to map out the foundation of chronic disease and persistent infections due to the immune system being disabled and made it his life work.[96] However, the use of what Traub discovered was applied to the destruction of life rather than the pursuit of health.

The entire phenomenon of immune tolerance, which those affected today might know by other names, such as long COVID, Chronic Lyme Disease, Chronic Fatigue Syndrome, Myalgic Encephalomyelitis, fibromyalgia, rheumatoid arthritis, Gulf War Illness, and all of the controversial forms of chronic disease that have become a stigma to the afflicted, are all forms of immunodeficiency brought about by a class of antigen with a certain lipid profile and its effects serve as the basis of the strategic biological weapons that disable the immune system. In other words, the antigen or surface protein is the weapon, the most crippling aspect of the agents Traub weaponized.

In many ways, this antigen served as a perversion of nature, an abomination of science, geared to its very worst ideal, using viruses and microbes as weapons to create complex diseases that were extremely hard to treat, very confusing to diagnose, and very expensive to manage. Furthermore, there was also the unsettling reality that much of the West's reliance on vaccines to deal with even the most minor infectious diseases were actually exacerbating and even bringing on the condition itself due to the same manner of burning out the immune system.

As it exhausted the immune system from repeated exposure to toxic antigen, the immune system eventually reaches a state of immune deficiency synonymous with *immune tolerance*.[97] The immune system cannot respond appropriately in a state of exhaustion, which allows the reawakening of dormant viruses which then go to work destroying the brain and body from head to toe, much like Traub's LCM virus in his Rockefeller mice.[98] The injection of foreign protein into his mice to reactivate LCM virus was no different than the injection of a spike protein or antigen used in numerous vaccines.[99]

While the infectious origins of Traub's immune tolerance were being largely ignored from the Western approach to public health, several had taken notice of what happened and how Traub's findings were disregarded. First, American virologist John Hotchin had praised Traub in his Monograph, *Persistent and Slow-Virus Infections*, with the opening page, "*to Erich Traub, who started the whole thing.*"[100] One of Traub's protégés during WWII, Zvonimir Dinter had also acknowledged Traub's discovery having been glossed over by the 1960 Nobel Prize, in Dinter's 1984 paper, "Personal Experiences with Erich Traub":

Traub, "who started the whole thing." [...]

TRAUB's talent soon began after he began research at Princeton, the Rockefeller Institute branch. The topic to which he dedicated his work in the first place was the behavior of lymphocytic choriomeningitis virus in mice. A number of communications that began in Science and continued in the

Journal of Experimental Medicine, and which are generally regarded as classical today, where "many pioneering series of investigations in many of the key biological properties of the virus were established." (1) When BURNET and MEDAWAR received the Nobel Prize in 1960 for their seminal immunological work, I, as a veterinarian and as TRAUB's colleague, would have liked to see that he, too, had participated in the prize, because what TRAUB already described in 1936 and 1939, was the mode of origin of the condition, which was later baptized as "immune tolerance" and which represented a pillar of Burnet's clone-selective theory (2). The American researcher HOTCHIN showed appreciation for TRAUB's dedication by giving him his monograph with the words: "To ERIC TRAUB who started the whole thing" (3).[101]

It was clear that Traub's findings on the science of immune tolerance in chronic persistent infections and the neurological disease that comes with it were conveniently being ignored by the establishment for all that it implied.[102] This kind of discovery would turn conventional medicine and immunology on its head, disrupting a very large and prestigious medical industrial complex. Needless to say, Traub's work and focus becomes a doorway to many other unfortunate aspects of modern science, medicine, and aspects of human nature.

Around this time in Erich Traub's career, he returned to the study of LCM virus, and in the years 1960-1963 he published some of his best papers on the chronic disease in persistent infections with LCM virus resulting in the complex phenomenon, *immune tolerance*.

Particularly noteworthy is Traub's 1960 paper, "Observations on immunological tolerance and 'Immunity' in mice infected congenitally with the virus of lymphocytic choriomeningitis (LCM)," because it is here we find some of the best descriptions of the stealth mechanisms that underlie many of the controversial chronic diseases plaguing Americans today, with patients who are very ill with some of the most debilitating symptoms yet their healthcare providers are finding no signs of illness, no antibodies to disease agents, and no abnormal bloodwork, and based on this, they deny the complaints of their patients as illegitimate or psycho-somatic:

> *Mice infected* [congenitally from mother to newborn] *with LCM virus carry large amounts of active virus in their blood and organs for many months and discharge considerable quantities of the agent with their secretions and excretions (11). This observa-*

tion indicates continuous multiplication of the virus in the organs of such animals, which look like normal individuals in spite of their chronic infection. [Maternal transmission of LCM] infection leads to a stable [parasitism] between virus and body. It was also observed that mice infected [in the womb] would develop practically no [LCM Virus] antibodies.

[...]

Attempts to demonstrate neutralizing antibodies in the [blood] of such animals using customary techniques gave essentially negative results.[103]

In this round of studies on LCM virus, Traub published further insight into the immunosuppression of LCM,[104] the affinity for the lymph nodes,[105] the lack of antibodies with no abnormal bloodwork,[106] the rapid acceleration of cancers like leukemia and lymphomatosis,[107] and he compared LCM virus to some of the murine cancer viruses.[108] He had already shown back in 1941, how LCM virus would accelerate a rapid spike in cancer from mice born infected from their mothers, demonstrating how LCM infections can maintain persistence through many successive generations cursing the health of future generations with slow chronic infections, neurological disease, and a massive rise in cancers.[109]

FAO ASSIGNMENTS IN IRAN AND TURKEY

After stepping down from the Tübingen institute, Erich Traub took on new assignments for the Food and Agriculture Organization (FAO) of the United Nations to setup an FMD laboratory at the Razi Institute of Serum and Vaccines in Tehran, Iran, lasting from 1963 to 1966.[110] Upon his arrival and setting up to study FMD in Iran, Traub voiced great pleasure in watching FMD spread like wildfire among the Iranian peasantry, freely spreading its pestilence unaffected by mass vaccination, indicating this may have been one of his weaponized strains of FMD Virus:

A study of serological variation of Foot-and-Mouth Disease (FMD) virus is particularly rewarding in a large country where the disease can spread rather freely, more or less unhampered by mass vaccination and sanitary measures, and where a considerable part of the flock owners still lead a nomadic life.[111]

He collaborated with several Iranian researchers on FMD virus for years beyond the mission, with Iranian counterparts like Abbass Shafyi,[112] H. Ramyar,[113] and G. K. Kanhai.[114] Upon further analysis, Traub's research in Iran had clear offensive weapons potential. In one paper with G. K. Kanhai, he lays out the implications of the work to include *"increase of potency of the causative agent," "virus adaptation to certain species of animals and escalation or decrease of infectivity and pathogenicity for other species," "different affinity of virus strains for certain cells (cardiac FMD)," "differences in susceptibility among individual animals of the same species," "persistent infection,"* among other factors.[115]

In earlier chapters I mentioned Traub having shown one of his Iranian counterparts how to adapt various pathogens, for example, rickettsia or blood parasites to new animal hosts using a coinfecting animal virus, which Kanhai tried out using the Sendai virus of the influenza group of viruses to adapt the *Babesia*-like blood parasite *Theileria parva* (East Coast Fever) to new animals it didn't previously infect, like hamsters.[116]

Traub would take another mission for the FAO to Turkey to assist them in the setup of an FMD lab there, which took him from 1969 to 1972.[117] He would then return to Germany to take up research at the University of Munich headed by director and former deputy under Traub's institute in Tübingen, Dr. Anton Mayr.[118] This time, he was back to the virus that started the whole thing, the virus of Lymphocytic Choriomeningitis (LCM).

BACK TO LCM VIRUS "WHO STARTED THE WHOLE THING"

On October 16, 1972, Traub gave an introductory speech at a symposium on LCM virus, *Lymphocytic Choriomeningitis Virus and Other Arenaviruses,* which had been held at the Heinrich-Pette-Institute for experimental virology and Immunology, at the University of Hamburg.[119] This would begin the final phase of Erich Traub's career in virology and he would focus specifically on the LCM virus for the remainder of his life.

In his introductory speech at the symposium, Traub made some interesting statements and might be considered a cryptic recollection of some of Traub's veiled achievements with LCM in biological weapons work. Traub mentioned that aside from the typical arboviruses (EEE, tick encephalitis, etc.), LCM virus could be transmitted by a variety of arthropods, such as mosquitoes, bed bugs, and ticks, while the LCM virus could also be grown in cultures of tick cells. He also mentioned the ability to transmit LCM virus with the parasitic nematode, *Trichinella spiralis.* The LCM virus itself he described as extremely labile, able to adapt to just about any situation and produce so many variants that it made reproducing any experimental work very difficult since it was always changing.

He then described the immune tolerance phenomenon and the chronic neurodegenerative disease that became more pronounced in each subsequent generation. He also notes that immune tolerant chronically infected mothers invariably gave birth to infected newborns who harbored and transmitted considerable quantities of virulent virus in their secretions and excretions, despite not showing any outward signs of disease and producing little to no antibodies:

> Congenitally infected mice look like normal individuals for many months, most of them for their entire life, in spite of the fact that they carry large amounts of virus in their organs and blood and discharge virus continuously in their nasal secretions, urine, feces, milk, and sperm. They have no effective mechanism for virus clearance. [bloodwork] is essentially normal. In contrast to mice with acute adult infection, they can readily pass the virus to normal mice by contact (nose to nose), with the milk or by sexual intercourse. In tolerant females every successive litter becomes infected congenitally, no matter whether the animal was mated with a normal male or a tolerant one. All embryos in each successive litter are infected.[120]

The mice born from infected mothers would look indistinguishable from healthy mice, develop no antibodies and remain infected for life. This might have been a favorable form of immunity if not for the fact that the lifelong infection was not harmless even if they appeared healthy, at first.

Traub observed that as the infected mice born from an immune tolerant mother would appear healthy and like other healthy uninfected mice, but eventually they began to show signs of chronic neurodegenerative disease, kidney, and organ damage, which had been thought to be partially of an autoimmune reaction for some, but also pointed out that the antigen accumulating in the organs and brain is likewise at play.

Another damaging effect of these persistent life-long infections with LCM virus in congenitally infected mice was that as they matured, they would develop cancers (leukemia, lymphomatosis) in increasing frequency with each subsequent generation, occurring far more frequently and at a younger age as the mice continued through generations, eventually causing cancer in approximately 1 in 2 mice (50%) in future generations:

The interaction between persistent LCM virus infection and leukemia in mice and, to a lesser extent, in guinea-pigs has been the subject of numerous publications. We reported in 1941 that lymphatic leukemia was more frequent and appeared at a younger age in persistently infected mice from the Princeton colony than in LCM virus-free controls derived from the same stock. Later, leukemia was also seen in 1 of 2 wild mice persistently infected with LCM virus which Dr. Haas had sent me from the U.S.A.[121]

Lastly, Traub addressed some of the scientists who in 1967 had contested immune tolerance because they were able to find evidence of some antibodies from immune tolerant mice. They rejected the idea of the immune system recognizing the virus as "*self*," since often the term was used in the context of the immune system's distinguishing between *self* and *non-self*, but the condition was more complex than this. It also had to do with the immune system being forcefully suppressed into tolerating harmful pathogens because it can't fight back, rather than tolerating them as though the immune system recognizes them as part of the *self*-tissue. Traub did not create the term immune tolerance, however, and he explained it more like it was an immune *paralysis*, but he suggested that these two sides are in some sense half right, as the underlying condition is marked more by active suppression of the immune system by antigen rather than merely the immune system recognizing the pathogens as the same as *self*-tissues, but in the early stages of life this may have been more the case since its own tissue is infected through the mother passed to the newborn, and when the immune system matures later in life it begins to recognize these infectious agents as something other than itself.[122]

FINAL ROUND OF LCM AND THE DEATH OF A BIOWEAPONEER

With a notable, eye-opening speech presented at the 1972 symposium on LCM virus, Traub was able to put the remainder of his life to further study of LCM virus. From 1974-1981, Traub would publish six more papers on LCM Virus. He would study the progression of the disease in the later generations of mice persistently infected, born with compromised immune systems, which had been baptized "*immune tolerance*."[123]

From 1975 to 1976, just as Lyme arthritis was in its early stages of being admitted and acknowledged as a disease, Traub was studying the neurodegenerative effects of LCM termed "*early and late onset disease,"* essentially a progressive central nervous system disease that would mirror the neurological disease seen in Lyme Disease.[124] Lyme disease involved not only spirochetes but also the onset of persistent viral infections in parallel to the spirochete infection, and the spirochetes caused immunosuppression and auto-immune-like reactions comparable to Lupus erythematosus.[125]

The spirochete infection reawakened dormant viruses already within the host during the early stages of infection and this is mirrored by the symptoms.[126, 127] LCM was the animal model of these dormant viruses, comparable to Epstein-Barr Virus (EBV) or Human Herpesvirus 6 (HHV-6), to name a few, and as the spirochetes shed toxic lipid proteins into the blood, it would disable the immune system and these sleeping viruses awaken from dormancy establishing chronic, persistent viral infections in the manner of Traub's LCM virus.[128, 129, 130]

These studies gave Traub a comparable model to the progression of his biological weapons ravaging the American population.[131] In 1976, he began to study the antigen content found in the brains of mice showing that mice accumulated viral antigen in their brains, and played a role in the central nervous system disease it produced.[132] He also studied the effects on the kidneys which often led to kidney disease (nephritis), and the feeding habits of the mice. He found that mice that ate less frequently lived longer than those that did not.[133]

In Traub's final two papers, Traub addressed some of the debates about the concept of *immune tolerance* in relation to chronic, persistent infections like LCM that actively suppress the immune system, since other researchers would occasionally find limited antibodies in these mice but it was sporadic and these would disappear and reappear.[134] It was later demonstrated that this occurs because of the antigen mutating and continuously changing its biochemical composition to evade the immune response, and this was known as *antigenic variation.*[135] It was the antigen leading the immune system in an endless game of cat and mouse. This exhausts and overwhelms the immune system into an inadequate state and a slow, chronic disease follows.[136]

Traub concluded his career demonstrating the reality of severe, life-long persistent infections causing slow, debilitating chronic diseases producing little to no antibodies, no abnormal bloodwork, and little to no outward inflammation. Traub conclusively proves how individuals can be quite sick yet appear healthy to their physicians.[137] His lifelong study of the LCM virus demonstrates that there is an entire spectrum of disease marked by immunosuppression rather than inflammation, and the auto-immune-like reactions were more

263

or less the effect of the antigen fusing and proliferating tissues, organs, and brain, so that the term *tolerance* does not entirely do justice, as it appears to be a state where the immune system is persistently overwhelmed by a virus for which the antigens actively suppresses the immune system into a state of burnout.[138]

Traub's final round with LCM virus contains many inconvenient truths with vast implications for the sad state of the public health system's response to persistent infections that caused immune tolerance, like Lyme disease, post-vaccinal syndromes, and the unnecessary stigma attached to chronic disease today.[139] Traub's scientific research would prove to the many health care providers denying the complaints of those with chronic diseases lacking antibodies and inflammation, that chronic immunosuppression and persistent infections go hand in hand, they are marked by an absence of antibodies, no abnormal bloodwork or immune cell count, and without visible inflammation.[140]

It would call to light the fact that antigenic material or spike protein used in routine vaccination does not imply a harmless process, while many antigens are themselves self-replicating agents and can accumulate in tissues, organs, and brains to a large degree.[141] It would call serious attention to the triple signature of Traub's strategic bioweapons – chronic disease, mental illness, and cancer – now ravaging American life and robbing the lives of loved ones, families, and friends, while prematurely smothering an otherwise long and prosperous future.

On May 17, 1985, Erich Traub passed away quietly in his sleep, at 78 years of age, concluding a lifetime of virus research and bioweaponeering. Traub had worn the hats of many superpowers, the Soviet Union, Britain, USA, and Nazi Germany, and likewise, as a skilled bioweaponeer. If they wanted weapons of war, he gave them all more than they bargained for…

Endnotes

1   Traub, E., Shafyi, A., Ewaldsson, B., & Kesting, F. Serological variation of foot-and-mouth disease virus in Iran (1963-1966). Bull Off Int Epizoot., 11, 2035-2050. (1966).

2   Traub, E. & L. Hilmer. Unterschiedliche Thermoresistenz des amerikansichen Pferdencephalitis-Virus in der viramischen Phase bei kunstlich infizierten Mausen. [Differential thermoresistence of the American equine encephalitis virus in the viraemic state phase in artificially infected mice]. Zbl Bakt. Orig. 165(8). 507-513. (1955). [Translated to English by A. Finnegan (2019)]

3   Traub, E. Ueber die Ausscheidung des EEE-Virus und das gelentliche Vorkommen von Kontaktinfektion bestimmter Art bei Mausen. [Secretion of the eastern equine encephalitis virus and occasional incidence of certain contact infections in mice]. Zbl Bakt. Orig. 166(6). 462-475. (1956). [Translated to English by A. Finnegan (2019)]

4   Traub, E. Uber die aktive Immunitat von Kuken aus virusinfizierten Eiern. [Active Immunity from Virus-infected Eggs]. Zentralbl. Bakt. Abt. I. Orig., 164, 4th ser., 412-423. (1955). [Translated to English by A. Finnegan (2019)]

5   Traub, E. Experimentelle Unterschungen uber die Immunitat der Huhner gegenuber der atypischen Geflugelpest (Newcastle-Krankheit). [Experimental Research on the Immunity of Chickens Against the Atypical Fowl Plague (Newcastle Disease)]. Monatsh. f. Prakt. Tierheil. 8, 153-167. (1956). [Translated to English by A. Finnegan (2019)]

6   Traub, E., & Kesting, F. Experiments on heterologous and homologous interference in LCM-infected cultures of murine lymph node cells. Archiv Fur Die Gesamte Virusforschung, 14(1), 55-64. doi:10.1007/bf01555163. (1964).

7   Traub, E. Specific Immunity as a factor in the Ecology of Animal Viruses. Perspectives of Virology: A Symposium. John Wiley & Sons, Inc. New York: Chapman and Hall. Ltd., London; pp. 160-183. (1959)

8   USDA, Plum Island Animal Disease Center (PIADC). Memorandum "Proposed Visit to Plum Island by Dr. Erich Traub," from R. A. Carlson, Administrative Officer, ARS, to M. S. Shahan, Director, Plum Island Animal Disease Laboratory, undated

9   Bundesforschungsanstalt für Viruskrankheiten der Tier, [travel records activity]. [Investigations against members of the Federal Research Center for Virus Diseases in Animals: Government official Hans Friedrich Melz and President Prof. Dr. Erich Traub], 1958 – 1963. (August 12, 1958). B 116/33791-B/116-33793. Bundesarchiv, Koblenz.

10   Ibid.

11   Ibid.

12   Traub, E. A booster effect of irradiated or formolized Newcastle disease virus upon the infectivity of active virus in the presence of chicken blood. National Naval Medical Center. Bethesda, MD. (1954) U.S. NAVY Project NM. NMRI Memorandum Report. Project NM 005 048.11.06

13   Ibid.

14   Traub, E. Produits vegetaux vecteurs du virus aphtheux. [Plant products and the spread of foot and mouth disease]. Bulletin de l'Office International des Epizooties; May. 42. 248-255. (1954). [Translated to English by A. Finnegan (2019)]

15   Traub, E. Uber die aktive Immunitat von Kuken aus virusinfizierten Eiern. [Active Immunity from Virus-infected Eggs]. Zentralbl. Bakt. Abt. I. Orig., 164, 4th ser., 412-423. (1955). [Translated to English by A. Finnegan (2019)]

16   Traub, E. & L. Hilmer. Unterschiedliche Thermoresistenz des amerikansichen Pferdencephalitis-Virus in der viramischen Phase bei kunstlich infizierten Mausen. [Differential thermoresistence of the American equine encephalitis virus in the viraemic state phase in artificially infected mice]. Zbl Bakt. Orig. 165(8). 507-513. (1955). [Translated to English by A. Finnegan (2019)]

17   Traub, E., Uber die Immunitat der weißen Maus gegenüber dem EEE-Virus. VII. Mit-teilung. Weitere Untersuchungen uber die Rolle der Interferenz bei der cerebralen Immunitat. [On the immunity of the white mouse to the EEE-virus. VII. Further investigations on the role of interference in cerebral immunity]. Z Immun Exp Ther. 122(3):229-38. (1961). [Translated to English by A. Finnegan (2019)]

18   Traub, E. & E. Reczko. Uber die Wirkung des Salvarsans auf die Influenzainfektion de Huhnerembryos. [On the Effects of Salvarsan on the Influenza Infection in Chick Embryos]. Z Immun exp ther. 112 (5-6). 420-33. (1955).

19   Dattwyler, R. J., & Halperin, J. J. (1987). Failure of tetracycline therapy in early lyme disease. *Arthritis & Rheumatism*, 30(4), 448–450. doi:10.1002/art.1780300414

20   Traub, E. & E. Reczko. Uber die Wirkung des Salvarsans auf die Influenzainfektion de Huhnerembryos. [On the Effects of Salvarsan on the Influenza Infection in Chick Embryos]. Z Immun exp ther. 112 (5-6). 420-33. (1955).

21   Traub, E. Ueber die Ausscheidung des EEE-Virus und das gelentliche Vorkommen von Kontaktinfektion bestimmter Art bei Mausen. [Secretion of the eastern equine encephali-tis virus and occasional incidence of certain contact infections in mice]. Zbl Bakt. Orig. 166(6). 462-475. (1956). [Translated to English by A. Finnegan (2019)]

22   Ibid.

23   Ibid.

24   Hotchin, John. Persistent and Slow Virus Infections. Karger, 1971

25   Federal Bureau of Investigation (FBI): RG 65 Erich Traub, (Declassified FBI Investiga-tions on the Loyalties of Erich Traub). NARA., Doc. # QO1-458431291, Doc. # QO1-458431291.

26   "Proceedings of Symposium on Vesicular Diseases : Plum Island Animal Disease Laboratory September 27-28, 1956 : Symposium on Vesicular Diseases (1957 : Plum Island, N.Y.) ." 1970. Internet Archive. [Washington, D.C.] : Agricultural Research Service, U.S. Dept. of Agriculture. January 1, 1970. https://archive.org/details/CAT31325716/page/40

27   Federal Bureau of Investigation (FBI): RG 65 Erich Traub, (Declassified FBI Investiga-tions on the Loyalties of Erich Traub). NARA., Doc. # QO1-458431291, Doc. # QO1-458431291.

28   Traub, E. Specific *Immunity as a factor in the Ecology of Animal Viruses. Perspectives of Virology: A Symposium.* John Wiley & Sons, Inc. New York: Chapman and Hall. Ltd., London; pp. 160-183. (1959)

29   Federal Bureau of Investigation (FBI): RG 65 Erich Traub, (Declassified FBI Investiga-tions on the Loyalties of Erich Traub). NARA., Doc. # QO1-458431291, Doc. # QO1-458431291.

30   United States, Department of Agriculture. (1970, January 1). Legislative history, public law 496 - 80th Congress, Chapter 229 - 2D session, S. 2038 : United States, Department of Agriculture, office of the general counsel. Internet Archive. https://archive.org/details/PL80496/page/n51/mode/2up

31   [Criminal proceedings against Melz and Professor Dr. Traub in front of the 1st Grand Criminal Chamber of the Tübingen District Court.] IA4, Bonn, December 21, 1959. [In-vestigations against members of the Federal Research Center for Virus Diseases in Animals: Government official Hans Friedrich Melz and President Prof. Dr. Erich Traub], 1958 – 1963. (August 12, 1958). B 116/33791-B/116-33793. Bundesarchiv, Koblenz.

32   Haagen, E. et al. "DEVELOPMENT IN TISSUE CULTURES OF THE INTRACELLULAR CHANGES CHARACTERISTIC OF VACCINAL AND HERPETIC INFECTIONS." The Journal of exper-imental medicine vol. 50,5 (1929): 665-72. doi:10.1084/jem.50.5.665

33   Haagen, E. (n.d.). Letter and report to the director of general medicine at the Reich Research Council concerning research [influenza, typhus, and epidemic jaundice]. Retrieved from   http://nuremberg.law.harvard.edu/documents/1173-letter-and-report-to-the-direc-tor?q=influenza# p.3 Evidence Code: NO-138 HLSL/Item No.: 1172

34   Crodel, Brigette. "Affidavit in Form of Questionnaire concerning Dr. Haagen's Typhus Experiments." Nuremberg Trials Project. Accessed August 22, 2019. http://nuremberg.law.harvard.edu/documents/232-affidavit-in-form-of-questionnaire?q=Typhus#p.10

35   Eberle, Henrik. "Ein Wertvolles Instrument": Die Universität Greifswald Im Nationalsozialismus. Bohlau Verlag, 2015.

36   Wolfram Fischer: Exodus of science from Berlin: questions - results - desiderata, Academy of Sciences in Berlin, p. 452.

37   Ibid.

38   [Criminal proceedings against Melz and Professor Dr. Traub in front of the 1st Grand Criminal Chamber of the Tübingen District Court.] IA4, Bonn, December 21, 1959. [Investigations against members of the Federal Research Center for Virus Diseases in Animals: Government official Hans Friedrich Melz and President Prof. Dr. Erich Traub], 1958 – 1963. (August 12, 1958). B 116/33791-B/116-33793. Bundesarchiv, Koblenz.

39   Geiss, E. & O. Weiss. Correspondence [Letter to Dr. Lübke at the Bundesministerium für Ernährung, Landwirtschaft und Forsten, about the misconduct at the Bundesforschungsanstalt für Viruskrankheiten der Tiere]. [Investigations against members of the Federal Research Center for Virus Diseases in Animals: Government official Hans Friedrich Melz and President Prof. Dr. Erich Traub], 1958 – 1963. (August 12, 1958). B 116/33791-B/116-33793. Bundesarchiv, Koblenz. [Translation to English by: A. Finnegan 2020]

40   Ibid.

41   [Investigations against members of the Federal Research Center for Virus Diseases in Animals: Government official Hans Friedrich Melz and President Prof. Dr. Erich Traub] 1958 – 1963. (August 12, 1958). B 116/33791-B/116-33793. Bundesarchiv, Koblenz. [Translation to English by: A. Finnegan 2020]

42   Carroll, M. C. (2004). Lab 257: The disturbing story of the government's secret Plum Island Germ Laboratory. New York: Morrow., pp. 10

43   Traub, E. [Letter to the Bundesminister für Ernährung, Landwirtschaft und Forsten regarding allegations of misconduct.] Tübingen, on May 31, 1959.. [Investigations against members of the Federal Research Center for Virus Diseases in Animals: Government official Hans Friedrich Melz and President Prof. Dr. Erich Traub], 1958 – 1963. (August 12, 1958). B 116/33791-B/116-33793. Bundesarchiv, Koblenz. [Translation to English by: A. Finnegan 2020]

44   [Criminal proceedings against Melz and Professor Dr. Traub in front of the 1st Grand Criminal Chamber of the Tübingen District Court.] IA4, Bonn, December 21, 1959. [Investigations against members of the Federal Research Center for Virus Diseases in Animals: Government official Hans Friedrich Melz and President Prof. Dr. Erich Traub], 1958 – 1963. (August 12, 1958). B 116/33791-B/116-33793. Bundesarchiv, Koblenz. [Translation to English by: A. Finnegan 2020]

45   [Criminal proceedings against Melz and Professor Dr. Traub in front of the 1st Grand Criminal Chamber of the Tübingen District Court.] IA4, Bonn, December 21, 1959. [Investigations against members of the Federal Research Center for Virus Diseases in Animals: Government official Hans Friedrich Melz and President Prof. Dr. Erich Traub], 1958 – 1963. (August 12, 1958). B 116/33791-B/116-33793. Bundesarchiv, Koblenz. [Translation to English by: A. Finnegan 2020]

46   [Prosecutor at the Stuttgart Regional Court 88 1036/58. Imprisonment for 1 .: next date of the examination on September 1, 1959 (sheet 279 d.A.).] [Investigations against members of the Federal Research Center for Virus Diseases in Animals: Government official Hans Friedrich Melz and President Prof. Dr. Erich Traub], 1958 – 1963. (August 12, 1958). B 116/33791-B/116-33793. Bundesarchiv, Koblenz. [Translation to English by: A. Finnegan 2020]

47   [reporting to the budget committee of the Bundestag on the results of the apparent examination of the institution and the criminal proceedings before the Grand Criminal

Chamber at the regional court in Tübingen. IA4-1559.2 - 102/59 Bonn, January 20, 1960]. [Investigations against members of the Federal Research Center for Virus Diseases in Animals: Government official Hans Friedrich Melz and President Prof. Dr. Erich Traub], 1958 – 1963. (August 12, 1958). B 116/33791-B/116-33793. Bundesarchiv, Koblenz. [Translation to English by: A. Finnegan 2020]

48   Bundesforschungsanstalt für Viruskrankheiten der Tier, [travel records activity]. [Investigations against members of the Federal Research Center for Virus Diseases in Animals: Government official Hans Friedrich Melz and President Prof. Dr. Erich Traub], 1958 – 1963. (August 12, 1958). B 116/33791-B/116-33793. Bundesarchiv, Koblenz..

49   [Investigations against members of the Federal Research Center for Virus Diseases in Animals: Government official Hans Friedrich Melz and President Prof. Dr. Erich Traub], 1958 – 1963. (August 12, 1958). B 116/33791-B/116-33793. Bundesarchiv, Koblenz. [Translation to English by: A. Finnegan 2020]

50   Weiss, O. & E. Geiss [Letter from employees Weiss and Geiss to the President of the Federal Audit Office about "questionable processes and facts" at the Federal Research Institute for Virus Diseases of Animals] [Investigations against members of the Federal Research Center for Virus Diseases in Animals: Government official Hans Friedrich Melz and President Prof. Dr. Erich Traub], 1958 – 1963. (August 12, 1958). B 116/33791-B/116-33793. Bundesarchiv, Koblenz. [Translation to English by: A. Finnegan 2020]

51   Traub, E. [Letter To the Federal Minister for Food, Agriculture and Forests and Federal Audit Office in reply to Letter from employees Weiss and Geiss to the President of the Federal Audit Office about "questionable processes and facts" at the Federal Research Institute for Virus Diseases of Animals] [Investigations against members of the Federal Research Center for Virus Diseases in Animals: Government official Hans Friedrich Melz and President Prof. Dr. Erich Traub], 1958 – 1963. (August 12, 1958). B 116/33791-B/116-33793. Bundesarchiv, Koblenz. [Translation to English by: A. Finnegan 2020]

52   Traub, E., & W.I. Capps. Report to the Government of Colombia on the Experiments with chick embryo-adapted foot-and-mouth disease virus. FAO Report Number: AN-EPTA 178 TA/272/S/2/, Accession Number: 050178. (1953)

53   Bundesforschungsanstalt für Viruskrankheiten der Tier, [travel records activity]. [Investigations against members of the Federal Research Center for Virus Diseases in Animals: Government official Hans Friedrich Melz and President Prof. Dr. Erich Traub], 1958 – 1963. (August 12, 1958). B 116/33791-B/116-33793. Bundesarchiv, Koblenz.

54   Testimony from employee (name unlisted) at the Bundesforschungsanstalt für Viruskrankheiten der Tier [Letter to the Bundesministerium für Ernährung, Landwirtschaft und Forsten, about the misconduct at the Bundesforschungsanstalt für Viruskrankheiten der Tiere]. [Investigations against members of the Federal Research Center for Virus Diseases in Animals: Government official Hans Friedrich Melz and President Prof. Dr. Erich Traub], 1958 – 1963. (August 12, 1958). B 116/33791-B/116-33793. Bundesarchiv, Koblenz. [Translation to English by: A. Finnegan 2020]

55   Weiss, O. & E. Geiss [Letter from employees Weiss and Geiss to the President of the Federal Audit Office about "questionable processes and facts" at the Federal Research Institute for Virus Diseases of Animals]. [Investigations against members of the Federal Research Center for Virus Diseases in Animals: Government official Hans Friedrich Melz and President Prof. Dr. Erich Traub], 1958 – 1963. (August 12, 1958). B 116/33791-B/116-33793. Bundesarchiv, Koblenz. [Translation to English by: A. Finnegan 2020]

56   Traub, E. Uber die Immunitat der weißen Maus gegenüber dem EEE-Virus. I-VIII. Z Immun Exp Ther. Volumes 117, 118, 121, 122. (1956-1961). [Translated to English by A. Finnegan (2019)]

57   Traub, E. Ueber die Ausscheidung des EEE-Virus und das gelentliche Vorkommen von Kontaktinfektion bestimmter Art bei Mausen. [Secretion of the eastern equine encephali-

tis virus and occasional incidence of certain contact infections in mice]. Zbl Bakt. Orig. 166(6). 462-475. (1956). [Translated to English by A. Finnegan (2019)]

58   Traub, E. & L. Hilmer. Unterschiedliche Thermoresistenz des amerikansichen Pferdencephalitis-Virus in der viramischen Phase bei kunstlich infizierten Mausen. [Differential thermoresistence of the American equine encephalitis virus in the viraemic state phase in artificially infected mice]. Zbl Bakt. Orig. 165(8). 507-513. (1955). [Translated to English by A. Finnegan (2019)]

59   Traub, E., & Schwöbel, W. Uber die Leistungsfahigkeit des intracerebralen Mausetestes und der Gewebekultur als Methoden zum Nachweis kleinster Megen von EEE-virus im Gewebe. [On the value of intracerebral inoculation and the tissue culture method for detecting smallest quantities of EEE-virus in tissue]. Z Immun Exp Ther., (1958). [Translated to English by A. Finnegan (2019)]

60   Traub, E., & W. Uhlmann. Versuche zur Prufung von Maul-und-Klauenseuche-Vakzinen an erwachsenen Mausen. [Testing foot and mouth disease vaccines on adult mice]. Monatshefte fur Tierheilkunde; 10:105-112. (1958). [Translated to English by A. Finnegan (2019)]

61   Traub, E., & Schwöbel, W. Versuche zur Ergundung des mangelhaften Immunisierungsvermögens von Maul-und-Klauenseuche-Vakzinen bei Schweinen [Attempts to clarify the reasons for poor immunogenicity of Foot-and-Mouth Disease in Swine]. Monatsh. F. Tierheil. 11. 1-13. (1958). [Translated to English by A. Finnegan (2019)]

62   PATTERSON, W C et al. "A study of vesicular stomatitis in man." Journal of the American Veterinary Medical Association vol. 133,1 (1958): 57-62.

63   Schmid, G P et al. "Newly recognized Leptospira species ("Leptospira inadai" serovar lyme) isolated from human skin." Journal of clinical microbiology vol. 24,3 (1986): 484-6. doi:10.1128/jcm.24.3.484-486.1986

64   Beller, K. Herzwasser und sonstige tierische Rickettsiosen [Heartwater and other animal rickettsioses]. Handbuch der Viruskrankheiten (Ed. E. Gildermeister, E. Haagen, O. Waldmann). Vol. 2, Section 7, chapter 3, pp. 606-623. (1939) [Translated to English by A. Finnegan, 2021]

65   HANSON, R P et al. "Human infection with the virus of vesicular stomatitis." The Journal of laboratory and clinical medicine vol. 36,5 (1950): 754-8.

66   PATTERSON, W C et al. "A study of vesicular stomatitis in man." Journal of the American Veterinary Medical Association vol. 133,1 (1958): 57-62.

67   FELLOWES, O N et al. "Isolation of vesicular stomatitis virus from an infected laboratory worker." American journal of veterinary research vol. 16,61 Part 1 (1955): 623-6.

68   Carroll, M. C. (2004). Lab 257: The disturbing story of the government's secret Plum Island Germ Laboratory. New York: Morrow., pp. 50-51

69   PATTERSON WC, MOTT LO, JENNEY EW. A study of vesicular stomatitis in man. J Am Vet Med Assoc. 1958 Jul 1;133(1):57-62. PMID: 13549332.

70   Committee on Human Resources. 1977. Biological Testing Involving Human Subjects by the Department of Defense, 1977: Hearings before the Subcommittee on Health and Scientific Research of the Committee on Human Resources, United States Senate, Ninety-Fifth Congress, First Session ... March 8 and May 23, 1977. S7-857 O. Washington: U.S. Govt. Print. Off. pp. 264-265, Retrieved from: https://archive.org/details/biologicaltestin00unit/page/264

71   JENNEY, E W et al. "Serological studies with the virus of vesicular stomatitis. I. Typing of vesicular stomatitis viruses by complement fixation." American journal of veterinary research vol. 19,73 (1958): 993-8.

72   PATTERSON WC, MOTT LO, JENNEY EW. A study of vesicular stomatitis in man. J Am Vet Med Assoc. 1958 Jul 1;133(1):57-62. PMID: 13549332

73   Ibid.

269

74   Baum, Stephen G., Andrew M. Lewis, Wallace P. Rowe, and Robert J. Huebner. 1966. "Epidemic Nonmeningitic Lymphocytic-Choriomeningitis-Virus Infection." *New England Journal of Medicine* 274 (17): 934–36. https://doi.org/10.1056/nejm196604282741704.

75   Bowen, G S et al. "Laboratory studies of a lymphocytic choriomeningitis virus outbreak in man and laboratory animals." *American journal of epidemiology* vol. 102,3 (1975): 233-40.doi:10.1093/oxfordjournals.aje.a112152

76   "Hamsters Killed To Prevent Spread Of Mild Meningitis." 1974. *The New York Times.* *The New York Times.* April 14, 1974. https://www.nytimes.com/1974/04/14/archives/hamsters-killed-to-prevent-spread-of-mild-meningitis-warning-issued.html

77   Brown, G C, and T P O'leary. "Fluorescent-antibody marker for vaccine-induced rubella antibodies." Infection and immunity vol. 2,4 (1970): 360-3. doi:10.1128/iai.2.4.360-363.1970

78   Pay, T W et al. "Production of rabies vaccine by an industrial scale BHK 21 suspension cell culture process." *Developments in biological standardization* vol. 60 (1985): 171-4.

79   Zhang, Jiayou et al. "Suspended cell lines for inactivated virus vaccine production." *Expert review of vaccines* vol. 22,1 (2023): 468-480. doi:10.1080/14760584.2023.2214219

80   "FATAL VIRUS FOUND IN WILD DUCKS ON L.I." 1967. The New York Times. The New York Times. December 26, 1967. https://timesmachine.nytimes.com/timesmachine/1967/12/25/93233480.html?pageNumber=26

81   "Duck Virus Enteritis an Old World Disease--in the New World : U.S. Agricultural Research Service Animal Health Division." n.d. Internet Archive. Accessed August 4, 2019. https://archive.org/details/CAIN709091593/page/n3

82   Carroll, M. C. (2004). *Lab 257: The disturbing story of the governments secret and deadly virus research facility.* New York: Morrow., pp. 35-38

83   "3.6 Million Fowl Killed in Drive To Halt a Deadly Avian Disease." n.d. *The New York Times.* *The New York Times.* Accessed August 5, 2019. https://timesmachine.nytimes.com/timesmachine/1972/06/16/79470954.html

84   Traub, E., Eine atypische Form der Geflügelpest in Hessen-Nassau. [The Atypical Form of Fowl Pest in Hessen-Nassau] Tierarztl Rundschau : 42-45. (1942a)

85   Todd, F. A., et al. "Proceedings of the 1956 Regional Meetings on Foreign Animal Diseases." U.S. Government Printing Office, Proceedings of the 1956 Regional Meetings on Foreign Animal Diseases, 1956. Retrieved from: https://archive.org/details/CAT10678014

86   Traub, E., & W.I. Capps. Report to the Government of Colombia on the Experiments with chick embryo-adapted foot-and-mouth disease virus. FAO Report Number: AN-EPTA 178 TA/272/S/2/, Accession Number: 050178. (1953)

87   RUSKA, H: Zur Frage der Potenzierung von Bakteriophagenlösungen durch Zerschäumen [On the question of the potentiation of bacteriophage solutions by foaming]. Kolloid-Zeitschrift 110 (1948), S. 175-177 [paper submitted in 1945, not published until 1948.]

88   Traub, E. Produits vegetaux vecteurs du virus aphtheux. [Plant products and the spread of foot and mouth disease]. Bulletin de l'Office International des Epizooties; May. 42. 248-255. (1954). [Translated to English by A. Finnegan (2019)]

89   Eberle, Henrik. "Ein Wertvolles Instrument": Die Universität Greifswald Im Nationalsozialismus. Bohlau Verlag, 2015.

90   Traub, E., & Capps, W. I. Experiments with chick embryo-adapted foot-and-mouth disease virus and a method for the rapid adaptation. National Naval Medical Center. Bethesda, MD. (1953) U.S. NAVY Project NM. NMRI Memorandum Report. Project NM 000 018.07

91   "Senior Scientist at Genentech : Oral History Transcript / 2002 : Yansura, Daniel G., 1950-." Internet Archive, www.archive.org/details/yansuragenentech00yansrich/page/50

92   "Recombinant DNA Research : Documents Relating to 'NIH Guidelines for Research Involving Recombinant DNA Molecules' V.5 1980 : National Institutes of Health (U.S.). Office of the Director." Internet Archive. [Bethesda, Md.] : U.S. Dept. of Health, Education, and Welfare, Public Health Service, National Institutes of Health ; Washington : For sale by the Supt. of Docs., U.S. Govt. Print. Off., January 1, 1976. https://archive.org/details/recombinantdnare-00nati_12, pp. 401

93   Norrby E. Nobel Prizes and Nature's Surprises. Singapore: World Scientific, 2013

94   Silverstein, Arthur M. "The curious case of the 1960 Nobel Prize to Burnet and Medawar." Immunology vol. 147,3 (2016): 269-74. doi:10.1111/imm.12558

95   Traub, E. Persistence of Lymphocytic Choriomeningitis Virus in Immune Animals and Its Relation to Immunity. Journal of Experimental Medicine, 63(6), 847-861. doi:10.1084/jem.63.6.847. (1936).

96   Traub, E. LCM Virus Research, Retrospect and Prospects. Lymphocytic Choriomeningitis Virus and Other Arenaviruses: Symposium held at the Heinrich-Pette-Institut für experimentelle Virologie und Immunologie, Universität Hamburg, October 16–18, 1972, 3-10. doi:10.1007/978-3-642-65681-1_1. (1973)

97   Traub, E. Serological Evidence for Antigenic Variation in Brains of Mice Infected Persistently with the Virus of Lymphocytic Choriomeningitis. Zentralblatt Für Veterinärmedizin Reihe B, 27(9-10), 806-822. (1980, 2010). doi:10.1111/j.1439-0450.1980.tb02035.x

98   Traub, E. Observations on "Late onset disease" and Tumor Incidence in Different Strains of Laboratory Mice infected Congenitally with LCM Virus I. Experiments with Random-bred NMRI Mice. Zentralblatt Für Veterinärmedizin Reihe B, 22(9), 764-782. (1975, 2010). doi:10.1111/j.1439-0450.1975.tb00643.x

99   Traub, E. A Filterable Virus Recovered from White Mice. Science, 81. (2099), 298-299. doi:10.1126/science.81.2099.298. (1935).

100   Hotchin, John. Persistent and Slow Virus Infections. Karger, 1971

101   Dinter, Z. Persönaliches, Begegnungen mit Erich Traub. Berl. Munch. Tier. Woch. 96. 70-72. (1984)

102   Silverstein, Arthur M. "The curious case of the 1960 Nobel Prize to Burnet and Medawar." Immunology vol. 147,3 (2016): 269-74. doi:10.1111/imm.12558

103   Traub, E. Observations on immunological tolerance and "Immunity" in mice infected congenitally with the virus of lymphocytic choriomeningitis (LCM). Archiv Fur Die Gesamte Virusforschung, 10(3), 303-314. doi:10.1007/bf01250677. (1960).

104   Traub, E., & Kesting, F. Further observations on the behavior of the cells in murine LCM. Archiv Fur Die Gesamte Virusforschung, 13(5), 452-469. doi:10.1007/bf01267789. (1963).

105   Traub, E. Multiplication of LCM virus in lymph node and embryo cells from non-tolerant and tolerant mice. Archiv Fur Die Gesamte Virusforschung, 11(4), 473-486. doi:10.1007/bf01241301. (1962).

106   Traub, E. Observations on immunological tolerance and "Immunity" in mice infected congenitally with the virus of lymphocytic choriomeningitis (LCM). Archiv Fur Die Gesamte Virusforschung, 10(3), 303-314. doi:10.1007/bf01250677. (1960).

107   Traub, E. Can LCM virus cause lymphomatosis in mice? Archiv Fur Die Gesamte Virusforschung, 11(5), 667-682. doi:10.1007/bf01243307. (1962).

108   Traub, E. & F. Kesting. Uber die naturliche Ubertragungsweise des Virus der lymphocytaren Choriomeningitis (LCM) bei Mausen und ihre Paralellen zum Ubertragungsmodus gewisser muriner Krebsviren. [On the natural mode of transmission of the virus of lymphocytic choriomeningitis in mice and its parallel to the mode of transmission of certain murine cancer viruses]. Zbl Bakt. Abt. I. Orig. Feb; 177:453-71. (1960). [Translated to English by A. Finnegan (2019)]

109   Traub, E. Ueber den Einfluß der latenten Choriomeningitis-Infektion auf die Ent-stehung der Lymphomatose bei weißen Mause [On the Influence of Latent Choriomeningitis Infection on the Development of Lymphomatosis in White Mice]. Zentrl. Bakt. I. Orig. 147 (16). 1-25. (1941). [Translated to English by A. Finnegan, 2019]

110   Traub, E., Shafyi, A., Ewaldsson, B., & Kesting, F. Serological variation of foot-and-mouth disease virus in Iran (1963-1966). Bull Off Int Epizoot., 11, 2035-2050. (1966).

111   Traub, E., Shafyi, A., Ewaldsson, B., & Kesting, F. Serological variation of foot-and-mouth disease virus in Iran (1963-1966). Bull Off Int Epizoot., 11, 2035-2050. (1966).

112   Traub, E., Hessami, M., & Shafyi, A. Indirect Complement Fixation in Foot-and-Mouth Disease. Zentralblatt Für Veterinärmedizin Reihe B, 15(4), 421-432. doi:10.1111/j.1439-0450.1968.tb00316.x. (1970, 2010).

113   Traub, E., & Ramyar, H. (1967). Lyophilizing foot-and-mouth disease virus at low drying temperature. Am J Vet Res, 126, 1605-1608.

114   Traub, E., & Kanhai, G. K. (1967, 2010). Behavior in Cattle of Iranian Strains of Foot-and-Mouth Disease Virus subjected to Serial Passage in Different Kinds of Cells*. Zentralblatt Für Veterinärmedizin Reihe B, 15(5), 518-524. doi:10.1111/j.1439-0450.1968.tb00326.x

115   Traub, E., Kanhai, G. K., & Kesting, F. Behavior of Foot-and-Mouth Disease Virus on Serial Passage in Different Kinds of Cells. A Contribution to Experimental Epidemiology at Cell Level*. Zentralblatt Für Veterinärmedizin Reihe B, 15(5), 525-539. (1967, 2010). doi:10.1111/j.1439-0450.1968.tb00327.x

116   Irvin, A D et al. "Cell fusion, using Sendai virus, to effect inter-species transfer of a cell-associated parasite (Theileria parva)." International journal for parasitology vol. 4,5 (1974): 519-21. doi:10.1016/0020-7519(74)90070-8

117   Traub, E., et al. Turkey: Vaccine Production. FAO Report Number: AGA-DP/TUR/69/533, Accession Number: 120100. (1972).

118   Traub, E. Demonstration, properties and significance of neutralizing antibodies in mature mice immune to lymphocytic choriomeningitis (LCM). Archiv Fur Die Gesamte Virusforschung, 10(3), 289-302. doi:10.1007/bf01250676. (1960).

119   Traub, E. LCM Virus Research, Retrospect and Prospects. Lymphocytic Choriomeningitis Virus and Other Arenaviruses: Symposium held at the Heinrich-Pette-Institut für experimentelle Virologie und Immunologie, Universität Hamburg, October 16–18, 1972, 3-10. doi:10.1007/978-3-642-65681-1_1. (1973)

120   Traub, E. LCM Virus Research, Retrospect and Prospects. Ibid., pp. 5

121   Traub, E. LCM Virus Research, Retrospect and Prospects. Ibid., pp. 9

122   Traub, E. LCM Virus Research, Retrospect and Prospects. Ibid., pp. 9-10

123   Traub, E. Demonstration, properties and significance of neutralizing antibodies in mature mice immune to lymphocytic choriomeningitis (LCM). Archiv Fur Die Gesamte Virusforschung, 10(3), 289-302. doi:10.1007/bf01250676. (1960).

124   Pachner, A R, and A C Steere. "The Triad of Neurologic Manifestations of Lyme Disease: Meningitis, Cranial Neuritis, and Radiculoneuritis." Neurology. U.S. National Library of Medicine, January 1985. https://www.ncbi.nlm.nih.gov/pubmed/3966001.

125   Kang, Insoo et al. "Defective control of latent Epstein-Barr virus infection in systemic lupus erythematosus." Journal of immunology (Baltimore, Md. : 1950) vol. 172,2 (2004): 1287-94. doi:10.4049/jimmunol.172.2.1287

126   Reik, L, A C Steere, N H Bartenhagen, R E Shope, and S E Malawista. "Neurologic Abnormalities of Lyme Disease." Medicine. U.S. National Library of Medicine, July 1979. https://www.ncbi.nlm.nih.gov/pubmed/449663

127   Tumminello, Richard, Lindsey Glaspey, Anita Bhamidipati, Patrick Sheehan, and

Sundip Patel. "Early Disseminated Lyme Disease Masquerading as Mononucleosis: A Case Report." The Journal of emergency medicine. U.S. National Library of Medicine, December 2017. https://www.ncbi.nlm.nih.gov/pubmed/29102094

128   DURAY, P. H., & STEERE, A. C. (1988). Clinical Pathologic Correlations of Lyme Disease by Stage. Annals of the New York Academy of Sciences, 539(1 Lyme Disease), 65–79. doi:10.1111/j.1749-6632.1988.tb31839.x

129   Sausen, Daniel G et al. "Stress-Induced Epstein-Barr Virus Reactivation." Biomolecules vol. 11,9 1380. 18 Sep. 2021, doi:10.3390/biom11091380

130   Traub, E. Observations on immunological tolerance and "Immunity" in mice infected congenitally with the virus of lymphocytic choriomeningitis (LCM). Archiv Fur Die Gesamte Virusforschung, 10(3), 303-314. doi:10.1007/bf01250677. (1960).

131   Traub, E. Observations on "Late onset disease" and Tumor Incidence in Different Strains of Laboratory Mice infected Congenitally with LCM Virus I. Experiments with Random-bred NMRI Mice. Zentralblatt Für Veterinärmedizin Reihe B, 22(9), 764-782. (1975, 2010). doi:10.1111/j.1439-0450.1975.tb00643.x

132   Traub, E., & Kesting, F. Age Distribution and Serological Reactivity of Viral Antigen in Brains of Mice Infected Congenitally with LMC Virus. Zentralblatt Für Veterinärmedizin Reihe B, 24(7), 548-559. (1975, 2010). doi:10.1111/j.1439-0450.1977.tb01024.x

133   Traub, E., & Kesting, F. Influence of Feeding on Development of Nephritis and on Breeding Efficiency in Mice Infected Congenitally with Different Strains of LMC Virus. Zentralblatt Für Veterinärmedizin Reihe B, 24(9), 722-727. (1975, 2010). doi:10.1111/j.1439-0450.1977.tb01045.x

134   OLDSTONE., M. B. A., and F. J. DIXON, 1967: Lymphocytic choriomeningitis: Production of antibody by "tolerant" infected mice. Science 118, 1193-1195.

135   Traub, E. Serological Evidence for Antigenic Variation in Brains of Mice Infected Persistently with the Virus of Lymphocytic Choriomeningitis. Zentralblatt Für Veterinärmedizin Reihe B, 27(9-10), 806-822. (1980, 2010). doi:10.1111/j.1439-0450.1980.tb02035.x

136   Traub, E. Factors Influencing Specific Antibody Formation in Mice Persistently Infected with LCM virus. Zentralblatt Für Veterinärmedizin Reihe B, 28(2), 133-145 (1980,2010). doi:10.1111/j.1439-0450.1981.tb01748.x

137   Traub, E. Observations on immunological tolerance and "Immunity" in mice infected congenitally with the virus of lymphocytic choriomeningitis (LCM). Archiv Fur Die Gesamte Virusforschung, 10(3), 303-314. doi:10.1007/bf01250677. (1960).

138   Traub, E. LCM Virus Research, Retrospect and Prospects. Lymphocytic Choriomeningitis Virus and Other Arenaviruses: Symposium held at the Heinrich-Pette-Institut für experimentelle Virologie und Immunologie, Universität Hamburg, October 16–18, 1972, 3-10. doi:10.1007/978-3-642-65681-1_1. (1973)

139   Dickson, K. "CRIMINAL CHARGE SHEETS JUNE 2017 Lobbying for a Hearing for Referral to the USDOJ for a Prosecution of the Lyme Disease Crimes." 2017. Published at: https://docs.wixstatic.com/ugd/47b066_01d68b1309ae457b81df1e06e6beae1e.pdf

140   Traub, E. Observations on immunological tolerance and "Immunity" in mice infected congenitally with the virus of lymphocytic choriomeningitis (LCM). Archiv Fur Die Gesamte Virusforschung, 10(3), 303-314. doi:10.1007/bf01250677. (1960).

141   Traub, E. Multiplication of LCM virus in lymph node and embryo cells from non-tolerant and tolerant mice. Archiv Fur Die Gesamte Virusforschung, 11(4), 473-486. doi:10.1007/bf01241301. (1962). "In later studies on tolerance by different groups of immunologists little or no attention has been paid to murine LCM, presumably, because the antigen involved is a selfreplicating agent."

Chapter Sixteen

TAINTED IMMUNITY

SOVIET & AMERICAN COOPERATION ON VACCINES IN THE COLD WAR

Political language is designed to make lies sound truthful and murder respectful, and to give an appearance of solidity to pure wind.
— George Orwell

As the Soviet Union began to launch its biological Day X against the West,[1] its direct actions were not always apparent, but it was learned that some of the most successful mass infections of a population, intentional or not, happened through the very technologies meant to prevent them – *vaccines* – so it logically follows that the Soviet Union realized it's potential for mass infection and the only way they could turn this into a channel of bioterrorism was through sabotage, and this could be done in several different ways.

First and most importantly, was through successful co-opting of American and Western scientists in the creation and production of vaccines.[2] Secondly, they could implant mass infection through the successful contamination of the animal tissues used to produce vaccines, which could be done by infecting the stock of animals to be used. This would have to employ stealth pathogens that were inapparent and lacked obvious signs of disease. They could infect the domestic animals like horses which are used for serum and vaccines.[3] They could set up an operation to infect the areas of the jungle where monkeys are sourced for cell cultures.[4] Exotic viruses of all kinds could be used to infect these animals in the wild and remain undetected while they are killed and processed to grow vaccine viruses which contain hidden, masked viruses that remain latent and infect all of the vaccine recipients and activate later.

Mass contamination has already happened with both polio vaccines,[5] first with the inactivated polio vaccine produced by Jonas

Salk, and the second vaccine produced by Albert B. Sabin and M. P. Chumakov. Both vaccines were contaminated by a carcinogenic virus, SV40. This virus acts just like Traub's LCM virus and passes down generations, causing neurological problems and cancers. The contaminated polio vaccines were given to 98 million Americans by 1960, infecting half of the U.S. population.[6]

The Soviet Union previously saw the value of this process, and this is likely the reason M.P. Chumakov met with Traub in 1947 at Insel Riems to talk about LCM Virus.[7] The Soviet Union developed a largescale bioweapons program to crush the West, all the while our scientists like Albert B. Sabin were teaming up with and getting cozy with their top bioweaponeers like M. P. Chumakov to make vaccines that would be given to American and Western civilians.[8]

The failures to allocate money and resources to assess biological espionage and Soviet biological warfare programs and capabilities were highlighted in a white paper by Katarzyna Zabrocka called "Under the Microscope: Why U.S. Intelligence Underestimated the Soviet Biological Weapons Program," showing there was a lack of prioritization on biological warfare intelligence from the start:

> Despite an increase in [biological warfare] intelligence priority by the [United States Central Intelligence Board] and the State Department (also stated in the referenced memorandum), it is important to note that the Defense Department did not raise the priority because it would compete with other requirements. As an example of Lowenthal's description of competing collection priorities described in the beginning of this section, certain issues in 1952 took precedence over [biological warfare] when it came to using limited resources for covert intelligence collection. [...]
>
> In summary, although it was clear in the early 50's that [biological warfare] intelligence collection was not prioritized, this was a deliberate choice by the Defense Department with consideration of the existing collection priorities and not blindness by the CIA (or other agencies and departments) to the necessity of more concrete [biological warfare] intelligence.[9]

As we mentioned previously quoting Igor V. Domaradskij's memoir, there had been, in existence, an ultra-secret, compartmentalized group of high-level military and Soviet Intelligence going back to the first generation of Soviet biological weapons that employed academicians and civilian scientists who could be used to bring their ambitions to realization, because as he mentioned in previous chapters, being a KGB informant would be a condition of foreign travel.[10]

We may recall once again, the Ex-KGB officer Alexander Kouzminov also mentioned in his memoir that the public health officials and prominent scientists in the West were a major target for Soviet operations and he described "Day X," in classified KGB files that meant a large-scale war of bioterrorism directed against Western civilians, explaining that they had been very successful in recruiting scientists in America to be operatives for the Soviet Union.[11] This could be far easier if the scientists were sympathetic to communism, which many of them were. We will see in this chapter, for example, how Jonas Salk was a member of several communist front organizations,[12] and Albert B. Sabin was sympathetic to communism and the Soviet Union.[13] These were the two scientists responsible for the polio vaccines.

I make no definite claims about Albert Sabin or Jonas Salk being foreign spies, but I will point out that much of what transpires in the following pages is highly suspect. The *useful pawn* is another possibility, but what you are about to read in the following pages is extremely suspicious and deserves serious investigation. However, we can show that the vaccine sabotage program of the Soviet Union brings us back to a little-known horse virus researched by Erich Traub at Insel Riems.

INSEL RIEMS AND EQUINE INFECTIOUS ANEMIA VIRUS (EIA)

In earlier chapters, I described Erich Traub's research on a highly immunosuppressive retrovirus called Equine Infectious Anemia Virus (EIA), to which very few antibodies could be made, and produced a slow-virus disease which eventually led to fatal disease, not unlike HIV.[14] In fact, the EIA virus is very closely related to HIV, as both are a lentivirus and classed as retroviruses, and also share antigens.[15] Like HIV, EIA uses reverse transcriptase and affects the T-cells (CD4).[16] Like HIV, EIA can be spread through re-used or shared needles.[17] Traub had begun working with EIA while at Giessen, and this work continued through WWII at Insel Riems.[18] When the Soviet Union took Insel Riems captive and after the facility was back to working order, evidence suggests the Soviets either tested the virus or saw how mass infections could result from the contamination of horse factories used to produce vaccines, giving them a diabolical strategy for mass infection of the West.[19]

When Traub left Insel Riems in 1948, the work on EIA accelerated and the Soviets earned a proficient understanding of the possibilities and ways in which it could be used. They gained greater insight on the stealth qualities as it spreads and contaminates animals used to make vaccines and serum, much like the events surrounding WWI described in the first few chapters.

Erich Traub had made several studies of Equine Infectious Anemia Virus with Karl Beller while at Giessen,[20] and sought to develop an antibody test to diagnose EIA with Werner Schäfer, but it was unsatisfactory since the virus was so immunosuppressive.[21] The virus was hard to diagnose and had a slow incubation period. This made diagnosis very difficult, and the Soviet Union had a very good idea of how problematic it could be in the production of vaccines because it had infected and contaminated several factories of horses in East and West Germany being used to produce serums and vaccines.[22]

In 1948, Zvonimir Dinter's bacteriology mentor from the University of Berlin, Joseph Fortner, published a lengthy paper about EIA having contaminated the horses at many horse factories producing vaccines and serum.[23] In this paper, he described how vaccine factories would often use the same needle on many horses and spread the infection to the rest of the horses. The problem was such a nightmare for the factories, that many would deny the diagnosis was EIA and continued operations, eventually learning from bitter experience, how much havoc the virus could reek if not properly addressed. An American Intelligence report shows that an investigation was launched into Insel Riems and their research on the combination of EIA, leukemia, and a sexually transmitted disease, *Lymphogranuloma*, a bacteria commonly found in AIDS patients:

> 1. It is reported that the Research institute on Riems Island, South of the Island of Rügen, does considerable research on leukosis (Leukose) of horses. Both the words Leukose and lymphogranuloma have been used in this connection, but source feels certain that this is a virus disease. He also stated that Riems uses a considerable number of young horses.
>
> 2. A horse butcher in Rostock stated that the Riems Institute's need of horses is unusually large. According to an official order, horses must be delivered to Riems for the procurement of red murrain (Rotlauf) vaccine* The butcher also delivers 500 kg of horse meat to Riems every week.
>
> [redacted] comment: Source states that in order to procure this vaccine it is not necessary to use live animals. He therefore doubts that the animals are sent to Riems for this purpose.[24]

The French HIV researcher Luc Montagnier found early cases of AIDS had a virus that was closely related to EIA rather than HTLV when he published "A new type of retrovirus isolated from patients presenting with lymphadenopathy and acquired immune deficiency syndrome: Structural and antigenic relatedness with equine infectious anaemia virus."[25] Secondly, another paper, "Equine infectious anemia virus gag and pol genes: relatedness to visna and AIDS virus," shows it was closely related to the HIV virus and to the visna virus of sheep.[26] It is interesting that a virus of sheep was brought up in connection to HIV and EIA, because Insel Riems was alternating serial passages of EIA between horses and sheep, published in "On four cases of the silent form of infectious anemia experimentally created by alternating passage horse-sheep-horse."[27] This would suggest that the EIA virus could have assimilated material from the visna virus in sheep giving it the properties of both.

There is no doubt that the Soviet Union understood these elements when they took what was learned from Insel Riems and began developing the largest, most ambitious biological weapons program, and it is certain that vaccine sabotage was among some of their most diabolical schemes developed from what was learned from Traub and his work up to that time. The Soviets could then master these techniques to employ silent, masked viruses that activated later, as valuable strategic biological weapons.

As for HIV, it has been put forward that the HIV virus could have originated in early polio vaccines and was put forward in a 1994 paper from the journal *Medical Hypotheses*, "Polio Vaccines and the Origin of AIDS," where it suggests the HIV virus could have come from the polio vaccines from the monkey tissues used.[28] In a 1992 article, "US Rethinks link between polio vaccine and HIV" had several years earlier stated the following on the possible link between the two:

> Most of the monkeys used to make early polio vaccine came from India, where none is known to be naturally infected with SIVs. It is possible that during the late 1950s some African green monkeys were used, but this cannot be proved. African green monkeys carry a type of SIV, but it is too unlike HIV genetically to have evolved into HIV between 1957 and the first undisputed appearance of the human virus in Africa.
>
> There are further problems. For example, the first confirmed case of AIDS has been traced back to 1958 in a Manchester seaman. He would have had to be infected with HIV some years before this. In addition, monkeys' kidney cells do

not normally support the growth of HIV. Also, the vaccine was given by mouth and HIV would be unlikely to survive in the gut.

Unless large numbers of monkeys from all species are tested for retroviruses, the 'missing link' may never be found. Meanwhile, the Wistar Institute has set up a committee to investigate the claims about Koprowski's vaccine. A spokesman confirmed last week that if samples of the vaccine could be found in the freezers, they would be tested for retroviruses.[29]

Evidence presented in this chapter suggests the "missing link" in this picture will not be found in monkeys, but instead in horses, as Equine Infectious Anemia Virus, from the horse serum added to produce the monolayer tissue cultures from monkey kidneys,[30] and all previous assessments of the possibility of HIV originating from polio vaccines never factored this into the equation since it did not occur to them that horse serum was used in the production of the monkey tissue cultures.

Traub had been working on this virus since 1942, and Insel Riems had been testing and modifying it since the Soviets occupied Insel Riems, and this older case described in 1958 is just after Insel Riems had been developing it since WWII. It was adapted to sheep, which could impart qualities from the visna virus of sheep.[31] Horse serum was mixed with the monkey kidney tissue cultures to produce the polio vaccines, described in "Monolayer Tissue Cultures I. Preparation and Standardization of Suspensions of Trypsin-Dispersed Monkey Kidney Cells,"[32] and could have also assimilated qualities of precursor simian viruses.

This would explain the relationship to all these other animal viruses of sheep, monkey, and so on. Insel Riems researchers Hubert Möhlmann and Heinz Röhrer conducted experiments that show EIA can be transmitted by oral ingestion and absorption in the gut.[33] Furthermore, since it would be exposed to considerable polio virus, it could also impart genetic material from polio, making it absorb in the gut far more easily since polio is so easily absorbed this way.

Because the entire question of Equine Infectious Anemia Virus and its relationship to HIV could be an entire book of its own, I will keep this short, but clearly the missing link and origins of the HIV virus might be solved with the aforementioned revelations of Insel Riems and Equine Infectious Anemia Virus, tying the virus back to Traub and the Soviet Union. Let us now proceed to cover Jonas Salk and the inactivated polio vaccine, followed by Albert Sabin and his

cozy relationship with M.P. Chumakov and other Soviet bioweaponeers during his years putting the oral polio vaccine on the market.
We will also be looking at the hemorrhagic fever viruses in further
depth.

JONAS SALK AND INACTIVATED POLIO VACCINE

Jonas Salk, the creator of the first polio vaccine, the inactivated polio vaccine, is described in *Polio: An American Story*, showing that
upon being subject to an extensive background check to clear him to
advise the U.S. Government, he was subsequently investigated by the
FBI for being associated with several communist front groups:

> As a consultant to the federal government, Salk was subject to a
> background check. Trouble came quickly. FBI agents regularly
> swapped information with staffers from the House Un-Ameri-
> can Activities Committee (HUAC), which kept extensive files
> on "subversive groups," complete with their publications and
> membership lists. As luck would have it, a HUAC report had
> once cited an obscure journal called Social Work Today as
> "pro-Communist." And Social Work Today had once lauded
> the good deeds of Jonas E. Salk, then an intern at Mount Sinai
> Hospital in Manhattan.
>
> Between 1948 and 1952, the FBI carried out more than
> four million of these federal background checks. In cases where
> "derogatory information" was found, the Civil Service Com-
> mission could order a full field investigation of the employee,
> an exhaustive procedure involving FBI offices throughout the
> country. In all, the bureau handled about 20,000 such probes,
> involving less than one percent of the federal work force. Salk
> got caught in this dragnet. Four FBI field offices took part in
> his investigation. Agents fanned out to interview friends, col-
> leagues, and neighbors. Others combed suspect publications
> and membership lists in search of his name. The first probes,
> conducted in 1950, linked Salk to several "pro-Communist"
> groups during his years at Mount Sinai and at the Universi-
> ty of Michigan. In 1941 he supposedly joined the "Commu-
> nist-controlled" American Labor Party. In 1946 he allegedly
> served as secretary-treasurer of the Independent Committee
> of the Arts and Sciences and Professions of Michigan, a group
> cited by HUAC, among others, as pro- Communist. In be-

tween, it was said, he had joined, contributed to, or appeared on the mailing lists of the National Council of American-Soviet Friendship, the American Association of Scientific Workers, the New York Conference for Inalienable Rights, and Russian War Relief — all "reliably reported" to be Communist fronts.[34]

The American Association of Scientific Workers is a group that has been brought up in numerous other investigations and congressional hearings on subversive groups active in the United States. Theodore Rosebury, who was a top scientist at Camp Detrick, active in the biological warfare program, was also a member of this group, and this can be found in an FBI investigation on bacteriological warfare.[35]

Initially Jonas Salk was tripped up from these associations, but a second FBI investigation was initiated and suddenly reversed his being a security threat and he was cleared to advise the U.S. Government.[36] The FBI, according to John Loftus, was significantly compromised, as Soviet moles in the FBI assisted Maclean in getting Traub cleared for the Paperclip program.[37]

At any rate, the inactivated polio vaccine was produced using monkey kidney cell cultures, but published work on the process for making these cell cultures shows that the monkey kidney cells were mixed with horse serum in making the final product,[38] and it was the horse virus EIA that the Soviet Union were so keenly concentrated on at Insel Riems in the early 1950s.[39] A 1946 publication by Traub's USDA colleague L.O. Mott shows that EIA had been suspected in rare human infections in the United States in 1946,[40] and like Foot-and-Mouth Disease, rare infections of man had been noted sporadically throughout the scientific literature.[41]

This polio vaccine was later found to be contaminated by another virus called SV40,[42] which has been shown to be oncogenic, that is, cancer causing.[43] When it became known that the polio vaccine was contaminated after being on the market for five years, the public health officials downplayed it as much as possible, claiming it was harmless, but eventually it was deemed cancer causing, even though there is still a concerted effort to convince the public to the contrary.

There was also the Cutter incident, where it was thought improperly inactivated polio vaccines were causing paralytic disease in the vaccine recipients. This was a major event at the time, and in *Polio: An American Story*, there is an unusual correspondence between Jonas Salk and John Enders, with the following exchange:

For Salk, the worst moment came in early May, as the Cutter incident was unfolding. At an emergency session at the NIH, he faced the wrath of the formidable John Enders, who had just returned from Stockholm with a Nobel Prize. Their relationship had been distant but cordial. Following a rare visit to Pittsburgh in 1953, Enders had written: "Jonas: your laboratory is indeed magnificent and the work going on worthy of the greatest praise." Now Enders told him: "It is quack medicine to pretend that this is a killed vaccine when you know it has live virus in it. Every batch has live virus in it."[44]

Enders must be referring to the fact that there really is no such thing as a killed virus. Insel Riems had shown, for example, binding mercury or any metal to bacteria or virus was *"highly reversible,"* and often the binding to metals occurred very unevenly.[45]

In 1956, the so-called "Cutter Incident" was contested by two papers with expert testimony of many top virologists, including Erich Traub, testifying about the inactivated polio vaccine, to say that there was no evidence that this company had done anything other than what they were told, and that in truth there was no reliable formula to guarantee inactivation because it did not happen like a first-order chemical reaction. That is to say, the inactivation process is highly unreliable and live, virulent virus is always possible to remain in the vaccine. More than this, these experts also testified to say that the vaccinated persons could shed considerable amounts of live, virulent virus after polio vaccination, and these experts thought this to be the most probable explanation for higher cases of polio in the placebo than the vaccinated, because the vaccinated were shedding and infecting the unvaccinated placebo cases.[46, 47]

As far as Jonas Salk is concerned, there is no definitive link to him being a foreign spy, but we can link him to communist front groups. Moreover, he published a book much later called *Survival of the Wisest*, to address overpopulation of the planet, voicing that something needed to be done about it, that scientific and medical advances that kept life going for many people was a threat to the planet because of overpopulation, as though he was hinting that letting them die was a viable solution if we cared about the planet:

> A major threat to the species is attributed to the increasing size of the human population, which, in turn, is ascribed to successes in science and technology. This "explanation" has evoked an attack upon science and the exploitation of its technology, to

the development of which are attributed many adverse effects upon the human species and upon other forms of life. "Polluters" who befoul the planet affect the "quality of life" and are regarded as a threat to the present and future equilibrium of the species and of the planet. Those who consider themselves on the side of Nature, and therefore of the human species, see others in opposition to both Nature and Man. Hence we are to be concerned not only with Man's relationship to Nature but with Man's relationship to himself.[48]

In the same book, he talks about how we are at the point where we can use RNA viruses to alter human biology, in an advantageous way, or a disadvantageous way,[49] not unlike the way SV40 acts in humans as a carcinogen. This book shows some of the psychopathic personality traits of Jonas Salk, which are quite disturbing, I may add, since I own a copy and have read the book in its entirety. Clearly, he had no qualms about mass infection and depopulation and probably had little more qualms about his vaccine being contaminated by such viruses like SV40, or HIV, which serve the very words coming out of his mouth in *Survival of the Wisest*.

ALBERT B. SABIN'S RISE TO PROMINENCE

Albert B. Sabin was born with the birth name Abram Saperstejn in Bialystok, a Russian-controlled section of Poland. When Albert was fairly young, he moved with his family to the United States in 1921 to avoid Jewish persecution. When he arrived, an uncle already in the United States, had ties to the powerful political organization, Tammany Hall, and Albert and his family were whisked away by fancy automobiles in a private reception by the organization.[50] Interestingly, Tammany Hall's Samuel Dickstein, a congressional representative in New York serving the House Committee on Un-American Activities (HCUA), was later found to be a paid spy for the NKVD.[51] At any rate, Sabin became a naturalized citizen in 1930 and changed his last name to Sabin and middle name to Bruce.

In 1933, he received a scholarship through the National Research Council Fellowship, travelled to Britain and attended the Lister Institute of Preventative Medicine in London for a year to study virology.[52] However, he returned in 1935, joining the Rockefeller Institute. He would begin working at the virus laboratory with Dr. Peter Olitsky, yet Olitsky was allegedly *"warned by several well-meaning persons"* that hiring Sabin would be a mistake, but he hired Sabin anyway.[53] While there Sabin met Max Theiler, a South African virologist who later won the Nobel Peace prize for his work on the Yellow Fever vaccine in Brazil with Hilary Koprowski, another friend of Sabin's, who had been a former scientist in Russian-controlled Poland.[54]

He joined the Rockefeller Institute just as Erich Traub was beginning his studies of LCM virus. Some years later in 1939, Sabin published a paper on a new mouse disease that was elucidated by intracerebral injections of yellow fever and Lymphocytic Choriomeningitis (LCM), called *Toxoplasma*.[55]

Sabin soon accepted a job at the University of Cincinnati children's hospital, with his own lab and allowed to research as he wished, and it is here that Sabin began to concentrate more on the polio virus, as he had been recruited to work for the National Foundation for Infantile Paralysis.[56] He took this job and began to focus more on the polio problem.

In the buildup to the Second World War, Sabin became an advisor to the Army and the War Department Service, before joining the military as a commissioned officer in the Army Medical Corps and the Armed Forces Epidemiological Board (AFEB).[57] Under the flexibility of this position, he was able to carry out research between overseas assignments, additional time at the University of Cincinnati, and other labs connected to the Rockefeller Institute where he worked on developing vaccines for Dengue Fever and Japanese B Encephalitis.[58]

After the war, Sabin began his work on the polio vaccine, with the help of Jonas Salk and Hilary Koprowski. Albert Sabin did not like having too many people working in his labs, and usually preferred to do things himself whenever possible. The Armed Forces Epidemiological Board (AFEB) provided funding for him to research various diseases he had been working on earlier in his career.[59]

On a side note, the reader may find it interesting that the polio virus was listed in the United States biological weapons stockpile as a biological warfare agent in the Canadian Ministry of Defence document on Operation Large Area Coverage.[60] The first polio epidemic in the United States was 1894,[61] right as activity with Foot-and-Mouth Disease Virus and other diseases were heating up between Germany, Britain, and the United States. Likewise, it is interesting that Foot-and-Mouth Disease Virus is so closely related to polio, in the family of *picornaviruses*. Plum Island published several articles on poliovirus and Foot-and-Mouth Disease Virus together in the 1990s comparing their proteins, such as, "Foot-and-Mouth Disease Virus and Poliovirus Particles Contain Proteins of the Replication Complex,"[62] and "Structure and Immunogenicity of Experimental Foot-and-Mouth Disease and

Poliomyelitis Vaccines."[63] Furthermore, since polio was absorbed in the gut, it is entirely plausible that polio could have tainted meat from infected livestock and thus bringing us back once again to the relevance of animals and animal disease in relation to human epidemics.

At any rate, in the wake of new polio epidemics, Sabin began to work on a live virus vaccine for polio, while Jonas Salk had been developing his inactivated vaccine. The two were bitter rivals, but each developed their respective vaccine. Sabin then turned to an unlikely friend from the Soviet Union when he was developing his oral polio vaccine, and that friend is M. P. Chumakov.

ALBERT B. SABIN COLLABORATION WITH M.P. CHUMAKOV

At some point after Joseph Stalin's death, M. P. Chumakov traveled to the United States with his wife Marina Voroshilova and several colleagues, and toured a number of American labs in what was considered the post-war period where the two enemies pretended to be open to each other. While this trip took place, it is said that Sabin and Chumakov became good friends, and Sabin decided to team up with Chumakov in developing a new vaccine for polio, even though it will be explained shortly, the Soviet Union had no plans to initiate a new polio vaccine and thought the Salk vaccine worked and saw no problems with it.[64]

Vetted by the FBI, Sabin was allowed to go to the Soviet Union and collaborate with Chumakov on an oral polio vaccine in June of 1953.[65] It is worth noting that around this time, Chumakov was also working on insects like ticks and mosquitoes, with such diseases as Tick encephalitis, Omsk Hemorrhagic Fever and Crimean-Congo Hemorrhagic Fever, Influenza, Q Fever, West Nile Virus, Lymphocytic Choriomeningitis (LCM), among others.[66]

The fact that Sabin sought to collaborate with a Soviet biological weapons expert like M. P. Chumakov and maintained cozy relationships with other Soviet bioweaponeers like V. M. Zhdanov,[67] Lev Zilber,[68] among others, is a question that deserves serious inquiry. These were bioweaponeers who tested their weapons on the Mongolians and Muslims in the far East for Stalin. Sabin would have certainly been in a position to know this information. At the time, the Soviets were secretly building a massive biological weapons program, sought to destroy the West with these weapons, and this is evident in Ken Alibek's memoir, *Biohazard: the Chilling True Story of the Largest Covert Biological Weapons Program in the World, Told from the inside by the Man Who Ran It.*[69]

V.M. Zhdanov, for example, was a known player in the Soviet biological weapons enterprise. This is explained in I. V. Domaradski's
memoir in the introduction by Alan P. Zelicoff:

> At its peak in the early 1980s, as many as one hundred thou-
> sand individuals – scientists, clinicians, administrators, and
> military personnel – were directly involved in this enterprise.
> Some of these were physicians and researchers internation-
> ally known for humanitarian work: V. M. Zhdanov, who first
> proposed the worldwide smallpox eradication campaign, also
> held a high position in the Soviet biological weapons (BW)
> program. [...] [70]

Dr. Albert B. Sabin was promoted as the hero of the polio era. [71]
He is credited as the scientist who eradicated polio from the United
States and the developing world, yet Sabin credits the Soviet Union
system and M.P. Chumakov for the success. [72] The Sabin-Cumakov
collaboration is alarming, first, because Chumakov was a key player in
the early expeditions with Dr. Lev Zilber, testing viruses and their tick
vectors for the biological warfare program. [73] Sabin also maintained
friendly communication with Lev Zilber, as records show. Both Zilber and Chumakov were involved in the early research expeditions
in 1938 on tick encephalitis and on hemorrhagic fever viruses that
produced fatal diseases related to Ebola and Marburg Virus. [74, 75]

In fact, Marburg Virus will come into focus in the following pages.
It can be said definitively that M. P. Chumakov was part of the Soviet
biological weapons program because the activities of his 1938 expedition with Lev Zilber are conclusively linked to biological warfare by
American Intelligence reports. [76] Sabin was also maintaining friendly
correspondence with a KGB agent in the World Health Organization,
Sergey Drozdov, and M.P. Chumakov's son Konstantin Chumakov
explains Drozdov was a KGB agent while showing that the KGB was
down in Africa in the 1950s:

> So and everybody knew at the time that Dresdoff[A] was one of
> those embedded KGB agents, because for instance, he spent
> several years in Africa in the '50s, working as a young doctor,
> and we know who these doctors were whom the Soviet Union
> sent to Africa. It was all KGB intelligence people. So then he
> went back to the Institute of Polio and he was -- he was doing
> solid science... [77]

[A]   Dresdoff here is spelled phonetically, he is referring to Sergey Drozdov

The Siberian research was among Chumakov's main areas of research, and this portion of research had been picked up in American intelligence reports involving Soviet biological warfare activities with ticks.[78] Next, as we look further into Chumakov's activities under the Soviet biological warfare program, he was doing an equal amount of work on other biological warfare agents, such as West Nile Virus (WNV), Q Fever, Crimean Congo Hemorrhagic Fever (CCHF), as well as exotic arboviruses of all kinds.[79]

Sabin left for Moscow in June of 1956 to work on the polio vaccine with Chumakov. Declassified U.S. intelligence files show that just one month after Sabin's arrival in Moscow to work on the polio vaccine, Chumakov was conducting field research on the biological warfare agent Q Fever.[80]

SOVIET INTEREST IN NEUROTROPIC VIRUSES & MONKEYS

Just several years earlier, in August of 1953, the Moscow Medical Military Institute began researching animal neuro-viruses that resembled polio and conducted experiments with monkeys to study human polio in chimps, monkeys, baboons, and green guenons. Knowing these kinds of primates would be used as source material for growing vaccine viruses, the Soviet Union began to apply some of Traub's stealth factors to new ventures, picked up in an American Intelligence report of a Soviet paper, "Animal Neurovirus Diseases Similar to Human Poliomyelitis":

> The absence of a satisfactory laboratory model of poliomyelitis makes the experimental study of this disease extremely difficult. At present, the only method of detecting the poliomyelitis virus is the experimental infection of monkeys or apes (obyez' yany) by means of virus-containing material obtained from the brains of dead human beings or the excrement of afflicted persons. The higher apes such as chimpanzees seem to be the most receptive to this method, followed by Javanese macaques, rhesus monkeys, hamadryas baboons, and green guenons, in that order. Increased interest in research pertaining to the study of the possibility of adapting the poliomyelitis virus to other species of animals is, therefore, understandable.[81]

According to Milton Leitenberg and Raymond A. Zalinskas in their work, *The Soviet Biological Weapons Program: A History*, the Soviet Union had a large vivarium, or monkey farm, where they kept extensive species of monkeys for research, which came into existence the same year Chumakov teamed up with Sabin to construct the oral polio vaccine, and just after American Intelligence picked up reports of extensive Soviet activity in the production and experimentation with animal neuro-infections that resembled human polio, with the same monkeys listed in the beginning of that report, would be the same monkeys identified as being maintained and kept at the vivarium:

> A vivarium was built at the institute as early as 1954 to house the many hundreds, perhaps thousands, of animals required for animal testing. Such testing allowed scientists to observe the results of experimental infections, pathogen propagation, prophylaxis methods, treatment regimes, and agent detection methods. Monkeys were especially valuable subjects, so the terrarium housed many types of primates, including African green monkeys, cynomolgus macaques, rhesus monkeys, chimpanzees, and baboons. In addition, the institute established a farm on an adjacent 11 hectares of land to grow produce required to feed the animals.[82]

As a Soviet virologist working on polio-like neuro-viruses at the Omsk Oblast, Chumakov worked directly with the top brass of power in the Soviet biological war machine, as a member of the Academy of Medical Sciences U.S.S.R., studying natural reservoirs for vector-borne diseases used in biological warfare.[83]

According to the former college Professor and director of the Chemical and Biological Weapons Non-Proliferation Program, the late Raymond A. Zilinskas, in his work, *The Soviet Biological Weapons Program and its Legacy in Today's Russia*, it was confirmed that the Academy of Medical Sciences was carrying out the research for the biological warfare program, including work on Q Fever, which Chumakov had been taking part, and was a member of the Academy.[84]

THE ADVENT OF THE SABIN-CHUMAKOV VACCINE

While Sabin and Chumakov finished the fine-tuning of their cooperative developments on oral polio vaccine (OPV), they began testing it in children in Mexico and the Soviet Union, and Jonas Salk and Hilary Koprowski assisted Sabin in his formulation of the OPV.[85] It was delivered as an oral suspension of live, attenuated polio virus in sugar cubes, given as the vaccine, produced in Moscow and

Sverdlovslk, among other countries who manufactured it, and from 1957-1960, they inoculated roughly 12 million children.[86]

After the initial trials, the Medical Military Institute started producing OPV on a large scale.[87] After it was given to many millions of people, it was shown to have been contaminated with the SV40 virus long after production,[88] and Chumakov suggested they switch to using green marmosets instead of the monkeys to solve the SV40 problem.[89] Three years after the polio vaccine had been deployed and given to millions of people, Chumakov was conducting further research into SV40 in OPV, with subsequent work cultivating the virus and studying it.[90]

The Sabin-Chumakov vaccine worked by giving the vaccine recipients "symptomless" cases, in other words, latent polio, and Magnesium chloride was added to the solution to increase thermostability, or heat resistance.[91] These infections, while seeming harmless at first, could play the same role as Traub's LCM virus and regain virulence in the future, which happens with live measles virus vaccines.[92] Reactivation of latent viruses is one of the many mechanisms in chronic Lyme-like diseases, and at the very heart of the various neuro-infections that resemble poliomyelitis.[93]

Other declassified reprints picked up by U.S. intelligence show that while Sabin was putting together this vaccine with Chumakov in the U.S.S.R., Chumakov was conducting an equal amount of field experiments and research on ticks, and tick-borne diseases relevant to biological warfare for the Academy responsible for biological warfare.[94, 95]

Additional aspects of this problem are highlighted in an article that appeared in Scientific American, "Birth of a Cold-War Vaccine," as it tells the story of the start of the Sabin-Chumakov collaboration on a vaccine for polio, the project came about after Chumakov took a trip to the United States, aided by colleagues whom the FBI suspected of being agents of the KGB.[96]

It was a fact back at that time, the Soviet scientists were not allowed to travel out of the Soviet Union unless they were sent for a very important reason serving the country. It was not a customary privilege to permit Soviet citizens, especially their best scientists, to leave the country, especially to travel to a rival country like the United States. Even more perplexing was that, on the rare occasion that this was granted, they would not allow both a husband and wife to embark on such a trip. One would have to stay behind, and this was done for collateral, to deter them from defecting from the Soviet Union.

Chumakov's trip to the United States was aided by his wife, Marina Voroshilova, and the colleagues he brought along were suspected KGB agents, and certainly not just scientists traveling about at leisure. Even Igor V. Domaradskij revealed in his memoir that those who take trips abroad as scientists, would become informants to the KGB or Soviet military as a condition of travel.[97]

As M.P. Chumakov's son, Konstantin Chumakov pointed out in retelling the story, the Soviet Union did not even need the Sabin vaccine, because they had the Salk vaccine and claimed it *"works just fine"*:

"Sabin publicly gave credit to my father and the Soviet system whose organization made such large trials possible," Konstantin says. "But I'm not sure my father ever told Sabin the true story of it. What actually happened – according to my father – went like this:

"My father couldn't get permission for a really big clinical trial. A lot of people in the Health Ministry were opposed to it. He was told, basically, 'We have the Salk vaccine, and it works fine, so there's no reason for you to test the live virus.' Well, my father decided to go around them.

"In the Soviet Union there was a higher authority – the Politburo [then known as the Presidium of the Central Committee], which consisted of a small group of Communist Party officials who could overrule everybody. At the time, Anastas Mikoyan was the Politburo member responsible for public health. Mikoyan was not a medical man — he was a political figure who went back to the revolution. But he and my father were well acquainted. Mikoyan may have appointed him to head the polio initiative in the first place." Refusing to accept the ministry's decision not to grant permission for the oral vaccine tests, Chumakov picked up one of the red telephones provided for the exclusive use of the most powerful people in the Kremlin – he was not among them – and dialed Mikoyan's number. As Chumakov related the story to his son, he got right to the point and asked Mikoyan's approval to proceed with the live virus vaccine tests.

"Are you sure this is a good vaccine, Mikhail?" Mikoyan asked.

"And that it's safe?"

"Yes," the virologist replied. "I'm absolutely sure."

"Then go ahead," Mikoyan said.

"That was it," says the younger Chumakov, whose account rings true with others familiar with the principals. "The only permission he had was verbal, over that Politburo hotline. Of course, the health minister was unhappy, but there was nothing he could do." [98]

From the very start of Sabin's cooperative effort with Chumakov, the circumstances of the project and the arrangements surrounding it are extremely suspicious, to say the least. In addition, the *Scientific American* article shows that the Soviet Union's public health ministers had no plans to initiate a new vaccine, so Chumakov wouldn't have been allowed to team up with Sabin without a special approval, and Chumakov wouldn't have taken all that time to try to work with Sabin on a new vaccine if he didn't have approval from the health ministry, who rejected Chumakov's request to test a new polio vaccine. Unless of course, his working with Sabin was approved by Soviet intelligence for another purpose.

Since Chumakov didn't have approval to create and test a new vaccine, it begs the question, why was Sabin taking trips to collaborate with Chumakov if they had not approved it? In order for Sabin to set foot in the Soviet Union to work with Chumakov at his Institute, he would have needed an approval by higher authorities and if it wasn't authorized by the health ministry to develop and test the new polio vaccine, then it was approved for some other reason by another authority.

M.P. Chumakov was willing to take a big chance by going around his superiors, using forbidden lines of authority and communication, in order to approve large-scale, experimental tests on Russian children in order to approve the Sabin-Chumakov vaccine for use in the Soviet Union. Perhaps he was so enthusiastic about his work that he put his career on the line, or it may just be that Chumakov was working a position of lower authority as a secret agent of the KGB, since his colleagues were already under the suspicion of American intelligence as agents of the KGB. [99]

In this light, the compulsive reaction to pick up that forbidden line may have been a line he was already familiar with using before. If he dialed Mikoyan on the red phone, he would have needed to know the correct number to get a hold of him, so knowing how to immediately get a hold of Mikoyan meant he knew the correct digits to reach him. It was not uncommon for KGB agents to be in positions that people like Chumakov held, and this reiterated in Ken Alibek's story, where certain personnel had additional powers and the authority of the KGB, while posing as common workers or average scientists.[100] Chumakov's history would support such an intelligence role, especially when it came to his work on some of the most dangerous viruses the world has ever seen, the hemorrhagic fever viruses, disease agents which eventually brought forth Marburg Virus and Ebola.

THE MARBURG VIRUS OUTBREAK & ORAL POLIO VACCINE PRODUCTION

In June of 2023, a Newsweek article was published about ticks carrying the Ebola-like hemorrhagic fever viruses were spreading West, in "Deadly Hemorrhagic Virus Spreading to New Countries, Scientists Warn." It states:

> "Some tick-borne infections, [such as] Crimean-Congo hemorrhagic fever, are highly likely to spread in the U.K. through our ticks at some point," James Wood, head of veterinary medicine at Cambridge University, said at the hearing.
>
> [Crimean-Congo hemorrhagic fever] is a viral disease caused by Nairovirus, spread via ticks, that has a fatality rate of between 10 and 40 percent, according to the World Health Organization (WHO). It is usually found in low levels across Africa, the Balkans, the Middle East and in Asia.[101]

The hemorrhagic fever viruses like Marburg Virus have a relevant context in relation to the polio vaccine, where the deadly Marburg Virus emerged in 1966, an older sibling to the more well-known and fatal Ebola virus.[102] In 1966, a deadly outbreak of a never-before-seen hemorrhagic fever virus happened at the Behringwerke lab in Marburg, West Germany while they were processing monkey tissues to make polio vaccines.[103]

The Marburg Virus was described and further assessed officially in a 1968 journal by former Reich scientist, Richard Haas, and several colleagues, published in "Production of Kidney tissue Cultures from African Green Monkeys, Experimentally Infected with the Causative Agent of Frankfurt-Marburg-Syndrome."[104]

The details surrounding the outbreak were described by the late Raymond A. Zilinskas and Milton Leitenberg and in their lengthy work on the Soviet biological weapons program, and becomes much more concerning and sinister in its implications, suggesting that the Soviet vaccine sabotage program had gone operational:

For years, urban legends have circulated about how the Soviet Union came into possession of hemorrhagic fever–causing viruses. One particularly common legend is that brave KGB agents entered the graveyards in Marburg an der Lahn, Germany, and at high personal risk dug up corpses of victims of Marburg virus disease to obtain tissue samples carrying the virus. This is implausible because there was an official strain exchange program between West Germany and the Soviet Union at the time.

The program was launched after Marburg virus was first discovered in 1967, when Marburg an der Lahn and Frankfurt am Main, Germany, as well as Belgrade, Yugoslavia, experienced outbreaks of a mysterious and deadly illness. Thirty-one people became sick, of whom seven died (there were six secondary cases). The source of the causative virus were subclinically infected African green monkeys that had been imported to Marburg/Frankfurt/Belgrade for research and to prepare poliovirus vaccines.

To head off any concern that its work with the new virus was an indication of a secret German BW program, in 1967 the German government gave a sample of the virus to Mikhail P. Chumakov, who was then the director of the USSR-AMN Scientific Research Institute of Poliomyelitis and Viral Encephalitides (now called the M. P. Chumakov Institute of Poliomyelitis and Viral Encephalitides) in Moscow. The Germans assumed that Chumakov's investigation would quickly determine that the virus could not have originated from a BW laboratory. Indeed, after Chumakov published an abstract of his initial work to characterize the virus, the Soviets did not lodge accusations of Germany having a secret BW program.[105]

The incident was treated as an accident, yet the Soviet Union immediately pointed fingers at West Germany, with none other than M.P. Chumakov there to grab this new Marburg Virus in order for West Germany to prove they didn't have a secret biological warfare program. However, it was M.P. Chumakov, in the years preceding the outbreak, conducting research on Omsk Hemorrhagic Fever in experimental infections of monkeys, research indicating he was looking into the feasibility of infecting tissue cultures of monkeys, in "Experimental Data on Investigating the Pathogenicity of Omsk Hemorrhagic Fever Virus for Monkeys," from 1965,[106] again in "Electron

Microscopic Study of the Morphology and Localization of Omsk Hemorrhagic Fever Virus in Cells of the Infected Tissue Culture," and again in "Study of interrelationship between the Omsk hemorrhagic fever virus and the cells of the sensitive tissue culture," both from 1965.[107] There are many more studies by Chumakov on these viruses going back to 1938, but this should suffice to show Chumakov was knee-deep in hemorrhagic fever research at the time.[108] This was all done in the years just before the Marburg Virus outbreak.

Sabin was informed of the outbreaks in written correspondences with both labs.[109] Strange it is that his partner Chumakov would be marching down to the institute to demand cultures of the virus to "assess" whether they had weaponized the agent, when the disease is closely related to the hemorrhagic fevers of Siberia and the Far East of the U.S.S.R.[110] Crimean-Congo Hemorrhagic Fever, was originally called Crimean Hemorrhagic Fever. This is a virus that appeared in the years of Chumakov and Zilber's tick expeditions in the far East, possibly dating back as far as 1932, shown in an Intelligence report, and states that the diseases termed hemorrhagic fevers had first been described in the Soviet Union.[111]

Strains were later found in Africa, and this is how it earned the name Crimean-Congo Hemorrhagic Fever.[112] Chumakov was overseeing the research on these viruses, and an intelligence report shows that Chumakov realized the infection was silent in animals.[113] At this time, the same report shows he was also testing filtrates of poliomyelitis taken from humans on the monkeys.[114]

The U.S.S.R. had several African expeditions ongoing in Northern Nigeria back in 1966, seen in Defense publications of a translation of Soviet research, "Arbovirus Infections of Monkeys Captured in the Jungles of Northern Nigeria," through the research carried out under authority of Chumakov by his colleagues, B. F. Somenov and B. A. Lapin, at the Institute of Poliomyelitis and Viral Encephalitides, submitted in Dec. 1966.[115] Moreover, Intelligence reports show an English translation of the Russian book *Virus Hunters*, establishing the relation of Crimean Hemorrhagic Fever Virus to Marburg Virus:

> There are several hemorrhagic fevers. There is Omsk hemorrhagic fever, Bolivian hemorrhagic fever, and quite recently - a new fever became known, i.e., Marburg fever. The world-renowned virologist M. P. Chumakov was invited from the Soviet Union to the [Federal Republic of Germany] to identify this fever. However, this is not enough. Startling facts have become known recently. As a result of joint efforts on the part of work-

ers of the Institute of Poliomyelitis and Virus Encephalitides of the Academy of Medical Sciences USSR and scientists of Yale University (D. Casals, et al.), in a short period it was possible to establish the fact that there is a relationship between the virus of Crimean hemorrhagic fever and the agent of Congo infection, which is widespread in Africa and some regions in India. There is no more doubt that these viruses are close relatives, and the fight against them should be waged from the positions developed in the USSR.[116]

Likewise, Lassa Fever Virus, another hemorrhagic fever related to the Crimean-Congo Hemorrhagic Fever, surfaces several years later in 1969 in West Africa and Nigeria.[117] Russian strains of Crimean Hemorrhagic Fever surface in the Congo in 1968, and the Marburg-infected monkeys came from Uganda, right near the Congo.[118] The fact that the Crimean Hemorrhagic Fever Virus surfaces in the Congo around this time is significant, indicating the Soviet Union was testing its weapons in Africa.[119] Scientific literature explains that Crimean Congo Hemorrhagic Fever disease is related to the Ebola and Marburg Hemorrhagic Fever disease.[120]

It is evident that after Chumakov was given the strain of Marburg Virus from West Germany, the Soviet Union immediately began to further weaponize it. We know this because Ken Alibek reveals in his memoir, they had a bioweapons program with the Marburg agent after obtaining it from the Marburg outbreak,[121] and this was first given to M. P. Chumakov, as Zalinskas and Leitenberg point out.[122] Moreover, Chumakov's Institute was active in the jungles of Africa in 1966, just a year before the outbreak, when Chumakov was concentrating heavily on hemorrhagic fever viruses producing a similar disease as Marburg Virus and its later cousin, Ebola Virus. This suspicious activity deserves further investigation.[123]

SUSPICIOUS ACTIVITY IN SOVIET COLLABORATION

As the SV40 problem began to plague the oral polio vaccine, Chumakov suggested that the manufacturers start using tissue cultures from green marmosets instead of African green monkeys (green guenons),[124] Chumakov can be found researching the feasibility of stealth viral infections of animal cell cultures in green marmosets some years later, with exotic arboviruses that even trained disease specialists have never even heard of. This was picked up in an American Intelligence report on the Soviet paper, "The Hemagglutinating

Properties and Cytopathic Activity of Some Little-Investigated Arbo-viruses."[125]

Alexander Kouzminov, a Russian defector and author of *Biological Espionage: Special Operations of the Soviet and Russian Foreign Intelligence Services in the West,* described massive KGB spy networks they allegedly had in big pharma, the public health system, and academic circles within the West. One of the channels he cites for waging bio-terrorism was vaccines. He mentions a secret shipping method called the VOLNA channel to send and receive biological materials like vaccines to and from their spies in the target or operating countries. He identifies the airline Aeroflot as being the airline they used for the VOLNA channel. He reveals a little background on the methodologies, stressing that anytime this method is used, they are to ship express and send a telegram to let them know. Kouzminov explains:

> Samples of biological materials and documents obtained by our special agents and Illegals were delivered to Moscow through two main channels. The first channel of delivery, the normal diplomatic bag, was used for sending secret documents to the department and, more seldom, samples of new drugs, pharmacological remedies, vaccines and other biological materials which could be preserved for a long time under normal conditions. The second channel was an urgent secret-delivery channel codenamed VOLNA (wave). This meant delivering the material via an international flight of the Soviet Aeroflot airline in the pilots' cabin, where one of the pilots was a KGB officer. This channel was always used in urgent situations when active biological materials were being sent by our people — for example, serums, virus vaccines, diagnostics, novel micro-organisms, strains of potentially dangerous pathogens, biotoxins, etc. The VOLNA shipment was preceded by a cipher telegram from the KGB rezidentura to our department with instructions specifying the flight that would be used. At whatever time this telegram came to the centre, the Directorate S duty officer had to inform one of us immediately about the parcel that was coming; VOLNA could not stand delay! [126]

Interestingly, in one cable from Sabin to Chumakov, they were using Aeroflot to send packages back and forth:

Letter Cable
Chumakov Poliomyelitis Institute 8th Street, Sokolinoi Gori

15 Moscow, U. S. S. R.
Can you send immediately 50 pieces of each type of poliovac-
cine candy refrigerated express via Aeroflot and Pan American
to Murray for check on potency in my laboratory prior to Moscow meeting. Please reply by cable. Best wishes.
Sabin [127]

In another cable, Sabin notifies Zhdanov of his trip to Russia,
bringing viruses that required immediate refrigeration, to be given to
bioweaponeers Zhdanov and Smorodintsev, who worked with Chumakov on the early hemorrhagic fevers and was part of the tick expeditions with Chumakov in 1937:

CABLE
Thursday, June 14, 1956 10:30 A. M.
Prof. Zhdanov Ministry of Health Moscow. U.S. S. R.
Glad to read paper on Present Status Living Attenuated Poliovi-
rus Vaccine Stop Leaving Riga June twenty 2215 Aeroflot 603
arrive Leningrad 0020 Stop Please notify Professor Smorodint-
sev Am bringing viruses requiring immediate refrigeration.
Sabin[128]

It is also interesting to note that in Sabin's correspondence to
Chumakov, it was done off-record through telegrams like Western
Union, and Sabin's exchanging viruses with Chumakov appears to be
before the exchange program existed.

Among other files, concerning activity can be found in correspondence between Albert Sabin, his American counterparts, and
M.P. Chumakov, where a breach of security for infectious material
took place, with a polio anti-serum #4, blood containing antibodies
used for research purposes, that was given to Sabin by Richard E.
Shope through M.P. Chumakov:

Dear Albert:
The serum that you left with me at the time of your last visit
has been tested by hemagglutination inhibition with the fol-
lowing results:
Antigen Titer of Serum
West Nile (Egypt), 4 units 1:640 +
Dengue, Hawaii, Type II 8 units 1:640 +
Dengue, Tr 1751, Type 2, 2 units 1:640 +
Yellow Fever, 5 units 1:20

Venezuelan EE, 4 units 0

The first dilution of serum in all cases was 1:10

These results are somewhat unexpected to say the least; the serum (it is presumably a monkey serum), undoubtedly has Group B anti-bodies. Now, is that due to the inoculation of the "type 4" polio; or had the animal been used previously for work with other viruses; or did it have Group B antibodies to begin with? [129]

The results followed with a letter to Chumakov from Sabin, April 14, 1956:

Dear Professor Chumakov:

First of all I want to thank you for the very nice letter you sent me before your departure from the United States and I also wish to tell you how greatly I enjoyed the visit of your group in Cincinnati.

When Dr. Shope returned from Russia he transmitted to me a vial of serum labeled "type 4 polio antiserum" which you very kindly sent along for me. I obtained it from him while I was visiting the Rockefeller Institute in New York and, unfortunately, during the handling of the vial the tip broke and all but 0.3 ml. of the serum leaked out into the cotton around it. Since my main interest was to determine whether by chance this virus might be related to the dengue group of viruses. I turned the small amount of residual serum over to Dr. Casals at the Rockefeller Institute because he had all the antigens available for immediate testing. Although I expected a completely negative result. I was very much surprised to learn from him only yesterday that he obtained the following results in a hemagglutination inhibition test using your serum and the antigens indicated below.

Antigen Titer of Serum

Dengue, Type I 1:640+

 Type 2 1:640+

West Nile (Egypt) 1:640+

Yellow Fever 1:20

Venezuelan, EE; 1:20 <10

Accordingly it becomes of considerable interest to know whether or not the serum that you sent me was a human serum or the serum of a monkey that might previously have been used for tests on Japenese B encephalitis or some other related virus.[130]

The *Scientific American* article discussing the Sabin and Chumakov collaboration states that M.P. Chumakov's son became the head of Vaccine Safety & Review at the FDA and has maintained that seat to the present day.[131] It was Dr. Sabin who vouched for young Chumakov and helped him get his foot in the door after various letters of recommendation by Sabin.[132,133] I make no claims about Konstantin Chumakov, but according to Konstantin, all the Valuable Russian scientists from Moscow University left the Soviet Union, and today fill high-level positions in academia and public health in the West:

> KC: [...] I mean the best testimony that everybody is here now doing extremely well. I mean practically all our graduates are now very highly successful American scientists. Some of them are Department Heads, Lab Chiefs, Full Professors, and it all came, everybody who came from this department are doing extremely well.
>
> LW: What about, I hope that the people who stayed in Russia are doing well, or is that your yardstick is that they're in the US?
>
> KC: Yeah, because in Russia, there is nobody who stayed. I mean I know a couple of guys who stayed there, but everybody else left...[134]

At another point in the interview, Konstantin talks about the penetration of the World Health Organization (WHO) by Soviet scientists working for the KGB, Sergey Drozdov, who worked directly with M. P. Chumakov, and went on to hold a prominent position at the World Health Organization.

Albert Sabin was in communication with Sergey Drozdov, numerous correspondence letters show. M. P. Chumakov was working with Drozdov at the time Sabin was collaborating with Chumakov, which Intelligence reports show Drozdov at Chumakov's Institute and publishing research with Chumakov.[135]

Clearly there were security breaches in the setup of global organizations like the World Health Organization (WHO), the Food and Agriculture Organization (FAO), and this would extend to the tripartite cooperation that tested and facilitated Western biodefense activities.[136] With Traub, the penetration of the FAO was already a success. Konstantin Chumakov made it clear that the WHO was also penetrated.

In summary, I make no definitive claims about Jonas Salk or Albert Sabin and their loyalties or motivations, but these past associations with communist front organizations, collaborations and cozy friendships maintained with serious players in the Soviet biological weapons program, are extremely suspicious, and I believe these facts should be presented to my readers. Clearly the Soviet Union successfully gained the trust of Western scientists and took part in a vaccine that would be administered to millions of Americans.

Why they would offer to help America defeat polio, while scheming in secret with the biggest biological weapons program the world has ever seen, with an intelligence program scheming to solicit spies and carry out Day X, largescale bioterrorism against innocent American civilians, contradicts the feigned cooperation to eradicate disease.[137] There is clearly more to this story. To conclude this work, I leave you with this quote by Erich Traub's protégé Werner Schäfer, a warning to the future of civilization, ironically reminding us of our moral responsibility in the part we play on this earth:

At the present time, when concentrated scientific activity is often directed toward the destruction and not toward the preservation of life, one might fear that the phrase "concentration is the prudence of life" will some day be inverted into "concentration is the stupidity of life." To avoid such an occurrence, scientific workers all over the world would do well to return to the ethics of the stoicist Seneca, who noted in his Naturales Quaestiones that "by exploration of the facts natural sciences base the moral life of man on a solid foundation; they liberate him from fear and let him recognize the glory and magnitude of divine creation."[138]

Endnotes

1   Kouzminov, Alexander. *Biological Espionage: Special Operations of the Soviet and Russian Foreign Intelligence Services in the West*. Manas Publications, 2006

2   United States Congress. "PREVENTING ANOTHER SV40 TRAGEDY: ARE TODAY'S VACCINE SAFETY PROTOCOLS EFFECTIVE? : Committee on Government Reform." 2003. Internet Archive. Government Publishing Office. November 13, 2003. https://archive.org/details/gov.gpo.fdsys.CHRG-108hhrg92772?q=SV40

3   Fortner, J. Die ansteckende Blutarmut der Einhufer in den Impfstoffwerken. [The infectious anemia in equines in the vaccine factories]. Berl Munch Tierarztl Wochenschr. May; 34 (5): 49-53. (1948)

4   Lapin, B. A. & B. F. Semenov. Arbovirus Infections of Monkeys Captured in the Jungles of Northern Nigeria. Voprosy Virusologiy. 755-757. 1967

5   United States Congress. "PREVENTING ANOTHER SV40 TRAGEDY: ARE TODAY'S VACCINE SAFETY PROTOCOLS EFFECTIVE? : Committee on Government Reform." 2003. Internet Archive. Government Publishing Office. November 13, 2003. https://archive.org/details/gov.gpo.fdsys.CHRG-108hhrg92772?q=SV40

6   Shah, Keerti, and Neal Nathanson. "Human Exposure To Sv40: Review And Comment." American Journal of Epidemiology, vol. 103, no. 1, 1976, pp. 1–12., doi:10.1093/oxfordjournals.aje.a112197 Retrieved from https://academic.oup.com/aje/article-abstract/103/1/1/151919?redirectedFrom=fulltext, or: https://www.scribd.com/document/409584571/Human-Exposure-to-SV40-Review-and-Comment-Carcinogens-in-Vaccines

7   Central Intelligence Agency (CIA) Intelligence Reports: THE BACTERIOLOGICAL RESEARCH INSTITUTE ON THE ISLAND OF RIEMS. CIA-RDP83-00415R002200020014-9. Central Intelligence Agency (CIA), Reading Room, 2011. Retrieved from: https://www.cia.gov/library/readingroom/document/CIA-RDP83-00415R002200020014-9

8   Swanson, William. "Birth of a Cold War Vaccine." *Scientific American*, vol. 306, no. 4, 2012, pp. 66–69., doi:10.1038/scientificamerican0412-66.

9   Zabrocka, K. (2013, May 22). Under the Microscope: Why US Intelligence underestimated the Soviet Biological Weapons Program. Honors Program in International Security Studies Center for International Security and Cooperation. Stanford University. Retrieved February 19, 2021, from: https://stacks.stanford.edu/file/druid:wk216hz5745/Zabrocka_Katarzyna_Thesis_Final.pdf

10   Domaradskij☒ Igor Valerianovich., and Wendy Orent. *Biowarrior: inside the Soviet/Russian Biological War Machine*. Prometheus, 2003., pp. 141-143

11   Kouzminov, Alexander. *Biological Espionage: Special Operations of the Soviet and Russian Foreign Intelligence Services in the West*. Manas Publications, 2006

12   Oshinsky, David M. *Polio: An American Story*. Oxford University Press, 2006.

13   Swanson, William. "Birth of a Cold War Vaccine." *Scientific American*, vol. 306, no. 4, 2012, pp. 66–69., doi:10.1038/scientificamerican0412-66.

14   Traub, E. & K. Beller. Untersuchungen uber die ansteckende Blutarmut der Pferde. Immunitatsversuche. [Immunization experiments in equine infectious anaemia]. Monatshefte fur Praktische Tierheilkunde; 3:193-206. (1942, 1951). [Translated to English by A. Finnegan (2019)]

15   Montagnier, L.; Dauguet, C.; Axler, C.; Chamaret, S.; Gruest, J.; Nugeyre, M.T.; Rey, F.; Barré-Sinoussi, F.; Chermann, J.C. (1984). A new type of retrovirus isolated from patients presenting with lymphadenopathy and acquired immune deficiency syndrome: Structural and antigenic relatedness with equine infectious anaemia virus. Ann. Virol. (Inst. Pasteur) Vol. 135(1), 119–134. doi:10.1016/S0769-2617(84)80046-5

16   McGuire, Travis C et al. "Cytotoxic T lymphocytes in protection against equine infectious anemia virus." *Animal health research reviews* vol. 5,2 (2004): 271-6. doi:10.1079/ahr200482

17   Fortner, J. Die ansteckende Blutarmut der Einhufer in den Impfstoffwerken. [The infectious anemia in equines in the vaccine factories]. Berl Munch Tierarztl Wochenschr. May; 34 (5): 49-53. (1948)

18   Central Intelligence Agency (CIA) Intelligence Reports: The State Research Institute at Riems; Microbiological Research. CIA-RDP83-00415R000900020012-6. Central Intelligence Agency (CIA), Reading Room, 2011. Retrieved from: https://www.cia.gov/library/readingroom/document/CIA-RDP83-00415R000900020012-6

19   Fortner, J. Die ansteckende Blutarmut der Einhufer in den Impfstoffwerken. [The infectious anemia in equines in the vaccine factories]. Berl Munch Tierarztl Wochenschr. May; 34 (5): 49-53. (1948)

20   Traub, E. & K. Beller. Untersuchungen uber die ansteckende Blutarmut der Pferde. Immunitatsversuche. [Immunization experiments in equine infectious anaemia]. Monatshefte fur Praktische Tierheilkunde; 3:193-206. (1942, 1951). [Translated to English by A. Finnegan (2019)]

21   Traub, E., et al. Komplementbindungversuche bei der ansteckenden Blutarmut der Pferde. [Complement-binding experiments on Infectious anemia of the horse]. Berl. Munch. Tierarztl Wochenschr. 134-135. (1941). [Translated to English by A. Finnegan, 2019]

22   Traub, E. Immunisation Contre Le Rouget du Porc par les Vaccins Adsorbés Concentrés [Immunization against Red Murrain by Concentrate Adsorbate Vaccines] Bulletin de l'Office International des Epizooties 22-35. (1949)

23   Fortner, J. Die ansteckende Blutarmut der Einhufer in den Impfstoffwerken. [The infectious anemia in equines in the vaccine factories]. Berl Munch Tierarztl Wochenschr. May; 34 (5): 49-53. (1948)

24   Central Intelligence Agency (CIA) Intelligence Reports: DBR Research Institute on Riems Island. CIA-RDP82-00457R007600420002-4. Central Intelligence Agency (CIA), Reading Room, 2001. Retrieved from: https://www.cia.gov/readingroom/document/cia-rdp82-00457r007600420002-4

25   Montagnier, L. et al. (1984). A new type of retrovirus isolated from patients presenting with lymphadenopathy and acquired immune deficiency syndrome: Structural and antigenic relatedness with equine infectious anaemia virus. Annales de l'Institut Pasteur / Virologie, Vol. 135(1), 119–134. doi:10.1016/S0769-2617(84)80046-5

26   Stephens, R., Casey, J., & Rice, N. (1986). Equine infectious anemia virus gag and pol genes: relatedness to visna and AIDS virus. Science, 231(4738), 589–594. doi:10.1126/science.3003905

27   Möhlmann, H. Uber vier durch Wechselpassage Pferd-Schaf-Pferd experimentell erzeugte Falle der stummen Form der infektiosen Anamie [On four cases of the silent form of infectious anemia experimentally created by alternating passage horse-sheep-horse].Archiv fur Experimentelle Veterinarmedizin; 10:709-712. (1956)

28   Elswood, B F, and R B Stricker. "Polio vaccines and the origin of AIDS." Medical hypotheses vol. 42,6 (1994): 347-54. doi:10.1016/0306-9877(94)90151-1

29   Brown, Phyllida. "US Rethinks Link between Polio Vaccine and HIV." New Scientist, 3 Apr. 1992, www.newscientist.com/article/mg13418151-900-us-rethinks-link-between-polio-vaccine-and-hiv/.

30   DULBECCO, R, and M VOGT. "Plaque formation and isolation of pure lines with poliomyelitis viruses." *The Journal of experimental medicine* vol. 99,2 (1954): 167-82. doi:10.1084/jem.99.2.167

31   Möhlmann, H. Uber vier durch Wechselpassage Pferd-Schaf-Pferd experimentell erzeugte Falle der stummen Form der infektiosen Anamie [On four cases of the silent form of

infectious anemia experimentally created by alternating passage horse-sheep-horse].Archiv fur Experimentelle Veterinarmedizin; 10:709-712. (1956)

32   Youngner, J. S. (1954). Monolayer Tissue Cultures I. Preparation and Standard-ization of Suspensions of Trypsin-Dispersed Monkey Kidney Cells.. *Experimental Biology and Medicine*, 85(2), 202–205. doi:10.3181/00379727-85-20830

33   Möhlmann, H. & H. Röhrer. Weitere experimentelle Untersuchungen zur Frage der naturlichen Ubertragungsweise der infektiosen Anamie der Pferde. [Further experimental investigations on the question of the natural transmission of infectious anemia in horses]. Experimentelle Veterinarmedizin; 1951. 5:6-13. (1951)

34   Oshinsky, David M. *Polio: An American Story*. Oxford University Press, 2006.

35   "FBI Files: Bacteriological Warfare ." n.d. Bacteriological Warfare in the United States. Internet Archive. Accessed July 30, 2019 (2 of 5), Retrieved from: https://archive.org/stream/BacteriologicalWarfareInTheUnitedStates/fbi_bw2#page/n95/mode/1up

36   Oshinsky, David M. *Polio: An American Story*. Oxford University Press, 2006.

37   Loftus, J. personal communications, 2018-2023

38   Youngner, J. S. (1954). Monolayer Tissue Cultures I. Preparation and Standardiza-tion of Suspensions of Trypsin-Dispersed Monkey Kidney Cells.. Experimental Biology and Medicine, 85(2), 202–205. doi:10.3181/00379727-85-20830

39   Röhrer, H. & H. Möhlmann. Experimenteller Beitrag zur Frage der naturlicheri Ansteckung bel infektioser Anamie der Pferde. [Experimental contribution to the question of the natural infection of infectious anemia in horses]. Monatsh. f. Vet. Med. 5: 79-182. (1950)

40   STEIN, C D, and L. O. MOTT. "Suspected equine infectious anemia in man." Veteri-nary medicine vol. 41,11 (1946): 385-8.

41   Fortner, J. Die ansteckende Blutarmut der Einhufer in den Impfstoffwerken. [The infectious anemia in equines in the vaccine factories]. Berl Munch Tierarztl Wochenschr. May; 34 (5): 49-53. (1948)

42   Sweet BH, Hilleman MR: The vacuolating virus, SV40 Proc Soc Exp Biol Med 105 420-427, 1960

43   Shah, Keerti, and Neal Nathanson. "Human Exposure To Sv40: Review And Comment." *American Journal of Epidemiology*, vol. 103, no. 1, 1976, pp. 1–12., doi:10.1093/oxfordjournals.aje.a112197 Retrieved from https://academic.oup.com/aje/article-ab-stract/103/1/1/151919?redirectedFrom=fulltext, or: https://www.scribd.com/docu-ment/409584571/Human-Exposure-to-SV40-Review-and-Comment-Carcinogens-in-Vac-cines

44   Oshinsky, David M. *Polio: An American Story*. Oxford University Press, 2006.

45   Ruska, H. Über die Bindung des Sublimats an Bakterien und Virus. Naunyn - Schmiedebergs Arch 204, 576–585 (1947). https://doi.org/10.1007/BF00245723

46   EYER, H et al. "Zum Gutachten über die Schutzimpfung gegen Poliomyelitis; Mit-teilung des wissenschaftlichen Beirats" [Expert testimony on preventive poliomyelitis vac-cination; report of the scientific advisory council]. Munchener medizinische Wochenschrift (1950) vol. 98,14 (1956): 492-6.

47   EYER, H et al. "Zum Gutachten über die Schutzimpfung gegen Poliomyelitis. 2" [Concerning the report on the poliomyelitis vaccination. 2]. Munchener medizinische Wo-chenschrift (1950) vol. 98,40 (1956): 1356-60.

48   Salk, Jonas Edward. *The Survival of the Wisest*. New York: Harper & Row, 1973

49   Ibid., pp. 43-44

50   Jiménez, Rose. "Biographical Memoir: Albert B. Sabin 1906-1993." National Acad-

emy of Sciences Memoirs, National Academy of Sciences, www.nasonline.org/publications/biographical-memoirs/memoir-pdfs/sabin-albert.pdf

51   Weinstein, Allen; Vassiliev, Alexander (March 14, 2000). The Haunted Wood: Soviet Espionage in America–The Stalin Era. Modern Library. pp. 140–150. ISBN 0-375-75536-5.

52   Jiménez, Rose. "Biographical Memoir: Albert B. Sabin 1906-1993." National Academy of Sciences Memoirs, National Academy of Sciences, www.nasonline.org/publications/biographical-memoirs/memoir-pdfs/sabin-albert.pdf

53   Jiménez, Rose. "Biographical Memoir: Albert B. Sabin 1906-1993." National Academy of Sciences Memoirs, National Academy of Sciences, www.nasonline.org/publications/biographical-memoirs/memoir-pdfs/sabin-albert.pdf

54   Vaughan, Roger. Listen to the Music: The Life of Hilary Koprowski. Place of Publication Not Identified: Springer, 2012.

55   Sabin, A. B. "MICE AS CARRIERS OF PATHOGENIC PLEUROPNEUMONIA-LIKE MICROORGANISMS." Science (New York, N.Y.). July 07, 1939. Accessed August 22, 2019. https://www.ncbi.nlm.nih.gov/pubmed/17818576.

56   Jiménez, Rose. "Biographical Memoir: Albert B. Sabin 1906-1993." National Academy of Sciences Memoirs, National Academy of Sciences, www.nasonline.org/publications/biographical-memoirs/memoir-pdfs/sabin-albert.pdf

57   "Sabin, Albert B. (Albert Bruce), 1906-." The Albert B. Sabin Papers, 1930-1993, 1939-1969, (University of Cincinnati, Health Sciences Library, Henry R. Winkler Center for the History of the Health Professions)

58   Jiménez, Rose. "Biographical Memoir: Albert B. Sabin 1906-1993." National Academy of Sciences Memoirs, National Academy of Sciences, www.nasonline.org/publications/biographical-memoirs/memoir-pdfs/sabin-albert.pdf

59   Ibid., pp. 17

60   Department of National Defence (Canada), Biological Warfare. OPERATION LAC correspondence. Tripartite Reports pp. 000232 http://data2.archives.ca/e/e443/e011063033.pdf

61   "Polio." History of Vaccines RSS, historyofvaccines.org/history/polio/timeline

62   Newman JFE, Brown F. Foot-and-Mouth Disease Virus and Poliovirus Particles Contain Proteins of the Replication Complex. Journal of Virology 1997 Oct;71(10):7657-62. Rec #: 7941

63   Twomey T, Newman JFE, Burrage T, Piatti PG, Lubroth J, Brown F. Structure and Immunogenicity of Experimental Foot-and-Mouth Disease and Poliomyelitis Vaccines. Vaccine 1995 Nov; 13(16):1603-10. Rec #: 7948

64   Swanson, William. "Birth of a Cold War Vaccine." Scientific American, vol. 306, no. 4, 2012, pp. 66–69., doi:10.1038/scientificamerican0412-66.

65   Swanson, William. "Birth of a Cold War Vaccine." Scientific American, vol. 306, no. 4, 2012, pp. 66–69., doi:10.1038/scientificamerican0412-66.

66   Central Intelligence Agency (CIA) Intelligence Reports: SCIENTIFIC ABSTRACT M.P. CHUMAKOV - N.M. CHUMAKOV. CIA-RDP86-00513R000509120005-9. Central Intelligence Agency (CIA), Reading Room, 2000. Retrieved from: https://www.cia.gov/library/readingroom/document/CIA-RDP86-00513R000509120005-9.pdf

67   Sabin, Albert B., and Albert Bruce. 2010. "Zhdanov, Viktor Mikhailovich -- 1956-62 -- Correspondence, Individual -- Letter, 1957-06-21." UC DRC Home. University of Cincinnati. University of Cincinnati Libraries. November 17, 2010. https://drc.libraries.uc.edu/handle/2374.UC/684952

68   Zilber, L. A. (1965, November 15). Zhdanov, Viktor Mikhailovich -- 1956-62 -- corre-

spondence, individual -- letter, 1965-11-15. UC Digital Resource Commons. https://drc.libraries.uc.edu/items/91be8142-1eab-4756-9db3-17ec032f96a2

69   Alibek, Ken, and Stephen Handelman. *Biohazard: the Chilling True Story of the Largest Covert Biological Weapons Program in the World, Told from the inside by the Man Who Ran It.* Dell Pub., 2000

70   Domaradskiĭ, I. V., and Wendy Orent. *Biowarrior: Inside the Soviet/Russian Biological War Machine.* Amherst, NY: Prometheus Books, 2003, pp. 13

71   Jiménez, Rose. "Biographical Memoir: Albert B. Sabin 1906-1993." National Academy of Sciences Memoirs, National Academy of Sciences, www.nasonline.org/publications/biographical-memoirs/memoir-pdfs/sabin-albert.pdf

72   Swanson, William. "Birth of a Cold War Vaccine." *Scientific American*, vol. 306, no. 4, 2012, pp. 66–69., doi:10.1038/scientificamerican0412-66.

73   Kisselev, Lev L., et al. "Lev Zilber, the Personality and the Scientist." Advances in Cancer Research, 1992, pp. 1–40., doi:10.1016/s0065-230x(08)60301-2.

74   Central Intelligence Agency (CIA) Intelligence Reports: USSR CONFERENCE ON TICK ENCEPHALITIS AND RELATED DISEASES. CIA-RDP80-00809A000700200170-9. Central Intelligence Agency (CIA), Reading Room, 2011. Retrieved from: https://www.cia.gov/readingroom/document/cia-rdp80-00809a000700200170-9

75   Central Intelligence Agency (CIA) Intelligence Reports: USSR WORK ON HEMORRHAGIC NEPHROSO-NEPHRITIS. CIA-RDP80-00809A000700240068-9. Central Intelligence Agency (CIA), Reading Room, 2011. Retrieved from: https://www.cia.gov/library/readingroom/document/CIA-RDP80-00809A000700240068-9

76   Central Intelligence Agency (CIA) Intelligence Reports: THE MILITARY MEDICAL ACADEMY IMENI KIROV. CIA-RDP82-00047R000400500002-8. Central Intelligence Agency (CIA), Reading Room, 2011. Retrieved from: https://www.cia.gov/readingroom/document/cia-rdp82-00047r000400500002-8

77   Walker, Lisa. Konstantin Chumakov Interview 2005. NIH History Office, National Institutes of Health (NIH), 25 Apr. 2013, https://history.nih.gov/archives/downloads/konstantinchumakov.pdf Accessed 30 Oct. 2019.

78   Central Intelligence Agency (CIA) Intelligence Reports: THE MILITARY MEDICAL ACADEMY IMENI KIROV. CIA-RDP82-00047R000400500002-8. Central Intelligence Agency (CIA), Reading Room, 2011. Retrieved from: https://www.cia.gov/readingroom/document/cia-rdp82-00047r000400500002-8

79   Central Intelligence Agency (CIA) Intelligence Reports: SCIENTIFIC ABSTRACT M.P. CHUMAKOV - N.M. CHUMAKOV. CIA-RDP86-00513R000509120005-9. Central Intelligence Agency (CIA), Reading Room, 2000. Retrieved from: https://www.cia.gov/readingroom/document/cia-rdp86-00513r000509120005-9

80   Ibid., pp. 12

81   Central Intelligence Agency (CIA) Intelligence Reports: ANIMAL NEUROVIRUS DISEASES SIMILAR TO HUMAN POLIOMYELITIS. CIA-RDP80-00809A000700170265-8 Central Intelligence Agency (CIA), Reading Room, 2011. Retrieved from: https://www.cia.gov/readingroom/document/cia-rdp80-00809a000700170265-8

82   Leitenberg, Milton, et al. *The Soviet Biological Weapons Program: A History*. Harvard University Press, 2012. pp. 96

83   Central Intelligence Agency (CIA) Intelligence Reports: SOVIET SCIENTIFIC MEDICAL MEETING AT TASEKENT. CIA-RDP80-00809A000700200208-7. Central Intelligence Agency (CIA), Reading Room, 2011. Retrieved from: https://www.cia.gov/readingroom/document/cia-rdp80-00809a000700200208-7

84   Zilinskas, Raymond A. "The Soviet Biological Weapons Program and Its Legacy

in Today's Russia." CSWMD Occasional Paper, no. 11, 2016, pp. 1–72., Retrieved from: http://www.inss.ndu.edu/Portals/68/Documents/occasional/cswmd/CSWMD_OccasionalPaper-11.pdf?ver=2016-07-18-144946-743

85   Swanson, William. "Birth of a Cold War Vaccine." *Scientific American*, vol. 306, no. 4, 2012, pp. 66–69., doi:10.1038/scientificamerican0412-66.

86   Central Intelligence Agency (CIA) Intelligence Reports: SCIENTIFIC ABSTRACT A.Y. CHUMAKOV - M.P. CHUMAKOV. CIA-RDP86-00513R000509120004-0. Central Intelligence Agency (CIA), Reading Room, 2011. Retrieved from: https://www.cia.gov/library/reading-room/document/CIA-RDP86-00513R000509120004-0

87   Central Intelligence Agency (CIA) Intelligence Reports: SCIENTIFIC ABSTRACT A.Y. CHUMAKOV - M.P. CHUMAKOV. CIA-RDP86-00513R000509120004-0. Central Intelligence Agency (CIA), Reading Room, 2011. Retrieved from: https://www.cia.gov/library/reading-room/document/CIA-RDP86-00513R000509120004-0

88   Chumakov, K. M., et al. "Some Oral Poliovirus Vaccines Were Contaminated with Infectious SV40 After 1961" Yearbook of Pathology and Laboratory Medicine, vol. 2007, 2007, p. 353., doi:10.1016/s1077-9108(08)70481-x

89   Central Intelligence Agency (CIA) Intelligence Reports: SCIENTIFIC ABSTRACT M.P. CHUMAKOV - N.M. CHUMAKOV. CIA-RDP86-00513R000509120005-9. Central Intelligence Agency (CIA), Reading Room, 2000. pp. 38-40. Retrieved from: https://www.cia.gov/reading-room/document/cia-rdp86-00513r000509120005-9

90   Central Intelligence Agency (CIA) Intelligence Reports: SCIENTIFIC ABSTRACT M.P. CHUMAKOV - N.M. CHUMAKOV. CIA-RDP86-00513R000509120005-9. Central Intelligence Agency (CIA), Reading Room, 2000., pp. 44 Retrieved from: https://www.cia.gov/reading-room/document/cia-rdp86-00513r000509120005-9

91   Central Intelligence Agency (CIA) Intelligence Reports: SCIENTIFIC ABSTRACT M.P. CHUMAKOV - N.M. CHUMAKOV. CIA-RDP86-00513R000509120005-9. Central Intelligence Agency (CIA), Reading Room, 2000., pp. 38-40. Retrieved from: https://www.cia.gov/readin-groom/document/cia-rdp86-00513r000509120005-9

92   Valsamakis, A, P G Auwaerter, B K Rima, H Kaneshima, and D E Griffin. 1999. "Altered Virulence of Vaccine Strains of Measles Virus after Prolonged Replication in Human Tissue." Journal of Virology. American Society for Microbiology. October 1999. https://www.ncbi.nlm.nih.gov/pmc/articles/PMC112900/

93   Central Intelligence Agency (CIA) Intelligence Reports: ANIMAL NEUROVIRUS DISEASES SIMILAR TO HUMAN POLIOMYELITIS. CIA-RDP80-00809A000700170265-8 Central Intelligence Agency (CIA), Reading Room, 2011. Retrieved from: https://www.cia.gov/library/readingroom/document/CIA-RDP80-00809A000700170265-8

94   Central Intelligence Agency (CIA) Intelligence Reports: SCIENTIFIC ABSTRACT M.P. CHUMAKOV - N.M. CHUMAKOV. CIA-RDP86-00513R000509120005-9. Central Intelligence Agency (CIA), Reading Room, 2000., pp. 38-40. Retrieved from: https://www.cia.gov/readin-groom/document/cia-rdp86-00513r000509120005-9

95   Central Intelligence Agency (CIA) Intelligence Reports: FR:CHUMAKOV M P TO:CHURSIN V M. CIA-RDP91-00403R000200550061-8. Central Intelligence Agency (CIA), Reading Room, 2016. Retrieved from: https://www.cia.gov/library/readingroom/document/CIA-RDP91-00403R000200550061-8

96   Swanson, William. "Birth of a Cold War Vaccine." *Scientific American*, vol. 306, no. 4, 2012, pp. 66–69., doi:10.1038/scientificamerican0412-66.

97   Domaradskij Igor Valerianovich., and Wendy Orent. Biowarrior: inside the Soviet/Russian Biological War Machine. Prometheus, 2003.

98   Swanson, William. "Birth of a Cold War Vaccine." *Scientific American*, vol. 306, no. 4, 2012, pp. 66–69., doi:10.1038/scientificamerican0412-66.

99   Swanson, William. "Birth of a Cold War Vaccine." *Scientific American*, vol. 306, no. 4, 2012, pp. 66–69., doi:10.1038/scientificamerican0412-66.

100   Alibek, Ken, and Stephen Handelman. *Biohazard: the Chilling True Story of the Largest Covert Biological Weapons Program in the World, Told from the inside by the Man Who Ran It.* Dell Pub., 2000.

101   Thomson, Jess. "Deadly Hemorrhagic Virus Spreading to New Countries, Scientists Warn." Newsweek, 20 June 2023, www.newsweek.com/disease-crimean-congo-hemorrhagic-fever-spreading-1807693

102   Shevtsova, Z. V. "Some Results of Investigating 'Marburg Virus' (Rhabdovirus Simiae)." Apps.dtic.mil. October 20, 1971. Accessed August 23, 2019. https://apps.dtic.mil/docs/citations/AD0743032

103   Alibek, Ken, and Stephen Handelman. *Biohazard: the Chilling True Story of the Largest Covert Biological Weapons Program in the World, Told from the inside by the Man Who Ran It.* Dell Pub., 2000, pp. 124

104   Maass, Günther, Johannes Müller, Norbert Seemayer, and Richard Haas. "Production Of Kidney Tissue Cultures From African Green Monkeys, Experimentally Infected With The Causative Agent Of Frankfurt-Marburg-Syndrome." *American Journal of Epidemiology* 89, no. 6 (1969): 681-90. doi:10.1093/oxfordjournals.aje.a120982.

105   Leitenberg, Milton, et al. *The Soviet Biological Weapons Program: A History.* Harvard University Press, 2012., pp. 92-93

106   Central Intelligence Agency (CIA) Intelligence Reports: FR:CHILIE N TO:CHUMAKOV V E. CIA-RDP91-00403R000100840014-9. Central Intelligence Agency (CIA), Reading Room, 2016. Retrieved from: https://www.cia.gov/library/readingroom/document/CIA-RDP91-00403R000100840014-9

107   Central Intelligence Agency (CIA) Intelligence Reports: SCIENTIFIC ABSTRACT M.P. CHUMAKOV - A.YE. CHUMAKOV. CIA-RDP86-00513R000509120003-1. Central Intelligence Agency (CIA), Reading Room, 2000. Retrieved from: https://www.cia.gov/library/readingroom/document/CIA-RDP86-00513R000509120003-1

108   Central Intelligence Agency (CIA) Intelligence Reports: USSR WORK ON HEMORRHAGIC NEPHROSO-NEPHRITIS. CIA-RDP80-00809A000700240068-9. Central Intelligence Agency (CIA), Reading Room, 2011. Retrieved from: https://www.cia.gov/library/readingroom/document/CIA-RDP80-00809A000700240068-9

109   Stojkovic, L. J. "Yugoslavia (Belgrade), Institute of Hygiene P.R. Serbia -- 1959-81 -- OPV Production, International -- Letter to Albert B. Sabin, 1967-10-04." UC DRC Home. March 07, 2011. Accessed August 23, 2019. https://drc.libraries.uc.edu/handle/2374.UC/699286

110   Bray, Mike. "Comparative Pathogenesis of Crimean-Congo Hemorrhagic Fever and Ebola Hemorrhagic Fever." SpringerLink, Springer Netherlands, 1 Jan. 1970, link.springer.com/chapter/10.1007/978-1-4020-6106-6_17. Accessed 19 June 2023.

111   Central Intelligence Agency (CIA) Intelligence Reports: USSR WORK ON HEMORRHAGIC NEPHROSO-NEPHRITIS. CIA-RDP80-00809A000700240068-9. Central Intelligence Agency (CIA), Reading Room, 2011. Retrieved from: https://www.cia.gov/library/readingroom/document/CIA-RDP80-00809A000700240068-9

112   David-West, T S et al. "Seroepidemiology of Congo virus (related to the virus of Crimean haemorrhagic fever) in Nigeria." *Bulletin of the World Health Organization* vol. 51,5 (1974): 543-6.

113   Central Intelligence Agency (CIA) Intelligence Reports: USSR WORK ON HEMORRHAGIC NEPHROSO-NEPHRITIS. CIA-RDP80-00809A000700240068-9. Central Intelligence Agency (CIA), Reading Room, 2011. Retrieved from: https://www.cia.gov/library/readingroom/document/CIA-RDP80-00809A000700240068-9

114   Central Intelligence Agency (CIA) Intelligence Reports. EXPEDITIONS FOR THE STUDY OF OMSK EPIDEMIC HEMORRHAGIC FEVER. CIA-RDP80-00809A000600330562-1. Central Intelligence Agency (CIA), Reading Room, 2011. Retrieved from: https://www.cia.gov/readingroom/document/cia-rdp80-00809a000600330562-1

115   Lapin, B. A. & B. F. Semenov. Arbovirus Infections of Monkeys Captured in the Jungles of Northern Nigeria. Voprosy Virusologiy. 755-757. 1967

116   Central Intelligence Agency (CIA) Intelligence Reports: SCIENTIFIC ABSTRACT TRUKHANOV, G. YA. - TRUSKOV, P. F. CIA-RDP86-00513R002203330002-6. Central Intelligence Agency (CIA), Reading Room, 2001, pp. 13-19. Retrieved from: https://www.cia.gov/reading-room/document/cia-rdp86-00513r002203330002-6

117   Monath, T P. "Lassa fever: review of epidemiology and epizootiology." Bulletin of the World Health Organization vol. 52,4-6 (1975): 577-92.

118   Werner Slenczka , Hans Dieter Klenk, Forty Years of Marburg Virus, The Journal of Infectious Diseases, Volume 196, Issue Supplement_2, November 2007, Pages S131–S135, https://doi.org/10.1086/520551

119   Casals, J. "Antigenic similarity between the virus causing Crimean hemorrhagic fever and Congo virus." Proceedings of the Society for Experimental Biology and Medicine. Society for Experimental Biology and Medicine (New York, N.Y.) vol. 131,1 (1969): 233-6. doi:10.3181/00379727-131-33847

120   Bray, Mike. "Comparative Pathogenesis of Crimean-Congo Hemorrhagic Fever and Ebola Hemorrhagic Fever." SpringerLink, Springer Netherlands, 1 Jan. 1970, link.springer.com/chapter/10.1007/978-1-4020-6106-6_17. Accessed 19 June 2023.

121   Alibek, Ken, and Stephen Handelman. Biohazard: the Chilling True Story of the Largest Covert Biological Weapons Program in the World, Told from the inside by the Man Who Ran It. Dell Pub., 2000

122   Leitenberg, Milton, et al. The Soviet Biological Weapons Program: A History. Harvard University Press, 2012., pp. 92-93

123   Bray, Mike. "Comparative Pathogenesis of Crimean-Congo Hemorrhagic Fever and Ebola Hemorrhagic Fever." SpringerLink, Springer Netherlands, 1 Jan. 1970, link.springer.com/chapter/10.1007/978-1-4020-6106-6_17. Accessed 19 June 2023.

124   Central Intelligence Agency (CIA) Intelligence Reports: SCIENTIFIC ABSTRACT M.P. CHUMAKOV - N.M. CHUMAKOV. CIA-RDP86-00513R000509120005-9. Central Intelligence Agency (CIA), Reading Room, 2000., pp. 38-40. Retrieved from: https://www.cia.gov/readingroom/document/cia-rdp86-00513r000509120005-9

125   Central Intelligence Agency (CIA) Intelligence Reports: SCIENTIFIC ABSTRACT YAKUBAYTIS, E.A. - YAKUBOVICH, V.S. CIA-RDP86-00513R002203620001-5. Central Intelligence Agency (CIA), Reading Room, 2001. Retrieved from: https://www.cia.gov/reading-room/document/cia-rdp86-00513r002203620001-5, pp. 43

126   Kouzminov, Alexander. Biological Espionage: Special Operations of the Soviet and Russian Foreign Intelligence Services in the West. Manas Publications, 2006., pp. 73-74

127   Sabin, Albert B. "Chumakov, Mikhail Petrovich -- 1960-69 -- Correspondence, Individual -- Letter, 1960-04-08." Received by M. P. Chumakov, Chumakov, Mikhail Petrovich -- 1960-69 -- Correspondence, Individual -- Letter, 1960-04-08, University of Cincinnati. University of Cincinnati Libraries, 6 Apr. 2010. The Albert B. Sabin Archives, http://www.drc.libraries.uc.edu/bitstream/handle/2374.UC/679119/chumakov_1960-69_032.pdf?sequence=1Aug. 28, 1990

128   Sabin, A. B. letter to V. M. Zhdanov -- Russian Trip, Notes and Data -- 1956 -- Corrspondence, OPV Miscellaneous -- letter, 1956-06-14. Received by V. M. Zhdanov. University of Cincinnati. Hauck Center for the Albert B. Sabin Archives, University of Cincinnati. University of Cincinnati Libraries, retrieved from: https://drc.libraries.uc.edu/items/01abc0b1-3e42-

4611-b3ae-858662d4e289

129   Casals, J. "U.S.S.R Visitors -- 1955-56 -- Correspondence, Polio -- Letter, 1956-04-12." UC DRC Home. May 04, 2011. Accessed August 23, 2019. https://drc.libraries.uc.edu/handle/2374.UC/690878

130   Sabin, Albert B. "U.S.S.R Visitors -- 1955-56 -- Correspondence, Polio -- Letter, 1956-04-14." UC DRC Home. May 04, 2011. Accessed August 23, 2019. https://drc.libraries.uc.edu/handle/2374.UC/690897

131   Swanson, William. "Birth of a Cold War Vaccine." *Scientific American*, vol. 306, no. 4, 2012, pp. 66–69., doi:10.1038/scientificamerican0412-66.

132   Sabin, Albert B., and Albert Bruce. "Chumakov, K.M. -- 1990-93 -- Correspondence, Individual -- Letter, 1992-03-04." UC DRC Home. May 04, 2011. Accessed August 23, 2019. https://drc.libraries.uc.edu/handle/2374.UC/679034

133   Chumakov, K.M. -- 1990-93 -- Correspondence, Individual -- letter, 1991-02-28. Received by Albert B. Sabin. University of Cincinnati. Hauck Center for the Albert B. Sabin Archives, University of Cincinnati. University of Cincinnati Libraries, https://drc.libraries.uc.edu/bitstream/handle/2374.UC/679031/chumakkm_1990-93_008.pdf?sequence=1

134   Walker, Lisa. Konstantin Chumakov Interview 2005. NIH History Office, National Institutes of Health (NIH), 25 Apr. 2013, https://history.nih.gov/archives/downloads/konstantinchumakov.pdf Accessed 30 Oct. 2019.

135   Central Intelligence Agency (CIA) Intelligence Reports: SCIENTIFIC ABSTRACT DROZDOV, SZ.G. - DROZDOV, S.V.. CIA-RDP86-00513R000411230001-9. Central Intelligence Agency (CIA), Reading Room, 2000. Retrieved from: https://www.cia.gov/readingroom/document/cia-rdp86-00513r000411230001-9

136   Department of National Defence (Canada), Operation LAC. Biological Warfare. www.Data2.archives.ca/e/e443/e011063033.pdf

137   Kouzminov, Alexander. *Biological Espionage: Special Operations of the Soviet and Russian Foreign Intelligence Services in the West*. Manas Publications, 2006.,

138   Schäfer, W."Structure of some animal viruses and significance of their components." *Bacteriological reviews* vol. 27,1 (1963): 1-17. doi:10.1128/br.27.1.1-17.1963

EPILOGUE

"TRY!" for it is a great word, though it musters only three letters. It is the story of every achievement, from great to small, that the world has ever seen.

– Paschal Beverly Randolph

This book was truly a work of an immense commitment, a commitment and obligation, as I realized my talent for study and investigation of the esoteric history of biological warfare was truly a gift, it was my obligation to serve humanity to give many answers to those who were ignored and left in the dark by the public health system, with actions taken by the State Department which caused almost unbelievable and bewildering consequences to the Nation as a whole, endangering their country and thus being disloyal and unfaithful to actual National Security, they hid their own blunders in the interest of National Security to avoid accountability and responsibility. Unfortunately, this is an all too familiar tendency in human nature, but it is not a condonable one. I hope that that this work assists in bringing those actions to light, to their shame, because shameful it truly is. I believe this is only the tip of the iceberg.

I used to call this book "the project that never ends," because it took me so many years and having to overcome so many obstacles and adversities to get this book into publication to reach you – the reader – and I cannot begin to describe the immense effort and sacrifice I made to do this book, I've had relationships sour over this book, with the level of commitment I put to it. I've had to deal with some of the most frustrating situations because of this book, it was a toil, but a toil that I was cut out to handle.

This story *needed* to be told. Far too many sick, chronically ill people out there have been looking for answers about their condition and disease, too sick and left to fend for themselves, having their disease denied by the public health system, because the tests used, are incompetent, and Traub showed this phenomenon with LCM virus and immune tolerance. I felt it was my duty to use my talents to tell the story of a reckless, heartless, and brutal form of warfare – *biological warfare* – a true perversion and inversion of nature. Fort Detrick scientist Theodore Rosebury said it correctly when he stated, "*If you want to understand biological warfare you must figuratively stand on your head. biological warfare is an upside-down science, an inversion of nature.*"

Here is a prime example – anyone who brings up in a public discussion, biological warfare activities, bioterrorism, or outbreaks originating from a lab – they are immediately ridiculed and called a *conspiracy theorist*, even in the face of evidence, but yet the public health system and biodefense have billions of taxpayer dollars pouring into their program to protect against that, warning us how we need to be ready for the next pandemic and protect against bioterrorism, yet they aren't ridiculed and called conspiracy theorists for suggesting it. Its an upside down science that calls for upside down responses to cover for its upside down activity.

The COVID-19 pandemic was another upside down situation that unraveled exactly as I predicted, because the spike proteins on SARS-CoV-2 cause the same immune tolerance condition, termed *long COVID*, and the public health system's story kept changing and changing and changing, yet I knew every step of the way what was going to happen and *did* happen, (I have the emails to prove it) because I am well-versed in Traub's immune tolerance and I understand how the disease works. The top brass in public health, I know they are not ignorant of how the condition works. They know, but they consciously choose to keep these facts to themselves because they have a political agenda to serve.

If I have learned anything in researching and learning the science of immune tolerance, it is this: modern science has little respect for actual science, actual truth, for science as it is in nature, rather than what it is for the special interests funding it. They can and do manipulate data, setup fraudulent studies to get whatever outcome they want in published research, its the reason why every scientific publication funded for a vaccine will invariably conclude that the vaccine worked great, had robust antibodies, and no side effects, regardless of its safety or effectiveness. It is a problem of extremely dishonest people running our system.

Greed, ego, prestige, status, profiteering, a need to fit in and feel relevant or important, herd mentality, fear of ridicule, are all too familiar traits of the human condition. It's not that complicated to realize. Modern science is using the guise of science to sell us a political machine, a system of ulterior political agendas using the name of science, yet it is anything but scientific when it comes to the truth of nature's mechanics. It is being used to hide blunders and fallacies, to hide aspects of this war, to sell us treatments and vaccines which often do far more harm than good, and it is being used to hide the aspects of biological science that everyone has a right to know. With the way this modern political scientific machine is set up, none of its members will serve their moral obligation to humanity and tell of its folly without being crucified by the political machine using the guise of science.

The more I analyze the mysteries of disease, the more I realize how extremely far off from the path leading to true health, healing, and harmony we are. What is that solution? I do not yet know, but it is clearly far from what is being done at the present time. We need entirely new paradigms, and the science of immune tolerance proves this to be so. I believe these facts will only become more and more apparent as time goes on, and from bitter experience will the public health system and the World Health Organization (WHO) take part in its own destruction the more they push a politically motivated system that has no problem using dishonesty. Evidence in my research suggests that the WHO was compromised, perhaps from its inception, but certainly when KGB put their agents like Sergey Drozdov in positions at the organization, and the Food and Agriculture Organization (FAO) was compromised with officers like Erich Traub.

It is a general rule that when a mess is ignored and not cleaned up, it only becomes a much bigger mess, and I believe that is what we have here – a mess that has been left to fester – and has only become a much bigger mess than anyone could imagine. My research suggests the possibility that not only has the U.N. been compromised from its early days, but the public health system and biodefense has too.

Quite frankly, I'm not sure what the solution to this problem is, but I can tell you this: the only way to find the solution is to Try! First, admit and understand the problem itself, know all that there is to know about this problem and the facts surrounding it, and only then will we be in any position to attempt a viable solution. I don't feel it is my duty to find the solution because literally all of my time had been dedicated to trying to explain all there is to know about the problem itself, the mechanics that surround it, and this includes knowing how the public health system and their "science" is misleading us. It means understanding the nature of the slick deceptions being served to us as truth and as science, when it is anything but scientific or true, but made to look so.

Those of us who are sick, we must not give up, we must not surrender to defeat, as defeated as we may feel at times, we must look for strength deep within, and do our very best to rebuild our life with

313

the obstacles and disabilities that afflict us. These diseases are highly demoralizing and force us to search for a strength deep within that we often never even realized we had. But it often comes with a Dark Night of the Soul, a time of extreme disillusionment and jadedness.

The slow poison to our society is found in these great imitator antigens and was a very effective method of destroying Western civilization. Thinking these antigens could be used effectively as vaccines is only further digging us into the grave. We have to ask ourselves why they can't see or identify the problem? The public health system wants to ignore the problem and relies on everyone being ignorant and oblivious to what is going on, and for the most part, this is still the case, but we all start somewhere, because I too, for a good while, was ignorant of the details and inner mechanics, but in being devastated by the effects of these antigens and the desire to know my disease and its inner truths was activated many years ago. Some of us are driven by the unwavering willpower, like the Divine is moving through us. Sometimes all it takes to effect change in the world is a few very effective people.

* * *

The allegory of Prometheus, who steals the fire of science and technology of the Divine from the Gods to give to human civilizations, these goods ended up in the hands of those who only wished to rule others with deceitful intentions and self-aggrandizement. Perhaps the fire just needs to be taken back from the self-proclaimed 'Gods' of today, that is, the figurative "priest-class" of those controlling war, science, and medicine, for their own ends and agendas and not for health, with tyrants still ruling today as it did in the days of old.

* * *

Consider this a declaration of the humanity all of us have within, to be inspired by the Fire of Truth, the Power of Gnosis, that is, Knowledge used correctly and converted to Wisdom, for the good of all, not for leverage over others, but instead, used as a means to empower all, the true ideal of what should be part of the Great Work we all do, restored to its moral context and blazing through the trials and tribulations of today, carrying the blazing torch of Truth and Goodwill through the Dark Ages once more, until we reach a better day and age through an honest and heartfelt effort to Try and deal with the problems of the Ages, we must carry onward, we may be happy yet... we must push onward and Try!

Index

search Institute for Virus Disease of Animals (Bundesforschungsanstalt fur Viruskrankheiten) 172
University of Wisconsin 20, 144, 186, 253, 254
U.S. Army Activity in the U.S. Biological Warfare Programs 176
USDA (United States Department of Agriculture) 27, 31, 35, 37, 89, 136, 138, 139, 141, 143, 144, 146, 158, 160, 165, 172, 174, 177, 182-188, 192, 193, 196-200, 202-209, 223, 229, 244-246, 248, 253-255, 265, 281
USDA – Bureau of Animal Industry (BAI) 31, 144

V

Vaccine-Serum Laboratory 56
Van Den Heuvel, Frederick "Freddy" 166
Van Houweling, C.D. 35, 200, 206
Venezuelan Equine Encephalitis (VEE) 14, 141, 151, 179, 187, 244
Verdon, Rachel 169, 205
Vesicular Stomatitis Virus (VSV) 19, 144, 185, 186, 244, 253, 254
Virology in Germany 124
Virus Hunters 294
Virus N 136, 149
von Braun, Werner 167
von Papen, Franz 38
von Steinmetz, Erich 39, 46
Voroshilova, Marina 285, 290

W

Waffenprüf 9 56, 57
Waldmann, Otto 95, 103, 107-110, 115-119, 125, 127, 135, 157, 158, 160, 193, 269
Warner, Richard E. 188, 194
Washington, George 26, 27
Washington Post 176, 178, 190, 215, 226, 232, 236, 242
Weber, Klaus 211
Wehmaier, Ms. 252
Weiss, Otto 247, 250, 251, 267, 268
Western Equine Encephalomyelitis Virus (WEE) 85, 187
West Nile Virus 66, 85, 86, 285, 287, 297, 298
Widening Circle, Widening Circle: A Lyme Disease Pioneer Tells Her Story, The 210
Wood, James 240, 292, 304
Worker's and Peasant's Red Army (RKKA) 56, 57
World Health Organization (WHO) 196, 241, 292, 299, 313
Wormser, Gary 218, 237, 243

Y

Yale Arbovirus Research Unit (YARU) 209
Yersinia pestis 59, 151

Z

Zabrocka, Katarzyna 78, 205, 275, 301
Zalinskas, Raymond A. 287, 295
Zelicoff, Alan P. 286
Zhdanov, V.M. 70, 71, 73, 78, 285, 286, 297, 304, 308
Zilber, Lev 69, 72-74, 78, 79, 285, 286, 294, 304, 305
Zilinskas, Raymond A. 135, 288, 292, 305
Zimmerman, Arthur 22, 39
Zuckert, Wolfram 221
Zwick, Wilhelm 81, 82, 89, 93, 100, 114

ACKNOWLEDGMENTS

I thank My family and friends for their continued support in the writing of this book. Mom, Dad, Evan, Lu, Noah, Lilah, my dog Lucy. I thank and send my love to Azeeza and her 3 sisters. I thank my source and book project friends, John Loftus, Crystal Bennett, Jody Savin, thank you for all the support and help with research materials and advice and suggestions. I also thank additional friends who put up with me before and through this writing, Jon-Michael Aiello, Dan Aiello, Al Kalil, Kartashev Vyacheslav (Masta Shake), Jake Perry, John V. D'apollo (May you Rest in Peace), Jill D'apollo, Jeannie Heroux, Kelly Merriman, Veronica Casillas, Bethany Wing, Jorge Rosado of Merauder. I thank other Lyme sufferers and activists, Jena Blair, Laura Hovind & TruthCures.org. I thank Kris Millegan and TrineDay. I thank my spiritual mentor Vashish ji and W.G.K. I thank Professor Richard B. Spence, Richard Grove and Autonomy, Mark Passio and the One Great Work Network, Marja West, Angie and Jim from Victurus Libertas channel, actor and friend Steve Shellen, thanks to Randy Williams at Old Colony. I thank John at the Rail Trail bike shop in Brewster for great philosophical discussions and advice about life! I thank Jennifer and Buttermilk the dog (Olive) from the bike trail. I thank all friends and fans of my other site, The Garden of Great Work, I thank music for keeping me sane, especially the following bands: Snot (R.I.P. Lynn Strait), Candiria, Dissection, Deftones, Cage the Elephant, Sublime, Lana Del Rey, Mayhem, At the Gates, Sepultura, Soulfly, Merauder, Cave In, and so many more. I also give thanks and love to my nightshade plants and to my pet scorpions Kali (R.I.P.), Saturnine (R.I.P.), Soulreaper (and her new scorplings). I thank Reverend Myron Heckman, Cindy Zweil, and the Bible Alliance Church for their forgiveness and welcoming friendship. I thank all who take the time to read my book and give a very important issue the attention it so deserves....